Medical Genetics at a Glance

Dorian J. Pritchard
BSc, Dip Gen, PhD, CBiol, MIBiol
Former Lecturer in Human Genetics
University of Newcastle-upon-Tyne
UK
Former Visiting Lecturer in Medical Genetics
International Medical University
Kuala Lumpur
Malaysia

Bruce R. Korf
MD, PhD
Wayne H. and Sara Crews Finley Professor of Medical Genetics
Chairman, Department of Genetics
University of Alabama at Birmingham
Alabama
USA

Second edition

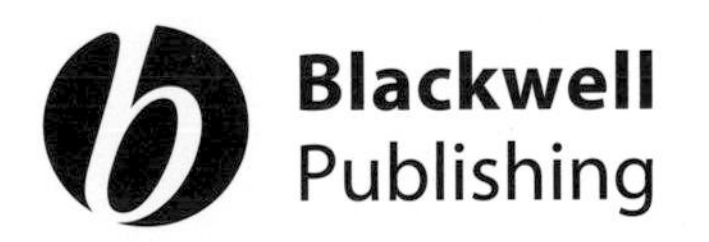

Published by Blackwell Publishing
Blackwell Publishing, Inc., 350 Main Street, Malden, Massachusetts 02148-5020, USA
Blackwell Publishing Ltd, 9600 Garsington Road, Oxford OX4 2DQ, UK
Blackwell Publishing Asia Pty Ltd, 550 Swanston Street, Carlton, Victoria 3053, Australia

First published 2003
Reprinted 2005, 2006
Second edition 2008

1 2008

Library of Congress Cataloging-in-Publication Data
Pritchard, D. J. (Dorian J.)
Medical genetics at a glance / Dorian Pritchard, Bruce R. Korf. – 2nd ed.
p. ; cm. – (At a glance series)
Includes bibliographical references and index.
ISBN 978-1-4051-4846-7 (alk. paper)
1. Medical genetics. 2. Developmental biology. I. Korf, Bruce R. II. Title.
III. Series: At a glance series (Oxford, England)
[DNLM: 1. Genetic Diseases, Inborn. 2. Chromosome Aberrations.
3. Genetics. QZ 50 P961m 2007]

RB155.P6965 2007
616′.042–dc22 2007006422

ISBN: 978-1-4051-4846-7

A catalogue record for this title is available from the British Library

Set in 9/11.5pt Times by Graphicraft Limited, Hong Kong
Printed and bound in Malaysia by KHL Printing Co Sdn Bhd

Commissioning Editor: Martin Sugden
Development Editor: Fiona Pattison
Editorial assistant: Robin Harries
Production Controller: Debbie Wyer
Artist: Jane Fallows

For further information on Blackwell Publishing, visit our website:
http://www.blackwellpublishing.com

The publisher's policy is to use permanent paper from mills that operate a sustainable forestry policy, and which has been manufactured from pulp processed using acid-free and elementary chlorine-free practices. Furthermore, the publisher ensures that the text paper and cover board used have met acceptable environmental accreditation standards.

Medical Genetics at a Glance

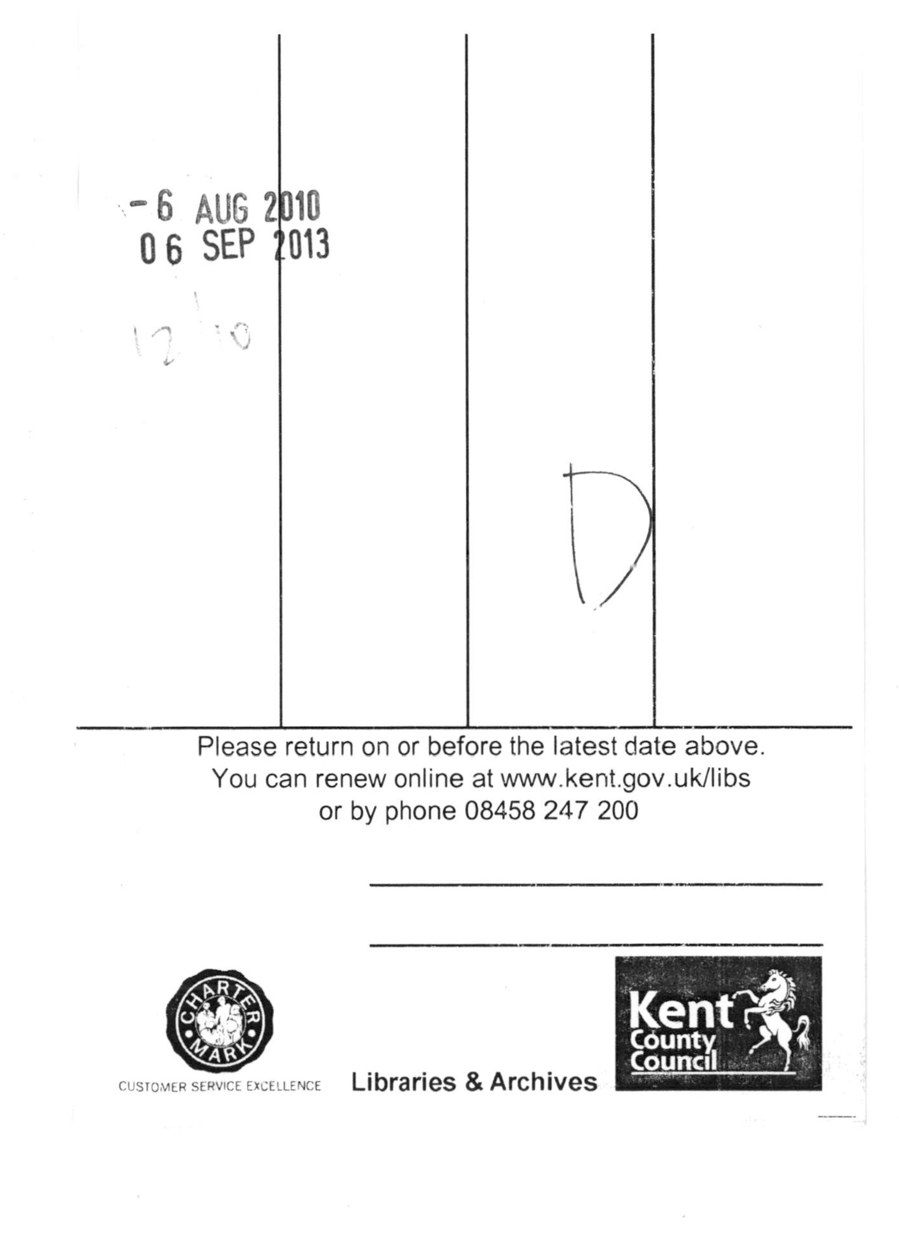

Contents

Preface to the first edition

This book is written primarily for medical students seeking a summary of genetics and its medical applications, but it should be of value also to advanced students in the biosciences, paramedical scientists, established medical doctors and health professionals who need to extend or update their knowledge. It should be of especial value to those preparing for examinations.

Medical genetics is unusual in that, whereas its fundamentals usually form part of first-year medical teaching within basic biology, those aspects that relate to inheritance may be presented as an aspect of reproductive biology. Clinical issues usually form a part of later instruction, extending into the postgraduate years. This book is therefore presented in three sections, which can be taken together as a single course, or separately as components of several courses. Chapters are however intended to be read in essentially the order of presentation, as concepts and specialised vocabulary are developed progressively.

There are many excellent introductory textbooks in our subject, but none, so far as we know, is at the same time so comprehensive and so succinct. We believe the relative depth of treatment of topics appropriately reflects the importance of these matters in current thinking.

Dorian Pritchard
Bruce Korf

Preface to the second edition

Reviewers of the first edition were generally impressed by the lucidity of the text, the clarity of the diagrams and the amount of information presented, but several pointed to a deficiency in clinical detail. This reflects a change in content of courses in medical genetics in recent years, especially following the sequencing of the human genome, and a trend towards increasing the emphasis on clinical correlations in basic science teaching.

In response, we have extended nine chapters of the first edition to 18, providing scope for fuller clinical accounts of the commoner genetic conditions and outline descriptions of less common disorders. We have written two new chapters on biochemical genetics, one on the embryonic definition of body pattern and one on ethical and social issues. To provide an element of self-assessment and some insight into the life of a medical geneticist, we have for the first time included 10 genetic case studies. A feature unique to this title is the method for using disease incidence in twins for estimating the penetrance of multifactorial conditions and the number of major causative genes. An innovation in the second edition is the use of coloured panels within the text to emphasize appropriate action in urgent situations.

The first edition is being used throughout the English-speaking world and has been translated into Chinese and Japanese, while Korean and Greek translations are in preparation. In keeping with this international readership, we stress clinical issues of particular relevance to the major ethnic groups, with information on relative disease allele frequencies in diverse populations.

We hope the introduction of full colour in the diagrams not only adds attraction, but also makes illustrated details more accessible and diagrams more memorable. More important, however, is the revision and updating of the text throughout and the introduction of nearly 50% more, largely clinical, material.

Dorian Pritchard
Bruce Korf

Acknowledgements

We thank thousands of students, for the motivation they provided by their enthusiastic reception of the lectures on which these chapters are based. We appreciate also the interest and support of many colleagues, but special mention should be made of constructive contributions to the first edition by Dr Paul Brennan of the Department of Human Genetics, University of Newcastle. We are most grateful also to Professor Angus Clarke of the Department of Medical Genetics, Cardiff University for his valuable comments on Chapter 61 and to Dr J. Daniel Sharer, Assistant Professor of Genetics, University of Alabama at Birmingham for constructive advice on our diagram of the tandem mass spectrometer. DP wishes to pay tribute to the memory of Ian Cross for his friendship and professional support over many years and for his advice on the chapters dealing with cytogenetics.

We thank the staff of Blackwell Publishing for their encouragement and tactful guidance throughout the production of this book and Jane Fallows for her tasteful presentation of the artwork.

Dorian Pritchard
Bruce Korf

List of abbreviations

A: adenine; blood group A.
AB: blood group AB.
abl: the Abelson proto-oncogene, normally on 9q, that participates in the Philadelphia derivative chromosome.
ACE: angiotensin-1 converting enzyme.
ACo-D: autosomal dominant
AD: autosomal dominant.
ADA: adenosine deaminase.
ADH: alcohol dehydrogenase.
AER: ridge of ectoderm along the apex of the limb bud.
AFP: α-fetoprotein.
AIP: acute intermittent porphyria.
ALDH: acetaldehyde dehydrogenase.
α_1-AT: α_1-antitrypsin.
APP: amyloid-β precursor protein.
AR: autosomal recessive.
ARMS: amplification refractory mutation system.
AS: Angelman syndrome; ankylosing spondylitis.
ASD: atrial septal defect
ASO: allele specific oligonucleotide.
ATP: adenosine triphosphate.
B: blood group B.
BAC: bacterial artificial chromosome.
BCAA: branched chain amino acid.
BCL: bilateral cleft lip.
***BCR*:** the breakpoint cluster region, normally on 22q that participates in the Philadelphia chromosome.
BLS: bare lymphocyte syndrome.
BMD: Becker muscular dystrophy.
BMI: body mass index.
BMP-4: bone morphogenetic protein 4.
bp: base pair.
BRCA1, BRCA2: breast cancer susceptibility genes 1 and 2.
C: cytosine; haploid number of single-strand chromosomes; number of concordant twin pairs.
2C: diploid number of single-strand chromosomes.
CAD: coronary artery disease.
CAH: congenital adrenal hyperplasia.
CATCH 22: cardiac defects, abnormal facies, thymic hypoplasia, cleft palate and hypocalcemia caused by microdeletion at 22q11.2.
CBAVD: congenital bilateral absence of the vas deferens.
cDNA: DNA copy of a specific mRNA.
CF: cystic fibrosis.
***CFTR*:** cystic fibrosis transmembrane conductance regulator; the cystic fibrosis gene.
CGD: chronic granulomatous disease.
CGH: comparative genome hybridization.
CHARGE: coloboma, heart defects, choanal atresia, retarded growth, genital abnormalities and abnormal ears.
CHD: congenital heart disease.
CL ± P: cleft lip with or without cleft palate.
CML: chronic myelogenous leukaemia.
CMV: *Cytomegalovirus.*
CNS: central nervous system.
CRASH: corpus callosum hypoplasia, retardation, adducted thumbs, spastic paraparesis and hydrocephalus due to mutation in the L1 CAM cell adhesion molecule.
CSF: cerebro-spinal fluid.
CT scan: computerized technique that uses X-rays to obtain cross-sectional images of tissues.
CVS: chorionic villus sampling.
CYP: cytochrome P450.
D: number of discordant twin pairs.
ddA (/T/C/G)TP: dideoxynucleotide A (T,C,G).
del: chromosome deletion.
ΔF508: the most common mutation causative of cystic fibrosis.
***der*:** derivative chromosome.
DHPR: dihydropteridine reductase.
DMD: Duchenne muscular dystrophy.
DNA: deoxyribonucleic acid.
DOPA: dihydroxyphenylalanine.
***dup*:** duplicated segment of a chromosome.
DZ: dizygotic, arising from two zygotes.
ELSI: the Ethical, Legal and Social Implications Program of the Human Genome Project.
ER: endoplasmic reticulum.
FAP(C): familial adenomatous polyposis (coli).
FCH: familial combined hyperlipidaemia.
FGF: fibroblast growth factor.
FGFR: fibroblast growth factor receptor.
FH: familial hypercholesterolaemia.
FISH: fluorescence *in-situ* hybridization.
FMR: a gene at Xq27.3 containing a CGG repeat, expansion of which causes Fragile-X disease.
FRAX: Fragile-X syndrome.
FSH: follicle stimulating hormone.
G: guanine.
G0, G1, G2: phases of the mitotic cycle.
G6PD: glucose-6-phosphate dehydrogenase.
GI: gastro-intestinal.
GLI3: a zinc finger transcription controlling protein.
GM: ganglioside.
GSD: glycogen storage disorder.
HAO: hereditary angioneurotic oedema.
HbA: normal allele for β-globin.
HbS: sickle cell allele of β-globin.
HGPRT/HPRT: hypoxanthine-guanine phosphoribosyl transferase.
HIV: human immunodeficiency virus.
HMGCoA: hydroxymethylglutaryl coenzyme A.
HMSN: hereditary motor and sensory neuropathy, Charcot–Marie–Tooth disease.
HNPCC: hereditary non-polyposis colon cancer.
hnRNA: heterogeneous nuclear RNA.
HoxA–D: Homeobox genes A–D.
***i*:** isochromosome.
ICSI: intra-cytoplasmic sperm injection.
IDDM: insulin dependent diabetes mellitus.
Ig: immunoglobulin.
***ins*:** inserted segment in a chromosome.
***inv*:** inverted segment of a chromosome.
IP: incontinentia pigmenti.

IQ: intelligent quotient
IRT: immunoreactive trypsin.
kb: kilobase (1000 bases).
λ_5: relative risk for a sib
LCHAD: long chain hydroxyacyl coenzyme A deficiency.
LDLR: low density lipoprotein receptor.
LEFTA/B: human equivalent of the gene Lefty-1/2.
LHON: Leber hereditary optic neuropathy.
LINES: Long interspersed nuclear elements
lod: 'Log of the odds'; the logarithm ($\log_{10}$) of the ratio of the probability that a certain combination of phenotypes arose as a result of genetic linkage (of a specified degree) to the probability that it arose merely by chance.
LSD: lipid storage disorder.
M: monosomy; mitotic phase of the cell cycle.
M1, M2: first, second divisions of meiosis.
MAPH: multiplex amplifiable probe hybridization.
Mb: megabase (1000 000 bases).
MCAD: medium chain acyl coenzyme A deficiency.
MELAS: mitochondrial encephalopathy, lactic acidosis and stroke-like episodes.
MEN: multiple endocrine neoplasia.
MERRF: myoclonic epilepsy with ragged red fibres.
MHC: major histocompatibility complex.
MIS: Müllerian inhibiting substance.
MND: Menkes disease.
MPS: mucopolysaccharidosis.
MRI: magnetic resonance imaging.
mRNA: messenger RNA.
MS: mass spectrometry; multiple sclerosis.
MS/MS: tandem mass spectrometry.
MTC: medullary thyroid carcinoma.
MZ: monozygotic, derived from one zygote.
N: haploid number of chromosomal DNA double-helices; in humans, 23.
NARP: neurodegeneration, ataxia and retinitis pigmentosa.
NOR: nucleolar organizer region.
NSD-1: nuclear SET domain 1; the gene at 5q35 responsible for Sotos syndrome.
NTD: neural tube defect.
NF1, NF2: neurofibromatosis types 1 and 2.
NHC protein: non-histone chromosomal protein.
NIDDM: non-insulin dependent diabetes mellitus.
O: blood group O.
OHD: 21-hydroxylase deficiency.
p: chromosomal short arm: symbol for allele frequency.
P: degree of penetrance.
p53: mitosis suppressor protein product of the gene, *TP53*.
PA: phenylalanine.
PAH: phenylalanine hydroxylase.
PCR: polymerase chain reaction.
PFGE: pulsed-field gel electrophoresis.
PGD: preimplantation genetic diagnosis.
PKU: phenylketonuria.
PNP: purine nucleoside phosphorylase.
Pol II: RNA polymerase II.
P-WS: Prader–Willi syndrome.
q: chromosomal long arm; symbol for allele frequency.
***r*:** ring chromosome.
rad: an absorbed dose of 100 ergs of radiation per gram of tissue.
ret: a proto-oncogene that becomes rearranged during transfection, initiating tumorigenesis.
RFLP: restriction fragment length polymorphism.
Rh: Rhesus.
RISC: RNA induced silencing complex.
RNA: ribonucleic acid.
RNAi: RNA interference.
rRNA: ribosomal RNA.
S: Svedberg unit; DNA synthetic phase of the cell cycle.
SCID: severe combined immunodeficiency disease.
Shh: sonic hedgehog, a gene concerned with body patterning.
SINES: short interspersed nuclear elements
siRNA: small interfering RNA.
SLE: systemic lupus erythematosus.
SLO: Smith–Lemli–Opitz syndrome.
SMA: spinal muscular atrophy.
snRNA: small nuclear RNA.
snRNP: small nuclear ribonucleo-protein; protein-RNA complex important in recognition of intron/exon boundaries, intron excision or exon splicing, etc.
***SRY*:** Y-linked male sex determining gene.
SSCP: single strand conformation polymorphism; study of DNA polymorphism by electrophoresis of DNA denatured into single strands.
STC: signal transduction cascade.
SVAS: supravalvular aortic stenosis.
T: thymine; trisomy.
T1DM; T2DM: type 1 and type 2 diabetes mellitus.
Taq: *Thermus aquaticus*.
***ter*:** terminal, close to the chromosome telomere.
TFM: testicular feminization, or androgen insensitivity syndrome.
TORCH: *Toxoplasma*, other, *Rubella*, *Cytomegalovirus* and *Herpes*.
***TP53*:** the gene coding for protein p53.
tRNA: transfer RNA.
ts: tumour suppressor
TSC: tuberous sclerosis.
U: uracil.
UCL: unilateral cleft lip.
UDP: uridine diphosphate.
VACTERL: as for VATER with cardiac and limb defects also.
VATER: vertebral defects, anal atresia, tracheo-oesophageal fistula and renal defects.
VCFS: velocardiofacial syndrome.
VNTR: variable number tandem repeat; usually applied to minisatellites.
VSD: ventricular septal defect.
WAGR: Wilms tumour, aniridia, genito-urinary anomalies and (mental) retardation.
XD: X-linked dominant.
XLA: X-linked agammaglobulinaemia.
XP: xeroderma pigmentosum.
XR: X-linked recessive.
YAC: yeast artificial chromosome.
ZIC3: a zinc finger transcription controlling protein.
ZPA: zone of proliferating activity.

1 Introduction and basic biology

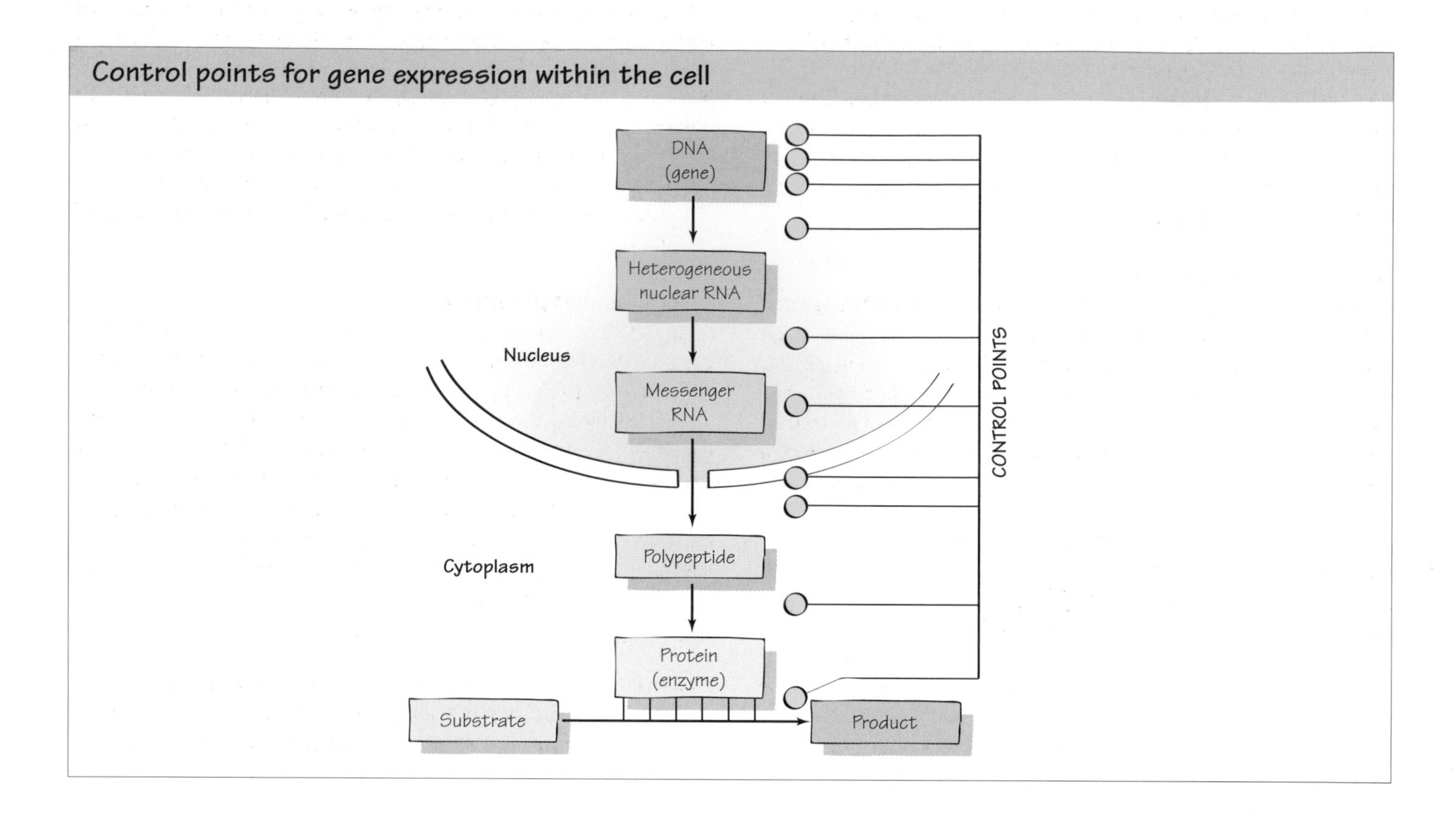

The case for genetics

Medicine is currently in a state of transformation, created by the convergence of two major aspects of technological advance. The first is the explosion in information technology, and the second the rapidly expanding science of genetics. The likely outcome is that within the foreseeable future we will see the introduction of a new kind of medicine, **individualized medicine**, tailored uniquely to the personal needs of each patient.

Clinicians currently use family histories and genetic testing to identify patients for further evaluation and for guidance on their management. Recognition of the precise (molecular) nature of a disorder enables correct interpretation of ambiguous symptoms. Some diseases, such as hypertension (high blood pressure), have many causes for which a variety of treatments may be possible. Identification of precise cause would allow clinicians to give personal guidance on the avoidance of adverse stimuli and enable precise targeting of the disease with personally appropriate medications. Progress along those lines has been slower than anticipated, but has now moved powerfully into related areas.

Pharmacogenetics is the study of differential responses to unusual biochemicals. For genetic reasons some individuals are hypersensitive to standard doses of commonly prescribed drugs, while others respond poorly. Genetic insight will guide physicians in the correct prescription of doses while discoveries in other areas of genetics are stimulating development of new kinds of medication. The field of **pharmacogenomics** involves the genetic engineering of pharmaceuticals. Human genes, such as those for insulin and interferon are introduced into microorganisms, field crops and farm animals and these species used as living factories for production of the human proteins. Genomics is also leading to the elucidation of molecular pathways of disease and the ability to target specific steps in these pathways.

In research into human diseases, **disease analogues** can be created in laboratory animals by targeted deletion of genes of interest. This approach has been used to create animal models for a wide variety of diseases such as cystic fibrosis and neurofibromatosis.

Some of these topics are outside the scope of this book, but the reader should have no doubt that the medicine of the future, the medicine he or she will practice, will rely very heavily on the insights provided by genetics.

Overview of Part 1

Although medical genetics is essentially about the transmission of harmful versions of genes from one generation to the next, it encompasses a great deal more. Part 1 covers the basic cellular, molecular and developmental biology necessary for its understanding.

The cell (Chapter 2)

Typically every cell in our bodies contains a pair of each of our genes and these are controlled and expressed in molecular terms *at the level of the cell*. During embryonic development cells in different parts of the body become exposed to different influences and acquire divergent properties, as they begin to express different combinations of the 20–25 000 gene pairs they each contain. Nevertheless, most cells have a similar basic structure and composition, as described in Chapter 2.

Genetic material (Chapters 3–5)

Most of the biochemical processes of our bodies are catalysed by enzymes and their amino acid sequences are defined by the genes. Genes are coded messages written into an enormously long molecule called **DNA**. This is elaborately coiled and in growing tissue is found alternately extended or tightly contracted.

The DNA is distributed between 23 pairs of homologous **chromosomes**. In a normal woman two of these are large **X-chromosomes**. A normal man also has 46 chromosomes, but in place of one X is a much smaller **Y**, that carries several genes, including the single gene responsible for triggering male development.

Gene expression (Chapters 6–8)

The means by which the information contained in the DNA is interpreted is so central to our understanding that the phrase: '*DNA makes RNA makes protein*'; or, more correctly, '***DNA makes heterogeneous nuclear RNA, which makes messenger RNA, which makes polypeptide, which makes protein***'; has become accepted as the '**central dogma**' of molecular biology. The production of the protein product of any gene can potentially be controlled at many steps (see figure).

Cell division and formation of eggs and sperm

(Chapters 9 and 10)

Body growth involves individual cells replicating their components, dividing in half, expanding and doing the same again. This sequence is called **the cell cycle** and it involves two critical events: **replication** of chromosomal DNA, and segregation of the duplicated chromosomes by **mitosis**.

A modified version of mitosis results in cells with only one, instead of two, sets of chromosomes. This is **meiosis**, which plays a critical part in the creation of the gametes.

Embryonic development (Chapters 11–13)

Fertilization of an egg by a sperm restores the normal chromosome number in the resultant **zygote**. This proliferates to become a hollow ball that **implants** in the maternal uterus. Development proceeds until birth, normally at around 38 weeks, but all the body organs are present in miniature by 6–8 weeks. Thereafter embryogenesis mainly involves **growth** and **differentiation** of cell types. At **puberty** development of the organs of reproduction is re-stimulated and the individual attains physical maturity. The period of 38 weeks is popularly considered to be 9 months, traditionally interpreted as three '**trimesters**'. The term '**mid-trimester**' refers to the period covering the 4th, 5th and 6th months of gestation.

Genotype and phenotype

Genotype is the word geneticists use for the genetic endowment a person has inherited. **Phenotype** is our word for the anatomical, physiological and psychological complex we recognize as an individual.

People have diverse phenotypes, partly because they inherited different genotypes, but an equally important factor is what we can loosely describe as 'environment'. This includes nutrients derived from the bodies of our mothers, growing space, our postnatal feeding and experience, sunlight, exercise, etc. A valuable concept is summarized in the statement: '*Phenotype is the product of interaction between genotype, environment and time*'; or:

Phenotype = Genotype × Environment × Time

Practically every aspect of phenotype has both genetic and environmental components. This is a point well worth remembering when we consider the possible causes of any disease, and an issue we address more closely in Part 2.

2 The cell

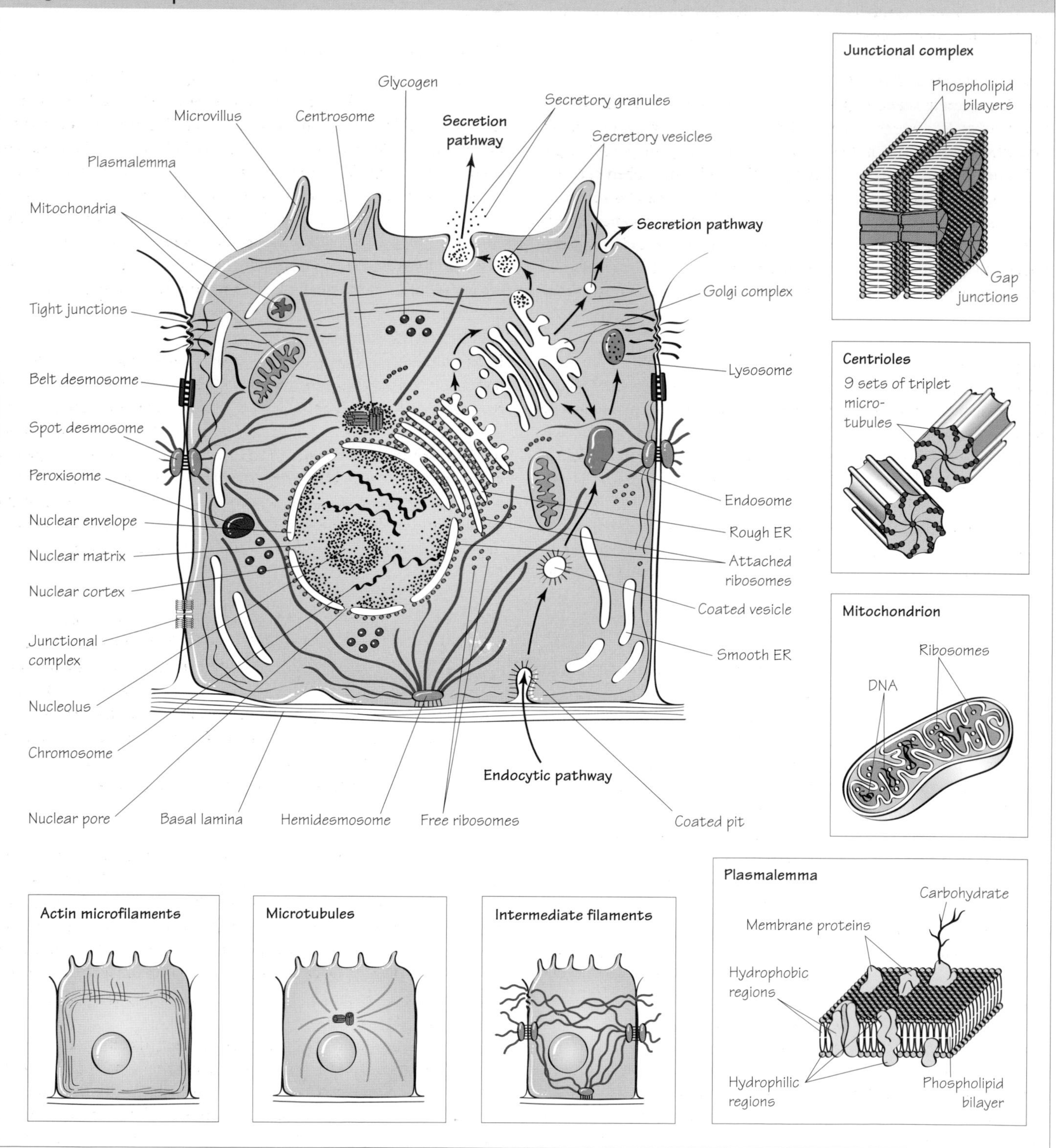

A generalized epithelial cell
Glycogen
Microvillus
Centrosome
Secretion pathway
Secretory granules
Secretory vesicles
Plasmalemma
Mitochondria
Secretion pathway
Golgi complex
Tight junctions
Lysosome
Belt desmosome
Spot desmosome
Peroxisome
Endosome
Nuclear envelope
Rough ER
Nuclear matrix
Attached ribosomes
Nuclear cortex
Coated vesicle
Junctional complex
Smooth ER
Nucleolus
Chromosome
Endocytic pathway
Nuclear pore
Basal lamina
Hemidesmosome
Free ribosomes
Coated pit
Junctional complex
Phospholipid bilayers
Gap junctions
Centrioles
9 sets of triplet micro-tubules
Mitochondrion
Ribosomes
DNA
Plasmalemma
Carbohydrate
Membrane proteins
Hydrophobic regions
Hydrophilic regions
Phospholipid bilayer
Actin microfilaments
Microtubules
Intermediate filaments

Overview

The cell is the basic functional component of the body. Its **nucleus** is both the repository of the vast majority of the genetic information of that individual and the centre of activity involving its expression. There are many different types of cell (e.g. epithelial, liver, nerve, etc.) and the several kinds of **organelles** and multitudes of soluble enzymes contained within their **cytoplasms** carry out the numerous differentiated aspects of metabolism characteristic of each cell type.

The plasma membrane

The **plasma membrane**, or **plasmalemma**, is a barrier to water-soluble molecules and defines the interface between the interior and exterior of the cell. It is basically a double, side-by-side array of phospholipid molecules forming a sheet of hydrophobic lipid sandwiched between two sheets of hydrophilic phosphate groups. Within the plasmalemma are a variety of proteins positioned with their hydrophobic regions within the lipid interior and their hydrophilic regions at either surface. **Microvilli** (singular: **microvillus**) are extensions of the apical plasmalemma that provide an increased surface for molecular exchange.

The nucleus

The genetic information is carried on the **chromosomes** (see Chapter 3) suspended in the **nuclear matrix**. This is a mesh of proteinaceous material densest close to the nuclear envelope where it is called the **nuclear cortex**.

The **nucleolus** is a morphologically distinct region within the nucleus specialized for production of **ribonucleic acid** components of the **ribosomes** (**rRNA**). A typical human nucleus contains a single large nucleolus, which at interphase (see Chapter 9) contains the **nucleolar organizer regions** of the acrocentric chromosomes (see Chapters 3 and 50).

The nucleus is bounded by a double membrane called the **nuclear envelope**, perforated by **nuclear pores**.

The cytoplasm

The **cytoplasm** consists of a gel-like a material called the **cytosol**. This contains deposits of glycogen, lipid droplets and free ribosomes (see Chapter 8) and is permeated by an array of interconnected filaments and tubules that form the **cytoskeleton**. The latter has three major structural elements: **microtubules**, **microfilaments** and **intermediate filaments**.

Microtubules are straight tubes built from alternating molecules of α- and **β-tubulin**. They radiate from a structure called the **centrosome**, which contains a pair of cylindrical structures called **centrioles** with a characteristic nine-unit structure. (Similar structures occur as **basal bodies** of cilia.) The microtubular network is important in the maintenance of cell shape, separation of the chromosomes during cell division and movement of cilia and sperm.

Microfilaments are double stranded polymers of the protein **actin** distributed mainly near the cell periphery and involved in cell movement and change of cell shape.

Intermediate filaments are tubular structures that link the desmosomes. They are composed of one of five or more different proteins, depending on cell type.

Mitochondria (singular: **mitochondrion**) are the largest and most abundant of the cytoplasmic organelles. Their main function is the production of energy through synthesis of ATP. They are semi-autonomous and self-replicating, each containing ribosomes and up to 10 or more copies of a circular strand of **mitochondrial DNA** carrying the mitochondrial genes (see Chapter 23). They contain the enzymes of the tricarboxylic acid (TCA) cycle and a major fraction of those involved in the oxidation of fatty acids.

Peroxisomes are partially responsible for detoxification of foreign compounds such as ethanol, but their major role is the oxidation of fatty acids.

The secretion pathway

The **endoplasmic reticulum** (**ER**) is a major site of protein and lipid synthesis and represents the beginning of the secretion pathway for proteins. It is a bulky maze of membrane-bound channels continuous with the nuclear envelope. Close to the nucleus it holds bound ribosomes and is known as '**rough ER**'. Away from the nucleus it lacks ribosomes and is called '**smooth ER**'. The ER also plays a role in neutralizing toxins.

Proteins synthesized in the ER are passed to the **Golgi complex** for further processing. This is a series of stacked, flattened vesicles. They are then collected in **storage vesicles** or **secretory vesicles** for **exocytosis**, i.e. release from the cell, in response to external stimuli.

Endocytosis

Endocytosis is the internalization and subsequent processing of constituents of the surrounding medium. Small particles are taken into vesicles by **receptor-mediated pinocytosis,** which involves internalization of surface bound material through formation of a **coated pit**. Larger particles are bound to membrane receptors and engulfed as **phagocytic vacuoles**; solutes are taken in by **fluid-phase pinocytosis**. The content of both pinocytic and phagocytic vesicles is usually delivered to the **lysosomes** for breakdown by enzymes called **lysozymes**. During this transfer the vesicles are sometimes referred to as **endosomes**.

Cell junctions

Tight junctions create a seal between the apical environment of epithelial cells and their basolateral surfaces. **Belt desmosomes** are elongated layers of fibres that assist in the binding together of adjacent cells, together with **spot desmosomes**, which are localized points of adhesion. **Hemidesmosomes** link epithelial cells to their basal lamina, which is a specialized derivative of the **extracellular matrix**. **Gap junctions** are grouped in **junctional complexes**. Each of these contains a pore permitting molecular communication between adjacent cells.

Medical issues

Several inherited diseases result from deficiencies in specific lysozymes, including Tay–Sachs, Fabry and Gaucher diseases (see Chapters 44, 45). Familial hypercholesterolaemia can result from failure of internalization of lipoprotein. Peroxisomes are absent in Zellweger syndrome, with malformed features, poor muscle tone, enlarged liver and renal cysts. Disorders of the mitochondria are listed in Chapter 23. A defective gap junction protein causes the X-linked form of Charcot–Marie–Tooth disease (see Chapter 22).

Many therapeutic drugs act on receptors located in the plasma membrane. Microtubule assembly is disrupted by the anti-cancer agents, *vincristine* and *vinblastine*, as well as *colchicine*, which is used to arrest cells at metaphase of mitosis (see Chapters 9, 50) for examination of the chromosomes. *Clofibrate*, used clinically to lower serum lipoprotein levels, acts by inducing formation of extra peroxisomes.

3 The chromosomes

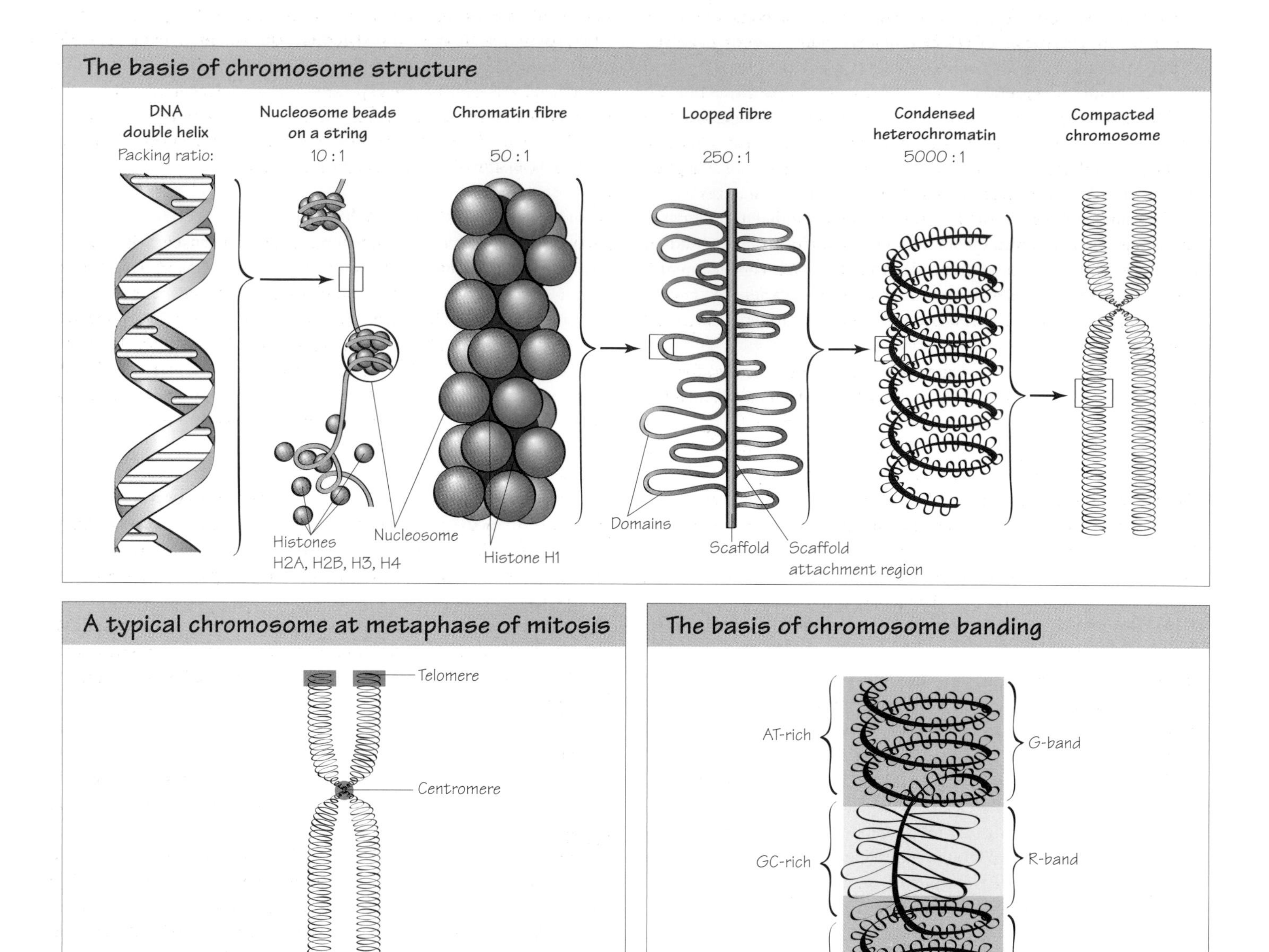

Overview

The word 'chromosome' means 'coloured body', referring to the capacity of these structures to take up certain histological stains more effectively than other cell structures. Each chromosome is composed of an extremely long molecule of DNA complexed with proteins and RNA to form a substance known as **chromatin**. They disperse throughout the nucleus during **interphase** of the cell cycle (i.e. when the cell is not dividing), but become compacted during **mitosis** and **meiosis** (see Chapters 9 and 10). DNA is packaged as chromosomes probably because packaging facilitates segregation of complete sets of genes into daughter cells at mitosis and packing into sperm heads following meiosis.

The staining properties of the chromosomes are utilized in diagnosis for their general visualization, for their individual identification and for the elucidation of chromosomal abnormalities. We can distinguish lightly staining regions designated **euchromatin**, from densely staining **heterochromatin**. Diagnostic aspects are dealt with in Chapters 23–27 and 50.

The genetic information, or **genome**, is carried in encoded form in the sequence of bases in the DNA (see Chapters 4–8). The vast majority of this information is in the nucleus, on chromosomes, but a small portion is in the form of naked loops of DNA within each mitochondrion in the cytoplasm. Nuclei are present in practically every cell of the body, the exceptions including red blood cells and the cells of the eye lens.

A typical human nucleus contains around 2 m of DNA divided between 23 pairs of chromosomes, giving an average of around 4 cm per chromosome. But prior to cell division this is reduced to less than 5 μm (0.005 mm) by intricate coiling and packing.

Chromatin structure

In each chromosome the DNA strand is wound twice around globular aggregates of eight histone proteins to form **nucleosomes**, the whole appearing as a **beaded string structure**. The proteins composing the **nucleosome core particle** are *two* molecules each of histones **H2A**, **H2B**, **H3** and **H4**. Histones are positively charged and so can make ionic bonds with negatively charged phosphate groups in the DNA. The amino acid sequences of histones show close to 100% homology across species, indicating their great importance in maintenance of chromatin structure and function. Each nucleosome accommodates about 200 base pairs of DNA and effectively reduces the length of the DNA strand to one-tenth.

The beaded string is then further coiled into a **solenoid**, or spiral coil, with 5–6 nucleosomes per turn, the structure being maintained by mediation of *one* molecule of histone **H1** per nucleosome. Formation of the solenoid decreases the effective length of the DNA strand by another factor of five, yielding an overall 'packing ratio' of about 50. This is the probable state of euchromatin at interphase in regions where the genes are not being expressed.

During mitosis and meiosis the chromosomes are condensed, a further 100-fold, achieving packing ratios of around 5000. The chromatin fibre is thought to be folded into a series of loops radiating from a central **scaffold** of **non-histone chromosomal proteins** (or **NHC proteins**) that bind to specific base sequences scattered along the DNA strand. Compaction of the chromosome probably involves contraction of these NHC proteins.

One of the most important of the scaffold proteins is **topoisomerase II**, a DNA-nicking-closing enzyme that permits the uncoiling of the two strands of the DNA double helix necessary for relaxation of DNA supercoils during replication or transcription (see Chapters 5 and 7). Topoisomerase II binds to **scaffold attachment regions** that are AT-rich (i.e. contain more than 65% of the bases A and T; see Chapter 4). It is believed that each loop may possibly act as an independent functional domain with respect to DNA replication or transcription.

The looped fibre is then further coiled to create the fully condensed heterochromatin of a chromosome at cell division.

Chromosome banding

Some parts of the compacted chromosome stain densely with Giemsa stain to create **G-bands**. These contain tightly packed, small loops because the scaffold attachment regions there are close together. They replicate late in S-phase (see Chapter 9) and are relatively inactive in transcription. Bands that stain lightly with Giemsa stain, **R-bands,** contain more loosely packed loops, are relatively rich in bases G and C and show most transcriptional activity. Differences between banding patterns of chromosomes allow their identification (see Chapter 50).

The centromere

When visible in early mitosis each chromosome is composed of two identical structures called **sister chromatids** connected at a **primary constriction**. This consists of a non-duplicated stretch of DNA called the **centromere** that duplicates during early anaphase of mitosis (see Chapter 9).

An organelle called the **kinetochore** becomes located on each side of each centromere in early prophase of mitosis and facilitates polymerization of **tubulin** dimers to form the **microtubules** of the **mitotic spindle**.

The telomeres

The term '**telomere**' refers to the specialized end of a chromosome. Specific telomeric proteins bind to this structure to provide a cap (see Chapter 5).

The telomeres have several probable functions: preventing the abnormal end-to-end fusion of chromosomes, ensuring complete replication of chromosome extremities, assisting with chromosome pairing in **meiosis** (see Chapter 10) and helping to establish the internal structure of the nucleus during interphase by linking the chromosomes to the nuclear membrane.

Euchromatin and heterochromatin

Euchromatin is compacted during cell division, but relaxes into an open conformation during interphase. In compacted chromosomes it constitutes the palely staining R-bands and contains the majority of the structural genes.

Heterochromatin is densely compacted at cell division and remains compacted at interphase. It is largely concentrated around the nuclear periphery and nucleolus and is relatively inactive in transcription. **Constitutive heterochromatin** is common to all cells of the body, while **facultative heterochromatin** varies, representing regions of the genome that are expressed differentially in the different cell types.

4 DNA structure

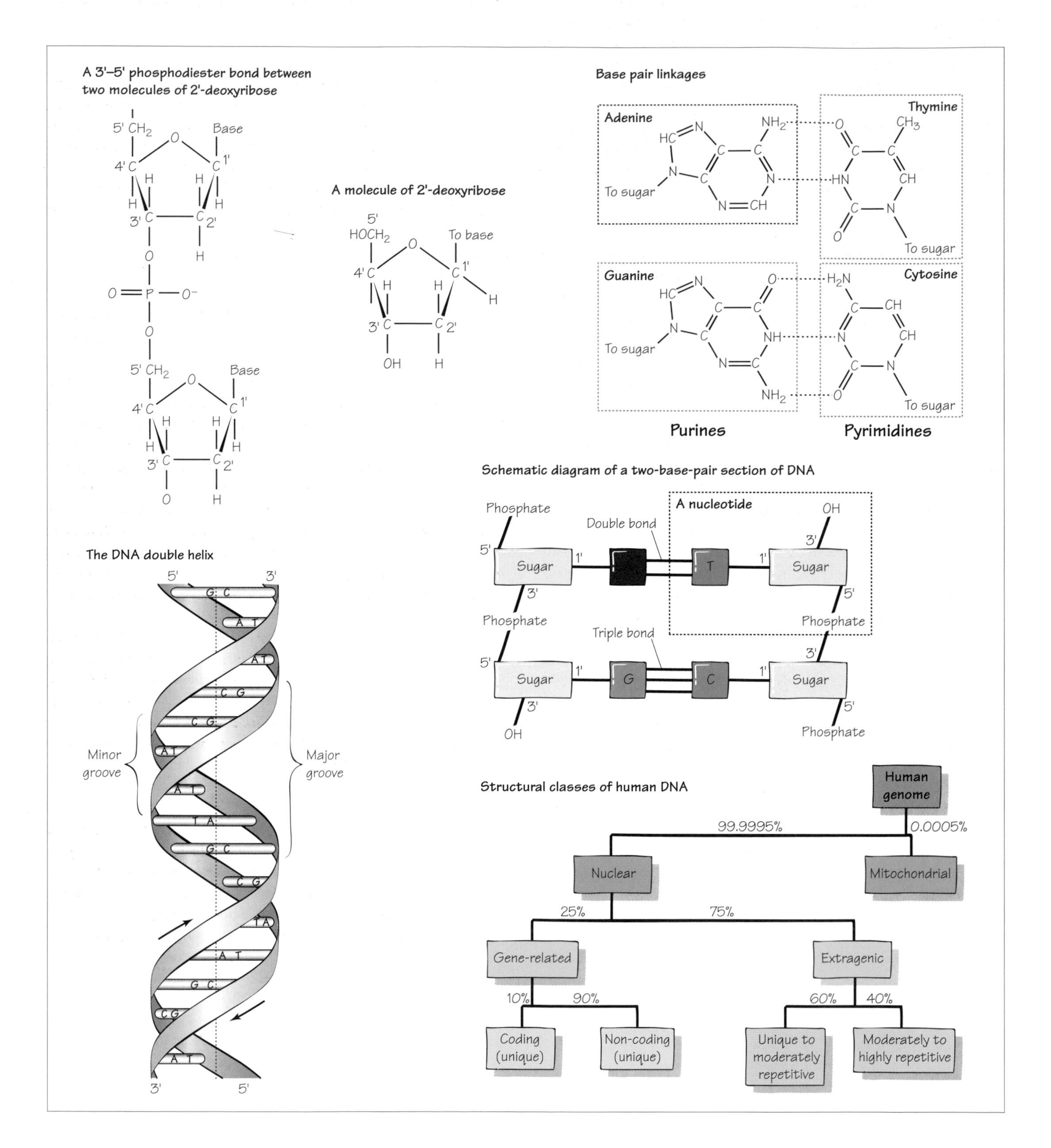

Overview

As we learnt in Chapter 3, the chromosomes are composed essentially of **DNA**, which contains coded instructions for synthesis of every protein in the body. DNA consists of millions of nucleotides within two interlinked, coiled chains. Each nucleotide contains one of four bases and it is the sequence of these bases that contains the coded instructions.

Each base on one chain is matched by a complementary partner on the other, and each sequence provides a template for synthesis of a copy of the other. Synthesis of new DNA is called **replication** (see Chapter 5).

The unit of length of DNA is the **base pair** (**bp**) with 1000 bp in a **kilobase** (**kb**) and 1 000 000 bp in a **megabase** (**Mb**). A typical human body cell contains nearly 7000 Mb of DNA.

The structure of DNA

We can imagine the structure of DNA as like an extremely long, flexible ladder that has been twisted right-handed (like a corkscrew) by coiling around a telegraph pole. Each 'upright' of the ladder is a series of **deoxyribose** sugar molecules linked together by phosphate groups attached to their 3′ ('three prime') and 5′ ('five prime') carbon atoms. At the bottom of one upright is a 3′ carbon atom carrying a free hydroxyl (–OH) group and at the top, a 5′ carbon carrying a free phosphate group. On the other upright this orientation is reversed.

The 'rungs' of the ladder are pairs of nitrogenous **bases** of two types, **purines** and **pyrimidines**. The purines are **adenine** (**A**) and **guanine** (**G**) and the pyrimidines are **cytosine** (**C**) and **thymine** (**T**). The bases are attached to the 1′ carbon of each sugar. Each unit of purine or pyrimidine base together with one attached sugar and one phosphate group constitute a **nucleotide**. A section of double stranded DNA is therefore essentially two linked, coiled chains of nucleotides. This **double helix** has a **major groove** corresponding to the gap between adjacent sections of the sugar-phosphate chains and a **minor groove** along the row of bases. There are 10 pairs of nucleotides per complete turn of the helix.

The pairs of bases of the 'rungs' are hydrogen-bonded together and since both A and T have two sites available for bonding while C and G each have three. *A always pairs with T on the opposite strand and C with G*. This **base pairing** (known as Watson–Crick base pairing) is very specific and ensures that the strands are normally precisely complementary to one another. Thus if one strand reads 5′-CGAT-3′, the complementary strand must read 3′-GCTA-5′ in the same direction, or 5′-ATCG-3′ if we obey the normal rule of describing the sequence from 5′ to 3′. The number of A residues in a section of DNA is therefore always equal to the number of T residues; similarly, the number of C residues always equals the number of G (Chargaff's rule).

The centromeres

Centromeric DNA contains short sequences of bases repeated many times 'in tandem array'. The sequences vary between chromosomes, but there are substantial regions of homology. The most important component is a 171-bp repeat called **alpha-satellite DNA**. This is AT-rich and contains a binding site for a protein contained within the **kinetochore**. The latter is responsible for assembly of the microtubules of the spindle apparatus.

The telomeres

In contrast to the centromeric repeats, telomeric sequences are the same in all human chromosomes and similar to those in other species. Human telomeric DNA consists of long arrays of tandem repeats of the sequence 5′-GGGTTA-3′ extending for several hundred bases on each chromosome end. Most of this is double-stranded, with 3′-CCCAAT-5′ on the complementary strand, but the extreme 3′ end is single-stranded and believed to loop around and invade the double helix several kilobases away. The triple-stranded structure so formed is stabilized by binding telomere-specific protein (see Chapter 5).

Structural classes of human DNA

The human *haploid* genome contains probably 20–25 000 nuclear genes, i.e. coding sequences and their associated control elements, in addition to 37 (including those for mitochondrial tRNA: see Chapters 6, 23) within the mitochondrial genome. However, *the nuclear genome represents no more than 3% of nuclear DNA*, the remainder having no coding function. This includes **introns** that interrupt the coding **exons** of most genes, plus the 75% of human nuclear DNA that is extragenic, i.e. outside or between the genes. Of the latter, 60% is of unique sequence or moderately repetitive, while 40% is moderately to highly repetitive.

The highly-repetitive fraction includes **microsatellite** and **minisatellite DNA**, which differ in the length of the repeat. Satellite DNA is so-called because its unusual AT : GC ratio gives it a buoyant density that differs from the bulk of the DNA. This causes it to separate out as a 'satellite band' when mechanically sheared whole DNA is subjected to density gradient centrifugation.

About 10% of the nuclear DNA consists of up to 500 000 copies of repetitive sequence DNA, the average size of the repeat units being ~ 800 bp, called **long interspersed nuclear elements**, or **LINES**. There are also about a million copies of a short repeat (~ 300 bp) known as *Alu* and ~ 400 000 of another of 130 bp called *MIR*, constituting together ~ 9% of the nuclear genome. The latter are called **short interspersed nuclear elements** or **SINES**.

Medical and legal issues

Microsatellite DNA is scattered throughout the genome and is useful for tracking the inheritance of disease alleles of genes to which they are closely linked. Minisatellite DNA is concentrated near the centromeres and telomeres, so is less useful for tracking genes, but since it is highly variable it is used for producing **DNA fingerprints**. These play an exceptionally important role in paternity testing and forensic identification (see Chapter 58).

5 DNA replication

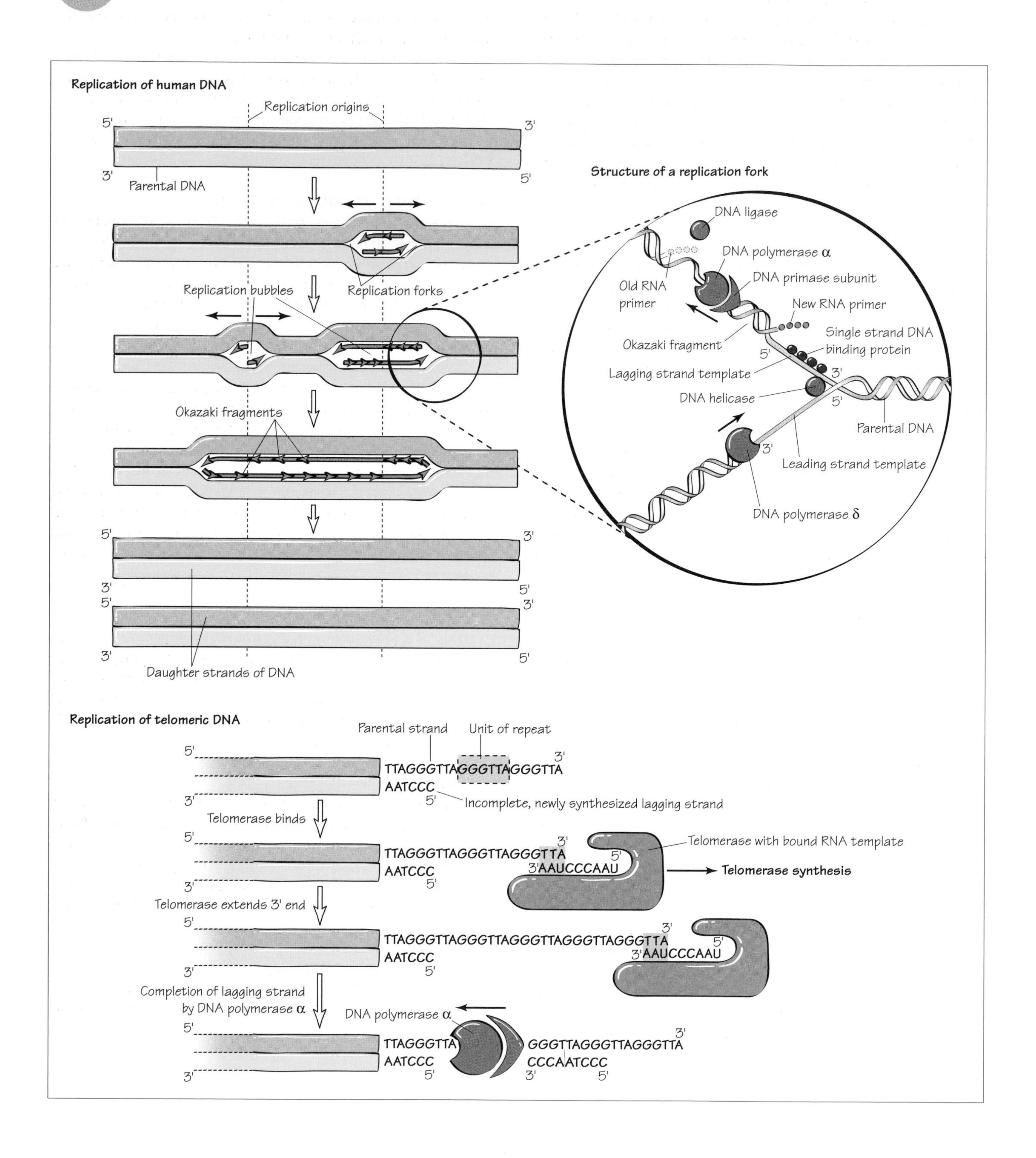

Overview

Cells multiply by the process of mitosis, but so that genetic information is not lost, the whole of the nuclear genome is first duplicated. This occurs during **S-phase** of the **cell cycle** (see Chapter 9). S-phase lasts about 8 hours. The DNA at the centromeres of the chromosomes is replicated in the middle of mitosis, just before chromosome segregation. Mitochondrial DNA is replicated out of phase with nuclear DNA.

Although the overall sequence of events during replication of nuclear DNA in higher organisms (eukaryotes) is similar to that in bacteria (prokaryotes), the details are subtly different. In eukaryotes replication takes place while the (nuclear) DNA remains in nucleosome configuration (see Chapter 3).

Replication

GC-rich sections of the DNA, recognizable as euchromatic R-bands in condensed chromatin (see Chapter 3), contain 'housekeeping genes' that operate in every cell. These sections replicate in early S-phase. The heterochromatic AT-rich G bands (see Chapter 3) contain few genes and replicate in late S-phase. Genes in AT-rich regions that code for differentiated properties and operate in some cells only, are found in facultative heterochromatin (see Chapter 3). This is replicated early in those cells in which the genes are expressed and late in those in which they are not.

The place on the DNA helix which first unwinds to begin replication is called the **replication origin**. Here the double strand is split open by a **helicase** enzyme to expose the base sequences. Replication proceeds along the single strands at about 40–50 nucleotides per second, simultaneously in both directions. In higher organisms there are many replication origins spaced about 50–300 kb apart. The resulting separations of the DNA strand are called **replication bubbles**, at each end of which is a **replication fork**.

New DNA is synthesized by enzymes called **DNA polymerases**, from **deoxyribonucleotide triphosphates** (**ATP**, **GTP**, etc.) which in the process are converted into monophosphate nucleotides (**AMP**, **GMP**, etc.). The release and hydrolysis of pyrophosphate from the triphosphates provides energy for the reaction and ensures it is virtually irreversible, making DNA a relatively very robust molecule.

All DNA polymerases can build new DNA only in the 5′ to 3′ direction, which means they must move along their **template strands** from 3′ to 5′. Replication can therefore occur continuously from the origin of replication along only one strand, called the **leading strand**. The other strand is called the **lagging strand** and, because of the orientation of the sugars, along this strand replication takes place only in short stretches. The new sections of DNA along the lagging strand are typically 100–200 bases long and are known as **Okazaki fragments**. Following their synthesis they are linked together by action of the enzyme **DNA ligase**. While awaiting replication the parental single-strand sequence of the lagging strand is temporarily protected by **single-strand binding protein** (or **helix destabilizing protein**).

Leading strand synthesis requires **DNA polymerase δ**; lagging strand synthesis uses a different enzyme, **DNA polymerase α**. The latter contains a **DNA primase** subunit that produces a short stretch of **RNA** (see Chapter 6), which acts as a primer for DNA synthesis. Replication of mitochondrial DNA occurs independently of that in the nucleus and utilizes a different set of enzymes, including the mitochondria-specific **DNA polymerase γ**.

The genome contains multiple copies of the five histone genes, from which copious quantities of histones are produced, especially during S-phase. These bind immediately onto the newly replicated DNA.

Since each daughter DNA duplex contains one old strand from the parent molecule and one newly synthesized strand, the replication process is described as **semi-conservative**.

Replication of the telomeres

Synthesis of DNA at the end of the lagging strand is problematical as DNA polymerase α needs to attach beyond the end of the sequence that is being replicated and work proximally, in the 5′-3′ direction. A specialized DNA synthetic enzyme called **telomerase** provides an extension of the lagging strand that enables this to happen.

Telomerase is a ribonucleoprotein that contains an RNA template with the sequence 3′-AAUCCCAAU-5′. This is complementary to one-and-a-half copies of the six-base telomeric DNA repeat, 5′-GGGTTA-3′ (see Chapter 4). The 3′-AAU of the RNA sequence of the telomerase binds to the terminal -TTA-5′ of the template lagging strand, leaving the rest of the RNA sequence exposed. Deoxyribonucleotides then assemble on this RNA template, extending the DNA repeat sequence by one unit. The telomerase then detaches and moves along to the new DNA terminal -TTA-5′, where the process is repeated. When a sufficiently long terminal repeat has been formed, DNA polymerase α attaches to the single-strand extension and assembles the complementary DNA strand in a proximal 5′-3′ direction back to the old end of the double strand, to which it becomes linked by the action of DNA ligase.

Repair systems

Occasionally a wrong base is inserted into a growing strand, but fortunately, healthy cells contain **post-replication repair enzymes** and **base mismatch proofreading systems** that correct such errors. These remove and replace the erroneously inserted bases, using the template strand as a guide. These repair systems utilize two additional DNA polymerases: β and ε (see Chapter 38).

Medical issues

Several cancer-predisposing conditions arise from defects in different aspects of the post-replication repair and mismatch repair systems. These include the chromosome breakage syndrome called **Bloom syndrome**, familial predisposition to breast cancer caused by mutations in the genes **BRCA1** and **BRCA2** and an autosomal dominant form of bowel cancer called **hereditary non-polyposis colon cancer** (**HNPCC**) (see Chapter 41).

One theory holds that telomeres are reduced in length at every round of mitosis and that the number of repeats they contain may play a role in limiting the number of times a cell can divide. On this theory, abnormally efficient, mutant telomerases may promote the indefinite growth of cancer cells by delaying telomere decay.

6 RNA structure

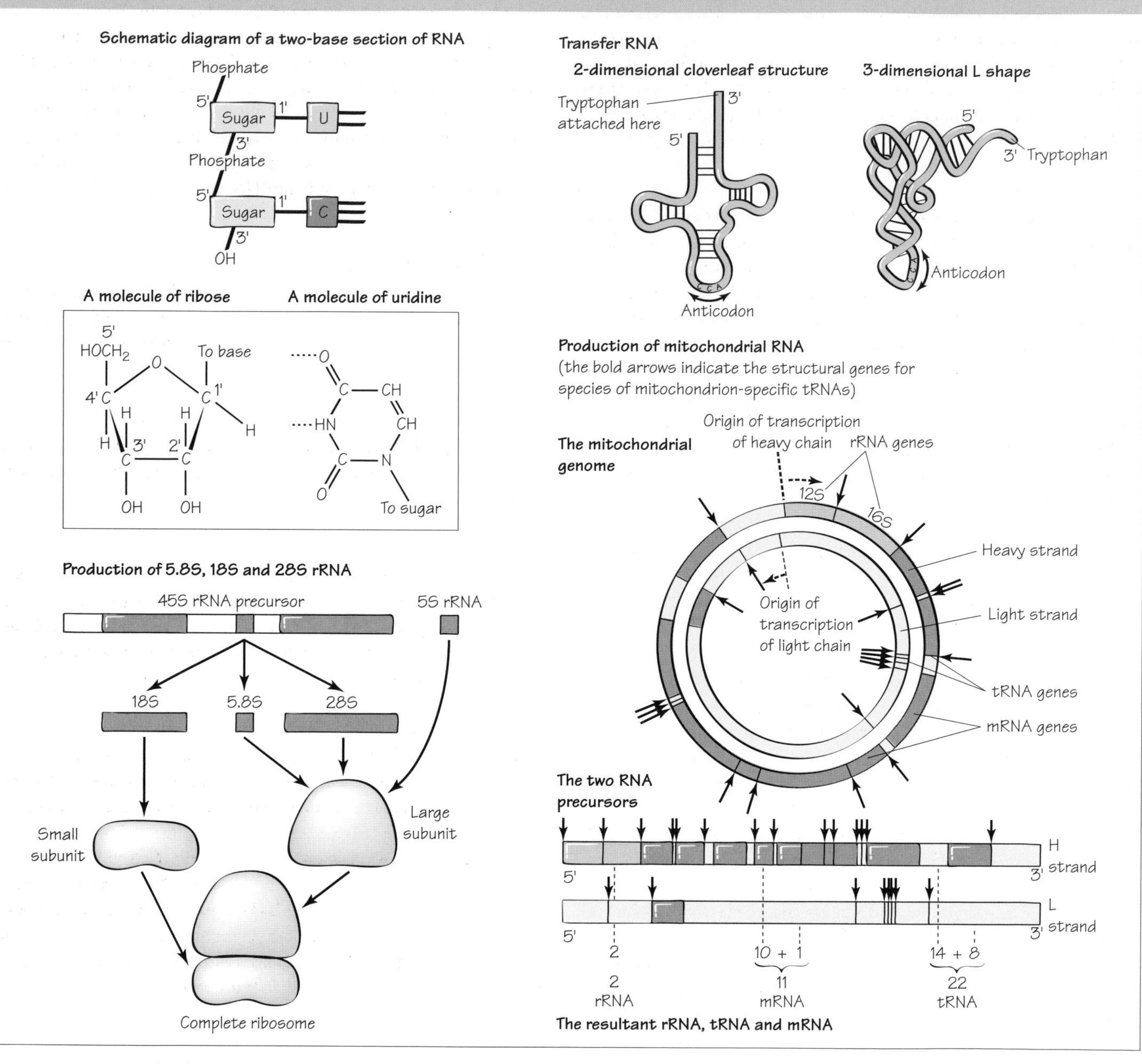

Overview

In Chapter 4 we learnt that DNA is the double-stranded nucleic acid that carries the genetic information we received from our parents and which we pass on to our children. **RNA** is a similar molecule that facilitates the expression of this genetic information within our own cells. The main differences between RNA and DNA are that RNA is (usually) single-stranded, **ribose** replaces deoxyribose and **uracil** replaces thymine. In **eukaryotes** (literally organisms with a 'true nucleus', i.e. higher organisms) RNA occurs as nine major types of molecule: **messenger RNA (mRNA)**, its precursor **heterogeneous nuclear RNA (hnRNA)**, **transfer RNA (tRNA)**, **ribosomal RNA (rRNA)**, **small nuclear RNA (snRNA)**, **small nucleolar RNA (snoRNA)**, **signal recognition particle RNA (srpRNA)**, **micro-RNA (miRNA)** and **mitochondrial RNA (mtRNA)**. Heterogeneous nuclear RNA is characteristic of eukaryotes and is not found in **prokaryotes** (literally 'before the nucleus,' e.g. bacteria and viruses). Some viruses use RNA in place of DNA for storage and transfer of genetic information between generations.

Heterogeneous nuclear and messenger RNA

Heterogeneous nuclear RNA and its derivative mRNA carry genetic information from the nuclear DNA into the cytoplasm.

There are as many species of hnRNA as there are genes, because hnRNA is the direct transcript of the coding sequences of the genome. They are transcribed from the DNA by the enzyme **RNA polymerase II**, or **Pol II**. Messenger RNA results from the processing of hnRNA, which includes the removal of non-coding **introns** and linking together of the coding **exons** (see Chapter 7). Messenger RNA therefore carries only the coding information of the corresponding species of each hnRNA, plus the flanking leader and trailer, so is considerably shorter.

Transfer RNA

Each molecule of tRNA consists of about 75 nucleotides linked together in a long chain that due to internal base pairing adopts a 'cloverleaf' structure, which then twists into an L shape. Transfer RNA is unusual in containing a variety of rarer bases in addition to C, G, A and U, and some of these are modified by methylation. The important feature of tRNA is that each 'charged' molecule carries an amino acid at its 3′ end, while on the middle 'leaf' of the cloverleaf structure are three characteristic bases known as the **anticodon**. The sequence of bases in the anticodon is specifically related to the species of amino acid attached to the 3′ terminus. For example, tRNA with the anticodon 5′-CCA-3′ carries the amino acid tryptophan and no other. It is this specific relationship that forms the basis of translation of the genetic message carried by mRNA (see Chapter 8).

Transfer RNA molecules are transcribed from their coding sequences in DNA by the enzyme **RNA polymerase III**, or **Pol III**. There are over 40 different tRNA subfamilies, each with several members.

Ribosomal RNA

Ribosomal RNA consists of several species usually referred to by their sedimentation coefficients in Svedberg units (S), deduced by their speed of centrifugation in a dense aqueous medium.

Each **ribosome** consists of one large and one small subunit. These contain many proteins derived by translation of mRNA, plus RNA that remains untranslated. The term 'ribosomal RNA' refers to the non-translated material. The small ribosomal subunit contains **18S rRNA** and the large subunit **5S**, **5.8S** and **28S rRNA**.

Ribosomal RNA is transcribed from DNA by two additional RNA polymerases. **Polymerase I** (**Pol I**) transcribes 5.8S, 18S and 28S, as one long **45S** transcript which is then cleaved into three sections, so ensuring they are produced in equal quantities. We each carry about 250 copies of the DNA sequence coding for the 45S transcript per haploid genome. These are in five clusters of tandem repeats on the short arms of Chromosomes 13, 14, 15, 21 and 22. These are known as the **nucleolar organizer regions** as their transcription and the subsequent processing of the 45S transcript occurs while they are held within the nucleolus.

There are about 2000 copies of the 5S rRNA gene in at least three clusters on Chromosome 1. These are transcribed by **Pol III** outside the nucleolus and imported for **ribosome** assembly, along with ribosomal proteins.

Ribosomal RNA contains around 95 **pseudo-uridine** sites created by isomerization of uridine through the agency of snoRNA.

Small nuclear RNA

The conversion of hnRNA into mRNA by the removal of introns occurs in the nucleus in RNA-protein complexes called **spliceosomes**. Each spliceosome has a core of three **small nuclear ribonucleo-proteins** or **snRNPs** (pronounced 'snurps'). Each snRNP contains at least one snRNA and several proteins. There are several hundred different snRNAs, transcribed mainly by Pol II, which are believed to be capable of recognizing specific ribonucleic acid sequences by RNA-RNA base pairing. The most important in hnRNA processing are U1, U2, U4/U6 and U5.

Small nucleolar RNA

Small nucleolar RNA is mostly involved in directing or guiding site-specific base modifications in rRNA and snRNA, e.g. methylation and pseudouridylation. Many snoRNA genes are within introns of other genes.

Signal recognition particle RNA

Signal recognition particle RNA recognizes the signal sequence on proteins destined for export and helps transport them across the plasma membrane.

MicroRNA

There are an estimated 200 human miRNA species, each about 22 bases long derived by ribonuclease H cleavage of double-stranded 'hairpin' RNA precursors corresponding to inverted repeats. These control translation of structural genes by binding to complementary sequences in the 3′ untranslated regions of their mRNA.

Mitochondrial RNA

Mitochondrial DNA is in the form of a continuous loop coding for 13 polypeptides, 22 tRNAs and two rRNAs (one 16S, the other 23S). Most genes are on one strand, the **heavy strand**, but a few are on its complement, the **light strand** and *both strands are transcribed*, as two continuous transcripts, by a **mitochondrion-specific RNA polymerase**. This enzyme is coded by a nuclear gene. The long RNA molecules are then cleaved to produce 37 separate RNA species and the mitochondrial ribosomal and transfer RNAs join forces to translate the 13 mRNAs. Many additional proteins are imported into the mitochondria from the cytoplasm, having been transcribed from nuclear genes.

Medical issues

Patients with **systemic lupus erythematosus** (see Chapter 43) have antibodies directed against their own snRNP proteins. One set of snRNA genes on Chromosome 15q is paternally imprinted and thought to play a role in **Prader–Willi syndrome** (see Chapter 21).

7 Production of messenger RNA

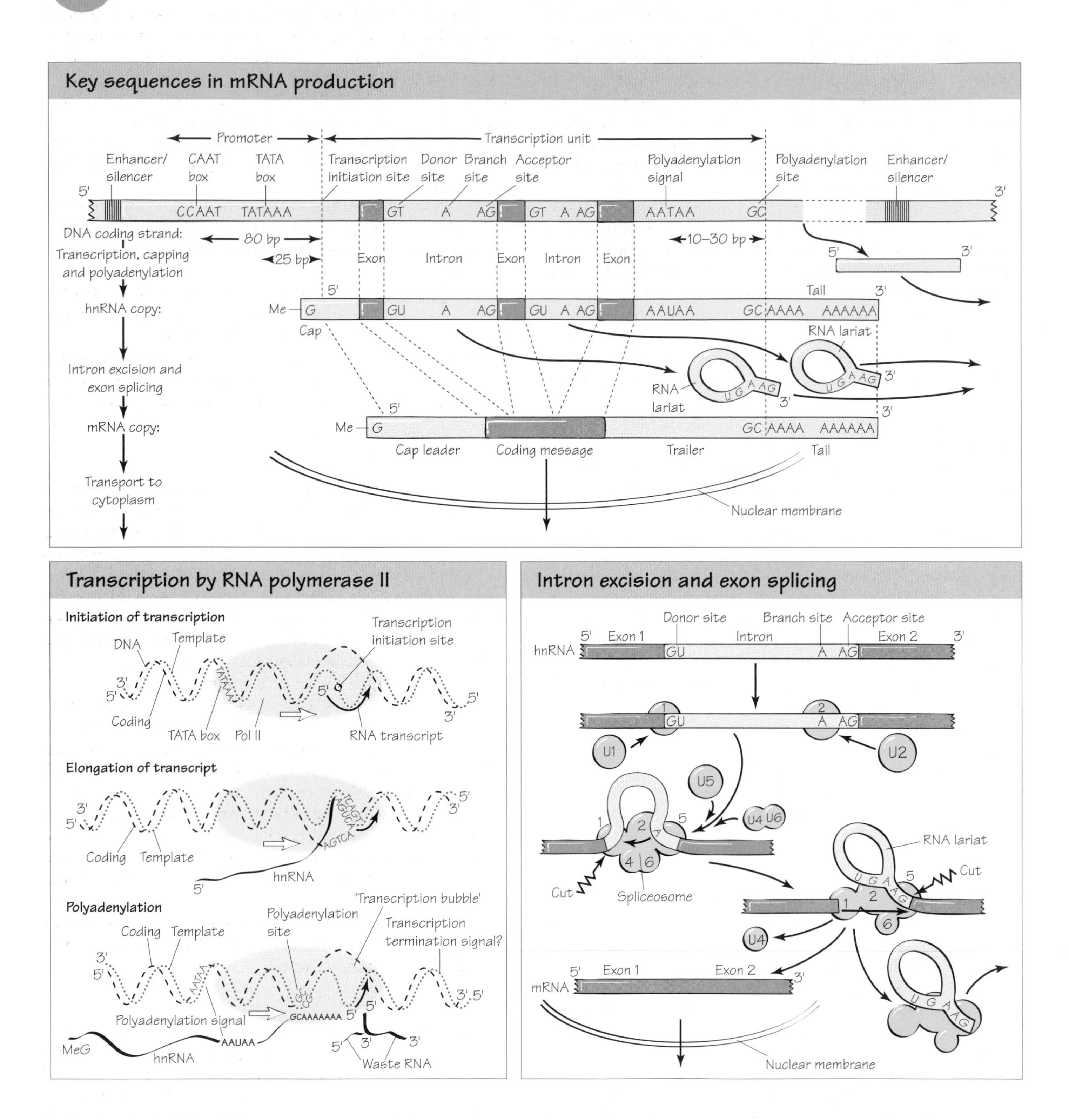

Overview

Most metabolic processes are catalysed by proteinaceous enzymes. Proteins are also the main structural components of the body and the amino acid sequences of all proteins are coded in the DNA. Conversion of the DNA-encoded information into protein involves transcription into an hnRNA copy, processing into mRNA, translation into polypeptide and elaboration into protein (see Chapter 8).

The structure of a gene

Eukaryotes differ from prokaryotes in that most of their genes contain redundant DNA that interrupts the coding sequences. These stretches of non-coding DNA are called **introns**, while the coding sequences are called **exons**. In both groups, outside the coding region are a **leader** and **trailer**, plus a variety of transcriptional control sequences.

Genes that code for protein are called 'structural genes' and their transcription is performed by RNA polymerase Pol II. A sequence just 'upstream' (i.e. 5′) of the coding sequence constitutes the **promoter**, which acts as a binding site for **transcription factors** that indicate where Pol II should begin its action.

Among proteins we can distinguish '**housekeeping proteins**' present in all cell types and '**luxury proteins**' produced for specialized functions. The promoters of genes that code for luxury proteins include a '**TATA box**', with a sequence that is a variant of 5′-TATAAA-3′ at about 25 bp upstream of the **transcription initiation site**. Genes that code for '**housekeeping proteins**' instead usually have one or more '**GC boxes**' in variable positions, containing a variant of 5′-GGGCGG-3′. Another common promoter element is the '**CAAT box**' (e.g. 5′-CCAAT-3′) at −80 bp and there are often also **enhancer** and **silencer** sequences some distance away, that bind controlling factors which interact with the promoter by looping of the DNA. Some 'luxury' genes have additional function-specific control elements.

'Downstream' (i.e. 3′) of the transcription initiation site is the **leader sequence**, which is not translated. The coding message follows, usually interrupted by one or more introns and followed by the non-coding **trailer**. At the end of the trailer is the **polyadenylation site** of variable sequence, but defined by 5′-AATAA-3′ (5′-AAUAA-3′ in the RNA transcript), 10–30 bases upstream.

Introns begin with the sequence **GT**A(/G)GAGT and end with a run of Cs or Ts preceding **AG**. The first **GT** (**GU** in the hnRNA) and the last **AG,** together with an **A** residue situated within a relatively standard sequence near the downstream end, are important in intron removal. The 5' site is known as the **donor** site, the 3' site is the **acceptor** and the A residue is the **branch site**.

In *prokaryotes* transcription stops at a specific point indicated by an inverted repeat in the trailer followed by a run of T residues. The adoption of a hairpin loop by base pairing in the mRNA copy brings transcription to an end. An analogous structure exists in histone gene trailers, but *no general transcription termination signal has been identified in eukaryotes.*

Transcription

Transcription is signalled by assembly of protein transcription factors at the promoter. A molecule of Pol II binds to this **transcription complex** and splits open the double helix. The complex, now including the enzyme, then moves downstream, rather like the slider down a zip, causing local unwinding and splitting, followed by reformation of the double helix as it proceeds, creating a 17-bp long **transcription bubble**. When it reaches the transcription initiation point it ejects one transcription factor, acquires another and begins to synthesize RNA.

Using the strand orientated in the 3′-5′ direction (from left to right) as a template, Pol II grabs ribonucleotides and links them in one by one to produce a complementary RNA sequence, orientated with reverse polarity (i.e. 5′ to 3′). In other words, by applying the rules of base pairing to the **template strand** it creates a precise RNA copy of the **coding strand**. The enzyme transcribes through leader, exons, introns and trailer, and (apparently wastefully!) proceeds indefinitely downstream (see above).

Transcription factors

Transcription factors are proteins that bind to promoter sequences and initiate transcription. Typically they contain an **activation domain** and a **DNA binding domain.** Activation domains are rich in glutamate and either aspartate or proline, which assist in the formation of the transcription complex. The DNA binding domains are of four types.

1 The leucine zipper. This is an α-helical stretch of amino acids with leucine residues at every seventh position, corresponding to every second turn of the helix. This allows pairs of helices to become enmeshed, with a splayed region at the end, believed to grip the DNA like a clothes peg.

2 The helix-loop-helix. This consists of two peptide α-helices linked by a long, flexible loop that permits their packing closely parallel to one another. They are thought to exert control by blocking other gene regulating proteins.

3 The helix-turn-helix. This motif is a feature of the homeobox (see Chapter 12). It consists of two short α-helices separated by an amino acid sequence too short for them to lie in the same plane.

4 The zinc-finger. This is a finger-like structure comprised of around 23 amino acids held by a tetravalent zinc ion, typically linked to four cysteine residues, or two cysteines and two histidines at the base of the finger.

RNA processing

As hnRNA transcripts are synthesized, they are covalently modified to mark them as coded messages for later translation into polypeptide. The 5′ end is first capped by addition of 7-methyl GTP in reverse orientation. When the polyadenylation site appears in the hnRNA strand, it is cleaved there and **poly-A polymerase** adds on 100–200 residues of adenylic acid to form the **poly-A tail**. Both the cap and tail probably protect the molecule from degradation, contribute to the 'passport' that allows its export to the cytoplasm and later provide a recognition signal for the ribosome, indicating its availability for translation.

On average, an hnRNA molecule may have about 7000 nucleotides which are reduced to about 1200 in the mRNA by removal of as many as 50 introns. Histone genes are exceptional in having no introns.

The ribonucleoprotein complexes that remove the introns are called **spliceosomes** and they contain several snRNA species (U1–U6), each complexed with specific proteins. U1 snRNP (i.e. ribonucleoprotein containing U1 snRNA) binds to the upstream splice site, guided by a complementary sequence in the U1 snRNA. U2 snRNP binds to the branch site, then becomes linked to the bound U1, causing a loop in the hnRNA. U2 then cuts the hnRNA immediately upstream of **GU** (see above) and joins that upstream cut end of the intron to the junction site, creating a **lariat** shape. The downstream end of the intron is then cut just beyond **AG**, releasing the RNA lariat, and the spliceosome brings together and joins the two exons.

Medical issues

Alternative RNA splicing occurs normally in some transcripts, notably in the production of antibodies (see Chapter 42), but many genetic disorders involve errors in RNA splicing. In **Gilbert syndrome** cerebral palsy and mental retardation relate to insertion of TA into the normal TATAA promoter of the gene for UDP-glycosyltransferase. *Alpha-amanitin* from the death cap mushroom, *Amanita phalloides*, blocks the action of Pol II. The antibiotic, *rifampicin* (*rifamycin*) blocks bacterial transcription by binding to the β-subunit of the bacterial RNA polymerase; *actinomycin* intercalates between G-C pairs.

8 Protein synthesis

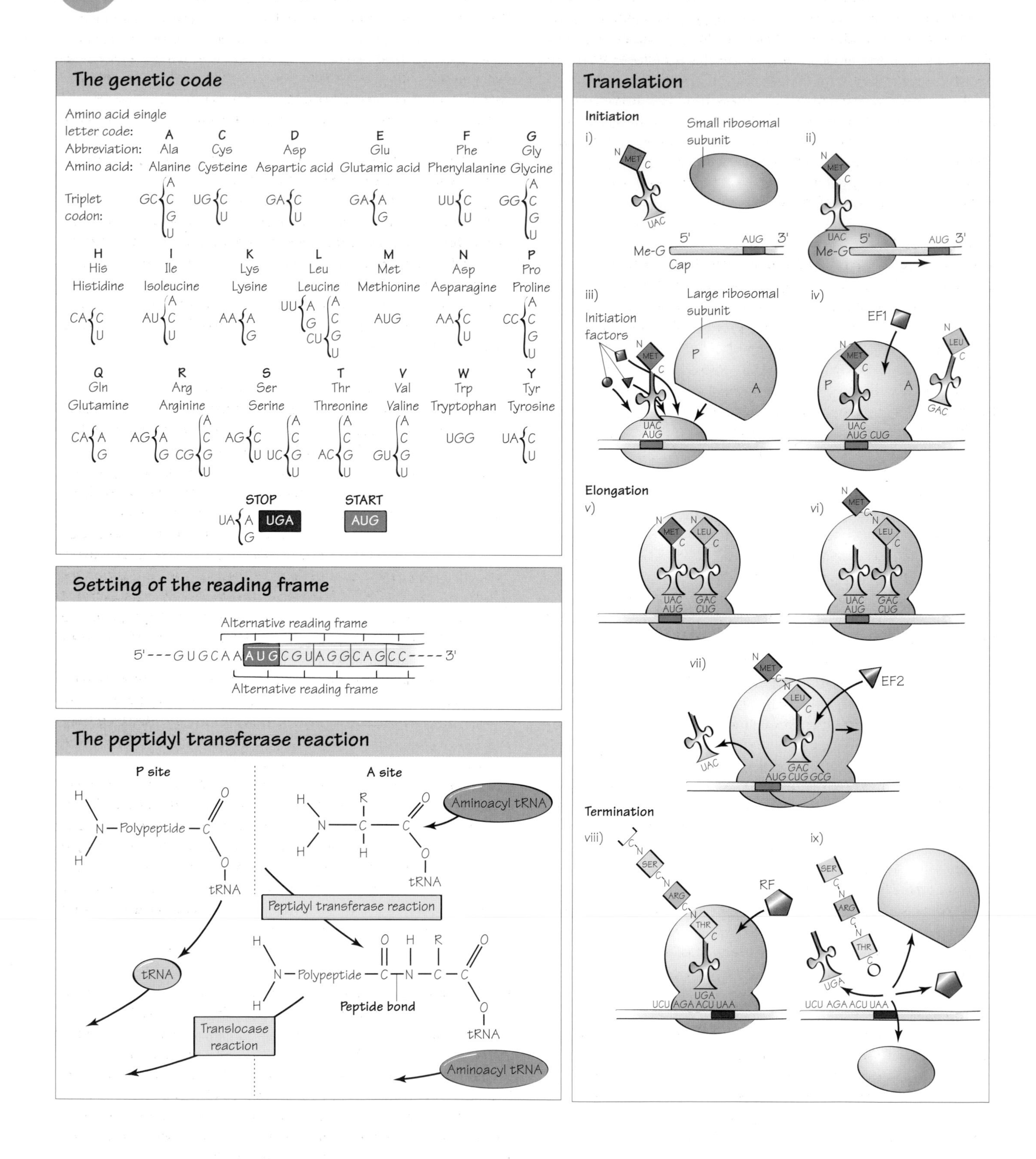

Overview

The main structural components of the body and most of its catalysts are **proteins**, each derived from one or more **polypeptides**. A polypeptide is a chain of amino acids, the sequence of which is determined by that of the bases in the corresponding mRNA, in accordance with '**the genetic code**'. Each amino acid is represented in mRNA by one or more groups of three bases called **triplet codons**, and their interpretation as polypeptide is called **translation**. Messenger RNA is translated from the 5′ to the 3′ end within cytoplasmic **ribosomes**. The resultant polypeptides are then modified into proteins. The functional properties of proteins derive largely from the active groups they display in their tertiary and quaternary conformations.

The genetic code

Translation requires transfer RNA molecules charged with amino acids appropriate to their anticodon sequences (see Chapter 6). Some amino acids are coded by several codons, only tryptophan and methionine by one each. Three of the 64 possible threefold combinations of A, C, G and U in the mRNA code for **STOP signals**: **UGA**, **UAG** and **UAA** (see 'The genetic code' in the figure). **AUG** codes for methionine and also acts as a **START signal**, simultaneously determining the amino- (or N-) terminal end of the polypeptide and selecting one of the three possible **reading frames** (see 'Setting of the reading frame' in the figure). The genetic code of mitochondrial DNA is slightly different.

Translation

Initiation

A small ribosomal subunit containing several **initiation factors** and methionyl tRNA charged with methionine binds to the 5′ cap on the mRNA, then slides along until it finds and engages with the first AUG sequence. The initiation factors are then released, a large ribosomal subunit binds to the small one and translation begins.

The large ribosomal subunit contains two sites, known as the **A site** (for aminoacyl) and the **P site** (for peptidyl). At the end of initiation the P site contains a charged met-tRNA with its anticodon engaged in the first AUG codon, while the A site is empty.

Elongation

The appropriate aminoacyl tRNA now becomes located in the A site, as dictated by the adjacent codon in the mRNA, with the help of a soluble **elongation factor** called **EF1**. The **peptidyl transferase reaction** then creates a **peptide bond** between the amino (-NH2) group of the amino acid at the A site and the carboxyl (-COOH) group of that at the P site, while the first tRNA is released.

The **translocase reaction** next promotes expulsion of the uncharged tRNA, moves the ribosome three bases along and translocates the growing peptide from A to P. This requires **elongation factor**, **EF2**.

Mitochondrial mRNAs are translated by mitochondria-specific tRNAs.

Termination

Elongation continues until a **STOP** codon enters the ribosome, all three being recognized by a single multivalent **release factor** (**RF**). This modifies the specificity of peptidyl transferase so that a molecule of water is added to the peptide instead. The ribosome is then released and dissociates into its subunits, so freeing the completed polypeptide.

Synthesis of an average polypeptide of 400 amino acids takes about 20 seconds.

As each ribosome vacates the messenger cap another attaches and follows its predecessor, creating a **polyribosome** or **polysome**. The mRNA usually survives for a few hours.

Protein structure

The amino acid sequence of a polypeptide defines its **primary structure**. The **secondary structure** is the three-dimensional form of parts of the polypeptide: the **α-helix**, the **collagen pro-α-helix**, or the **β-pleated sheet**.

Tertiary structure is the folded form of the whole polypeptide, composed of different secondary structures.

Quaternary structure is the final native conformation of a multimeric protein, e.g. **haemoglobin** is composed of two **α-globin** monomers, **two β-globin** monomers, one molecule of **haem** and an atom of ferrous iron. **Collagen fibres** are cables of many triple-helices, each formed as a rope of three pro-α-helices.

Structure is frequently maintained by **disulphide bridges** between cysteine residues on adjacent strands while enzymic properties depend on the distribution of charged groups.

Post-translational modification

Post-translational modification includes removal of the N-terminal methionine and cleavage. Association occurs between similar or different polypeptides, or with **prosthetic groups** such as haem.

Polypeptides destined for extracellular secretion are first **glycosylated** in the rough endoplasmic reticulum and Golgi apparatus. Their selection involves a **signal peptide** near the N terminus that binds to a cytoplasmic **signal recognition particle** consisting of cytoplasmic **7SL RNA** and six specific proteins. This links them to a receptor in the membrane of the endoplasmic reticulum. As it is synthesized the polypeptide is transferred through the membrane; when its carboxyl terminus emerges, the signal peptide is cleaved off. Polypeptides are transported to the Golgi apparatus in vesicles that bud off the endoplasmic reticulum (see Chapter 2).

Glycosylation is usually **N-linked**, involving addition of a common oligosaccharide to the side chain -NH_2 group of asparagine, as in the production of **antibodies** and **lysozymes**. **O-linked** oligosaccharides are attached to the -OH group on the side chain of serine, threonine or hydroxylysine, as with *secreted* ABO blood group antigens.

Other modifications include **hydroxylation** of lysine and proline, important in creation of the collagen pro-α-helix, **sulphation** of tyrosine, as a signal for compartmentalization and **lipidation** of cysteine and glycine residues, necessary for anchoring them to phospholipid membranes. **Acetylation** of lysine in histone H4 modifies its binding to DNA. Protein kinases **phosphorylate** serine and tyrosine residues, and can regulate enzymic properties, as in the **proto-oncogene signal transduction cascade** (see Chapter 40).

Medical issues

I-cell disease is due to deficiency in glycosylation of lysozymes. *Ricin* from castor beans blocks EF2; diphtheria toxin blocks translocase.

Many antibiotics target translation specifically ***in prokaryotes***. These include *erythromycin* which disrupts translocase, *chloramphenicol*, which interferes with peptidyl transferase, *tetracycline* which prevents binding of aminoacyl tRNAs, *puromycin*, which mimics an aminoacyl tRNA and *streptomycin*, which binds to the small ribosomal subunit. Human mitochondria have an evolutionary affinity with bacteria and some antibiotics interfere with mitochondrial function.

9 The cell cycle

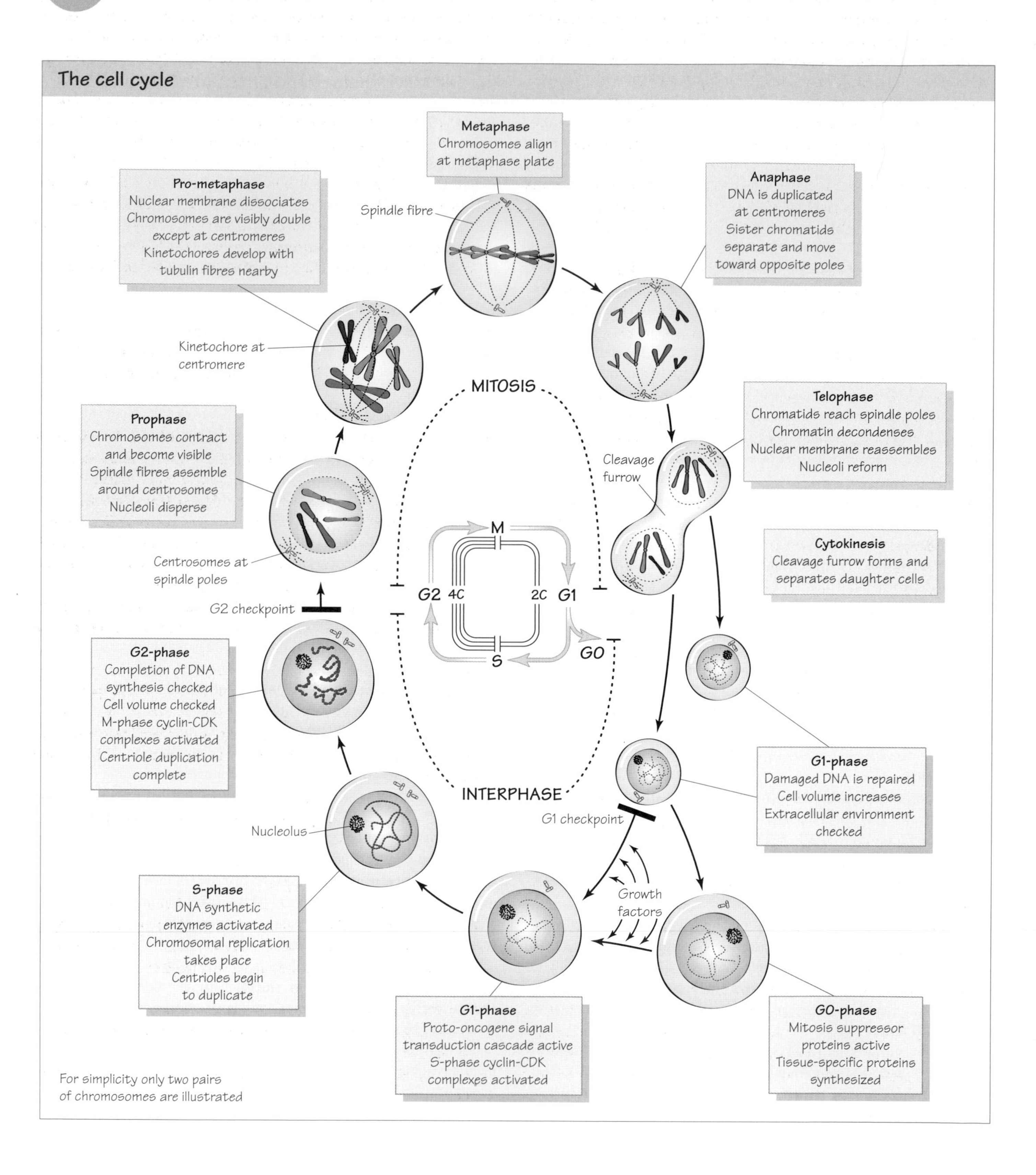

Overview

The body grows by increase in cell size and cell number, the latter by division, called **mitosis**. Cells proliferate in response to extracellular **growth factors**, passing through a repeated sequence of events known as **the cell cycle**. This has four major phases: **G1**, then **S**, **G2** and lastly the **mitotic** or **M-phase**. This is followed by division of the cytoplasm and plasma membrane to produce two identical daughter cells. G1, S and G2 together constitute **interphase**. The chromosomes are replicated during the **DNA synthetic** or **S-phase** (see Chapter 5). Most body cells are not actively dividing and are arrested at **'G0'** within G1.

Typically M-phase occupies between a half and 1 hour of a cycle time of about 20 hours. Normal (as distinct from cancer) human cells can undergo a total of about 80 mitoses, depending on the age of the donor.

The biochemistry of the cell cycle

The cell cycle is driven by alternating activation and deactivation of key enzymes known as **cyclin-dependent protein kinases**, or **Cdks**, and their cofactors called **cyclins**. This is performed by phosphorylation and dephosphorylation by other phosphokinases and phosphatases, specific cyclin-Cdk complexes triggering specific phases of the cycle. At appropriate stages the same classes of proteins cause the chromosomes to condense, the nuclear envelope to break down and the microtubules of the cytoskeleton to reorganize to form the mitotic spindle.

G1-phase

G1 is the gap between M- and S-phases, when the cytoplasm increases in volume. It includes the **G1 checkpoint** when damage to the DNA is repaired and the cell checks that its environment is favourable before committing itself to S-phase. If the nuclear DNA is damaged, a protein called **p53** increases in activity and stimulates transcription of protein **p21**. The latter binds to the specific cyclin-Cdk complex responsible for driving the cell into S-phase, so inactivating it and arresting the cell in G1. This allows sufficient time for the DNA repair enzymes to make good the damage to the DNA. If p53 is defective the unrestrained replication that ensues allows that line of cells to accumulate mutations and a cancer can develop. For this reason, p53 is known affectionately as **'The guardian of the genome'**.

G0-phase

Mammalian cells will proliferate only if stimulated by **extracellular growth factors** secreted by other cells. These operate within the cell through the **proto-oncogene signal transduction cascade** (see Chapter 40). If deprived of such signals during G1 the cell diverts from the cycle and enters the **G0** state. Cells can remain in G0 for years before recommencing division.

The G0 block is imposed by **mitosis-suppressor proteins** such as the **retinoblastoma (Rb) protein** encoded by the *normal* allele of the retinoblastoma gene. These bind to specific regulatory proteins preventing them from stimulating the transcription of genes required for cell proliferation. Extracellular growth factors destroy this block by activating G1-specific cyclin-Cdk complexes, which phosphorylate the Rb protein altering its conformation and causing it to release its bound regulatory proteins. The latter are then free to activate transcription of their target genes and cell proliferation ensues.

S-phase

The standard number of DNA double-helices per cell, corresponding to the diploid number of single-strand chromosomes, is described as **2C**. The 2C complement is retained throughout G1 and into S-phase, when new chromosomal DNA is synthesized and the cell becomes 4C. From the end of S-phase, through G2 and into M-phase each visually detectable chromosome contains two DNA molecules, known as **sister chromatids**, bound tightly together. In human cells therefore, from the end of S-phase to the middle of M there are 23 pairs of chromosomes (i.e. 46 observable entities), but 4C (92) nuclear DNA double-helices.

Mitosis involves sharing identical sets of chromosomes between the two daughter cells, so that each has 23 pairs and is 2C in terms of its DNA molecules. *G1, and G0 are the only phases of the cell cycle throughout which 46 chromosomes correspond to 2C DNA molecules.*

The replication of DNA during S-phase is described in Chapter 5.

G2-phase

A second checkpoint on cell size occurs during G2, the gap between S-phase and mitosis. In addition the **G2 checkpoint** allows the cell to check that DNA replication is complete before proceeding to mitosis.

Mitosis or M-phase

1 Prophase. The chromosomes, each consisting of two identical chromatids, begin to contract and become visible within the nucleus. The spindle apparatus of tubulin fibres begins to assemble around the two centrosomes at opposite poles of the cell. The nucleoli disperse.

2 Pro-metaphase. The nuclear membrane dissociates. Kinetochores develop around the centromeres of the chromosomes. Tubulin fibres enter the nucleus and assemble radiating out from the kinetochores and linking up with those radiating from the centrosomes.

3 Metaphase. Tension in the spindle fibres causes the chromosomes to align midway between the spindle poles, so creating the **metaphase plate**.

4 Anaphase. The centromeric DNA shared by sister chromatids is duplicated, they separate and are drawn towards the spindle poles.

5 Telophase. The separated sister chromatids (now considered to be chromosomes) reach the spindle poles and a nuclear membrane assembles around each group. The condensed chromatin becomes diffuse and nucleoli reform.

6 Cytokinesis. The cell membrane contracts around the mid-region between the poles, creating a **cleavage furrow** which eventually separates the two daughter cells.

The centrosome cycle

At G1 the pair of centrioles associated with each centrosome separate. During S-phase and G2 a new daughter centriole grows at right angles to each old one. The centrosome then splits at the beginning of M-phase and the two daughter centrosomes move to opposite spindle poles.

Medical issues

For karyotype analysis (see Chapter 50) dividing cells can be arrested at metaphase with the drug *colchicine*.

The drug *taxol* prevents spindle disassembly and is used in the treatment of cancer.

10 Gametogenesis

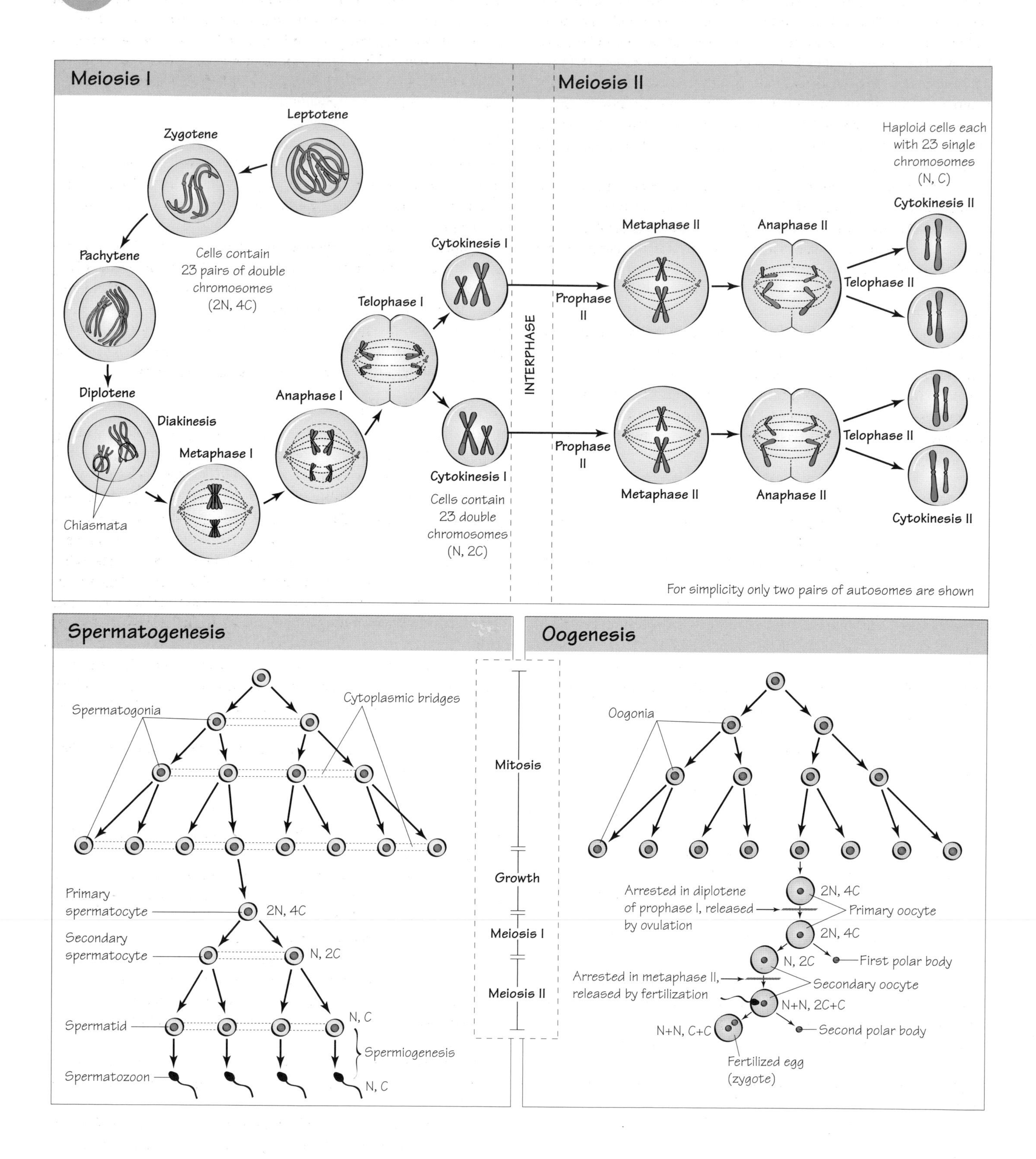

Overview

Each body cell contains two sets of chromosomes, one from the mother and one from the father. They are described as 2N or **diploid**. The sperm and ova contain only one set of chromosomes and are said to be 1N or **haploid**. The process by which the diploid number is reduced to haploid during the formation of the germ cells is called **meiosis**. In terms of the number of centromeres, this involves a **reductional division** followed by an **equational division** known as **Meiosis I** and **Meiosis II**. In men meiosis occurs by the pattern, seen in most diploid species, but in women there are several differences.

Crossing-over between maternally and paternally derived chromosomes ensures reshuffling of the genetic information between each generation. At **fertilization**, fusion of the haploid chromosome complement of the sperm with that of the ovum restores the chromosome number to diploid in the zygote.

Meiosis I

Meiosis I has similarities with mitosis, but is much more complex and extended in time. Primary spermatocytes and primary oocytes enter meiosis following G2 of mitosis, so they each have a diploid set of chromosomes (2N), but each of these contains replicated DNA as sister chromatids (i.e. are 4C; see Chapter 9). Prophase I involves reciprocal exchange between maternal and paternal chromatids by the process of **crossing-over**.

Prophase I

1 Leptotene. The chromosomes appear as long threads attached at each end to the nuclear envelope.

2 Zygotene. The chromosomes contract, pair with and adhere closely to (or '**synapse** with') their homologues. This normally involves precise registration, gene for gene throughout the entire genome. In primary spermatocytes X- and Y-chromosomes synapse at the tips of their short arms only.

3 Pachytene. Sister chromatids begin to separate, the double chromosome being known as a **bivalent**. The chromosome pair represented by four double helices is called a **tetrad**. One or both chromatids of each paternal chromosome crosses over with those from the mother in what is known as a **synaptonemal complex**. Every chromosome pair undergoes at least one crossover.

4 Diplotene. The chromatids separate except at the regions of crossover or **chiasmata** (singular: **chiasma**). This situation persists in all **primary oocytes** until they are shed at **ovulation**.

5 Diakinesis: the reorganized chromosomes begin to move apart. Each bivalent can now be seen to contain four chromatids linked by a common centromere, while non-sister chromatids are linked by chiasmata.

Metaphase I, anaphase I, telophase I, cytokinesis I

These follow a similar course to the equivalent stages in mitosis (see Chapter 9), the critical difference being that, instead of non-sister chromatids being segregated, pairs of reciprocally crossed-over sister chromatids joined at their centromeres are distributed to the daughter cells.

At the end of Meiosis I, secondary spermatocytes and secondary oocytes contain 23 chromosomes (1N), each consisting of two chromatids (i.e. 2C).

Meiosis II

There is a transient interphase, during which no chromosome replication occurs, followed by a prophase, metaphase, anaphase, telophase and cytokinesis. These resemble the equivalent phases of mitosis in that pairs of chromatids (bivalents) linked at their centromeres become aligned at the metaphase plate and are then drawn into separate daughter cells following replication of the centromeric DNA.

At the end of Meiosis II the cells contain 23 chromosomes (1N), each consisting of a single chromatid (1C).

Male meiosis

Spermatogenesis includes all the events by which spermatogonia are transformed into spermatozoa and takes about 64 days. Cytokinesis is incomplete throughout, so that each generation of cells remains linked by cytoplasmic bridges.

A diploid **primary spermatocyte** undergoes Meiosis I to form two haploid **secondary spermatocytes**. These both undergo Meiosis II to produce four haploid **spermatids**. The spermatids become elaborated into **spermatozoa** during **spermiogenesis**. This includes: (i) formation of the acrosome containing enzymes that assist with penetration of the egg; (ii) condensation of the nucleus; (iii) shedding of most of the cytoplasm; and (iv) formation of the neck, midpiece and tail.

Female meiosis

Oogenesis begins in the fetus at 12 weeks, but ceases abruptly at about 20 weeks, the **primary oocytes** remaining at diplotene of prophase I until ovulation, this suspended state being called **dictyotene**.

Ovulation begins at puberty and usually only one oocyte is shed per month. Under stimulation by hormones a primary oocyte swells accumulating cytoplasmic materials. At completion of Meiosis I these are inherited by one daughter cell, the **secondary oocyte**. The other nucleus passes into the **first polar body**, which usually degenerates without further division. Meiosis I is completed rapidly then, after a pause, the secondary oocyte is shed into the uterine, or Fallopian, tube.

Meiosis II stops at metaphase until entry of a sperm. It then completes division, producing a large haploid **ovum** pro-nucleus, which fuses with the sperm pro-nucleus, and a very small **second polar body**, which degenerates.

The whole process takes from 12 to 50 years, depending when fertilization takes place.

The significance of meiosis

1 The diploid chromosome content of somatic cells is reduced to haploid in the gametes.

2 Paternal and maternal chromosomes become reassorted with a potential for 2^{23} (= 8 388 608) different combinations, excluding recombination *within* chromosomes.

3 Reassortment of paternal and maternal alleles *within* chromosomes creates an infinite potential for genetic variation between gametes.

4 The *randomness* of reassortment of paternal and maternal alleles during meiosis (and at fertilization) ensures the applicability of probability theory to genetic ratios and the general validity of Mendel's laws (see Chapter 15).

5 The frequency of crossover between genes *within* chromosomes allows the relative positions of gene to be mapped (see Chapters 36 and 37).

6 Errors sometimes occur at chromosome pairing and crossing-over, which can produce **translocations**, as well as at their separation or **disjunction**, which can lead to **aneuploidy** (see Chapters 24 and 25).

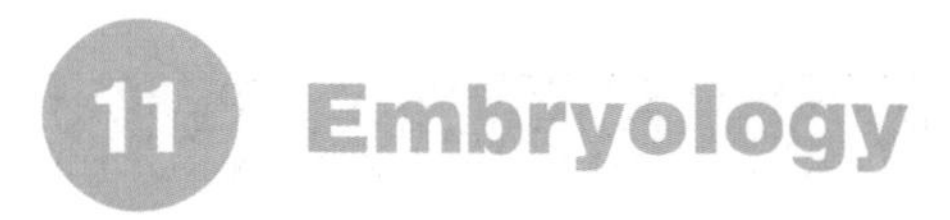

11 Embryology

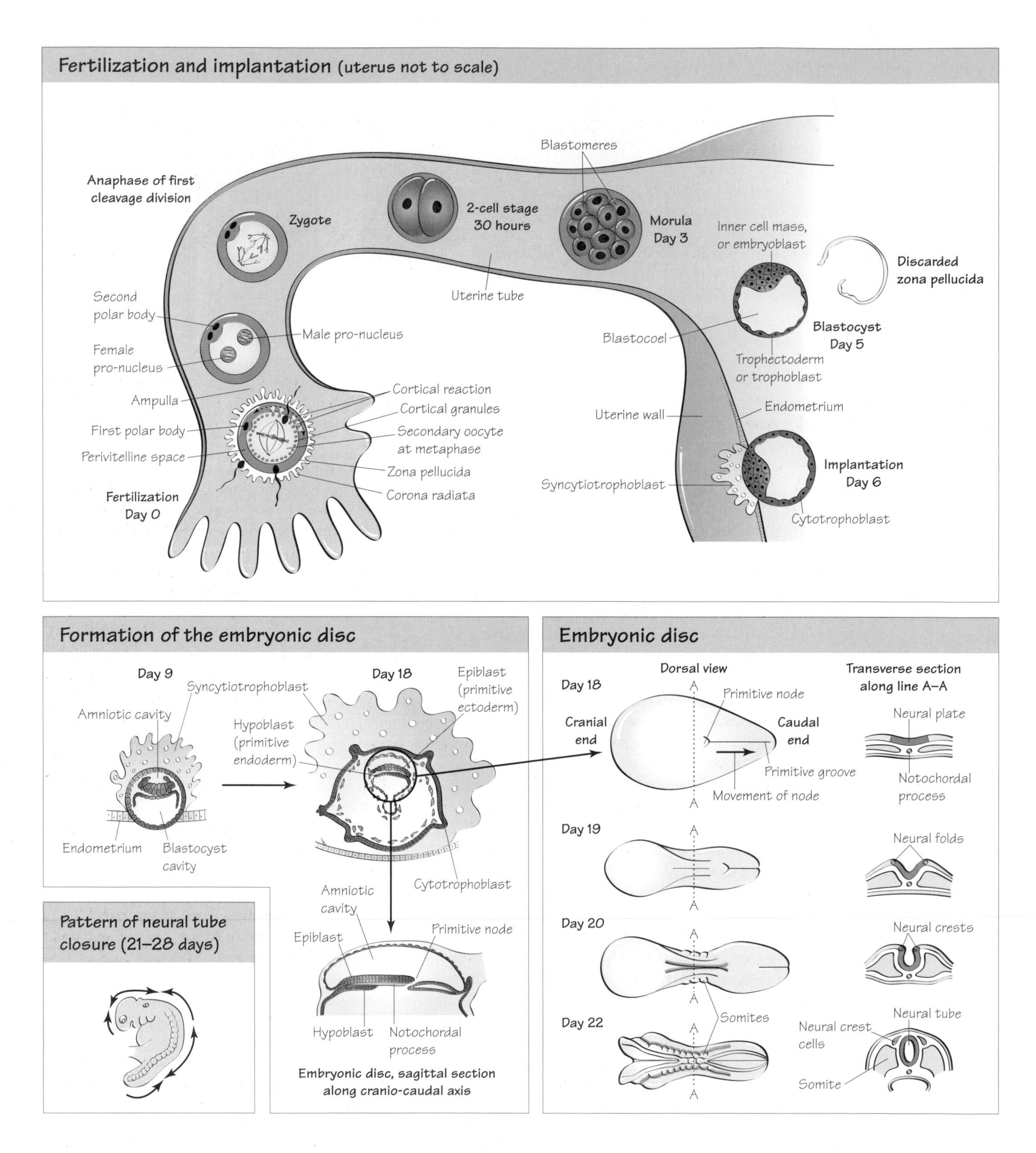

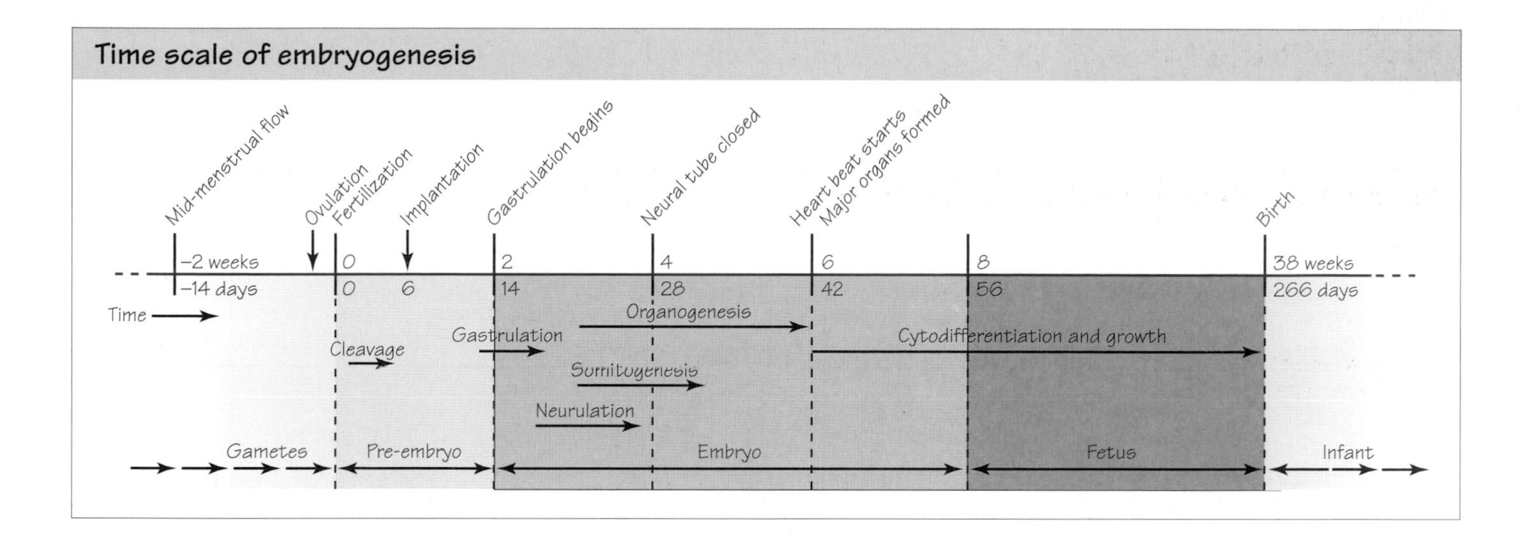

Overview

Fertilization by a sperm initiates **embryogenesis**. Mitosis ensues and the **pre-embryo** implants in the uterus. The **embryo** proper develops from a few internal cells, through creation of three **embryonic germ layers**. **Organogenesis** involves interactions between these and is completed by 6–8 weeks. During the subsequent period of **growth** and **cytodifferentiation** the individual is called a **fetus**.

The pre-embryo (days 0–14)

The secondary oocyte is shed into the peritoneal cavity and directed into the adjacent **uterine** (Fallopian) **tube**, where fertilization must take place within 24 hours. The sperm performs four functions: (i) *stimulation of metaphase II in the secondary oocyte*; (ii) *restoration of the diploid number of chromosomes*; (iii) *initiation of cleavage*; and (iv) *determination of sex*.

The sperm passes through the **corona cells** on the oocyte surface and adheres to the **zona pellucida**. The **acrosome** in the sperm head then releases enzymes that digest a tunnel through the zona pellucida, allowing the sperm to pass into the **perivitelline space** and fuse with the oocyte membrane. The sperm head is then engulfed by the oocyte and entry of more sperm prevented by a rapid **cortical reaction**. The oocyte nucleus completes metaphase II, expels the second polar body and maternal and paternal **pro-nuclei** fuse to form the **zygote**.

Mitosis of the pre-embryo is called **cleavage** and the resultant **blastomeres** are smaller after each division. The 16-cell **morula** passes down the uterine tube aided by peristalsis and ciliary movement. A space called the **blastocoel** forms off-centre in the morula to create the **blastocyst**, which swells and bursts from the zona pellucida. Two different cell types are now recognizable, the flattened **trophectoderm** cells of the outer **trophoblast** and an eccentrically placed **inner cell mass** or **embryoblast**.

On day 6 the blastocyst implants in the endometrium lining the uterus. Some trophoblast cells fuse to form the invasive **syncytiotrophoblast**, the remainder constituting the **cytotrophoblast**. The blastocyst now takes nourishment from the mother and grows rapidly as it sinks further into the endometrium.

The inner cell mass exposed ventrally to the blastocoel flattens to form the **primitive endoderm**, or **hypoblast**, while the remainder forms the **primitive ectoderm**, or **epiblast**, within which develops the **amniotic cavity**. The double-layered disc called the **embryonic disc** forms from the epiblast and hypoblast at 7–12 days, *from which the embryo proper develops*.

The embryo (weeks 2–8)

Gastrulation is the process which creates the **embryonic mesoderm** and initiates activity of the embryo's own genes. The **primitive streak** first appears in the epiblast at the caudal (tail) end of the embryonic disc, extends towards its centre and then develops the **primitive groove** in its amniotic (i.e. dorsal) surface. At the cranial (head) end of this develops a mass of cells called the **primitive** (or **Hensen's**) **node**.

Epiblast cells migrate across the disc, through the primitive groove and into the space above the hypoblast. These become the embryonic mesoderm, creating the three **germ layers**: **ectoderm** from the epiblast, **mesoderm**, and **endoderm** from the hypoblast together with some epiblast cells that merge with it. Mesoderm cells that migrate anteriorly and accumulate in the midline form the **notochordal process**, which later extends caudally.

The epiblast thickens to form the **neural plate** and a **neural fold** arises on either side of the central axis. These curve over, contact and from 22 days fuse in five separate movements to create the **neural tube**, which later becomes the spinal cord. Along the dorsal edges of the neural folds are the **neural crest cells** that migrate out to give rise to several cell types, including nerve, bone, supporting structures of the heart, adrenalin-secreting and pigment cells.

As the primitive node moves caudally down the midline, blocks of mesoderm on either side rotate to create 42–44 pairs of segmental **somites**, the most caudal 5–7 of which subsequently disappear (see Chapter 12).

The fetus (weeks 8–38)

The ectoderm is the origin of the outer epithelium and CNS and, with mesoderm, peripheral structures such as limbs; mesoderm forms muscles, circulatory system, kidneys, sex organs and together with endoderm, the internal organs; endoderm gives rise to the gut and digestive glands. The rudiments of all the major organs are formed through 'inductive' tissue interactions by about 6 weeks, when the heart starts beating. Thereafter development mainly involves increase in the number and types of cells. Birth normally occurs at 38 weeks.

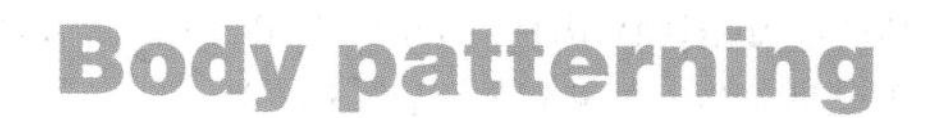

12 Body patterning

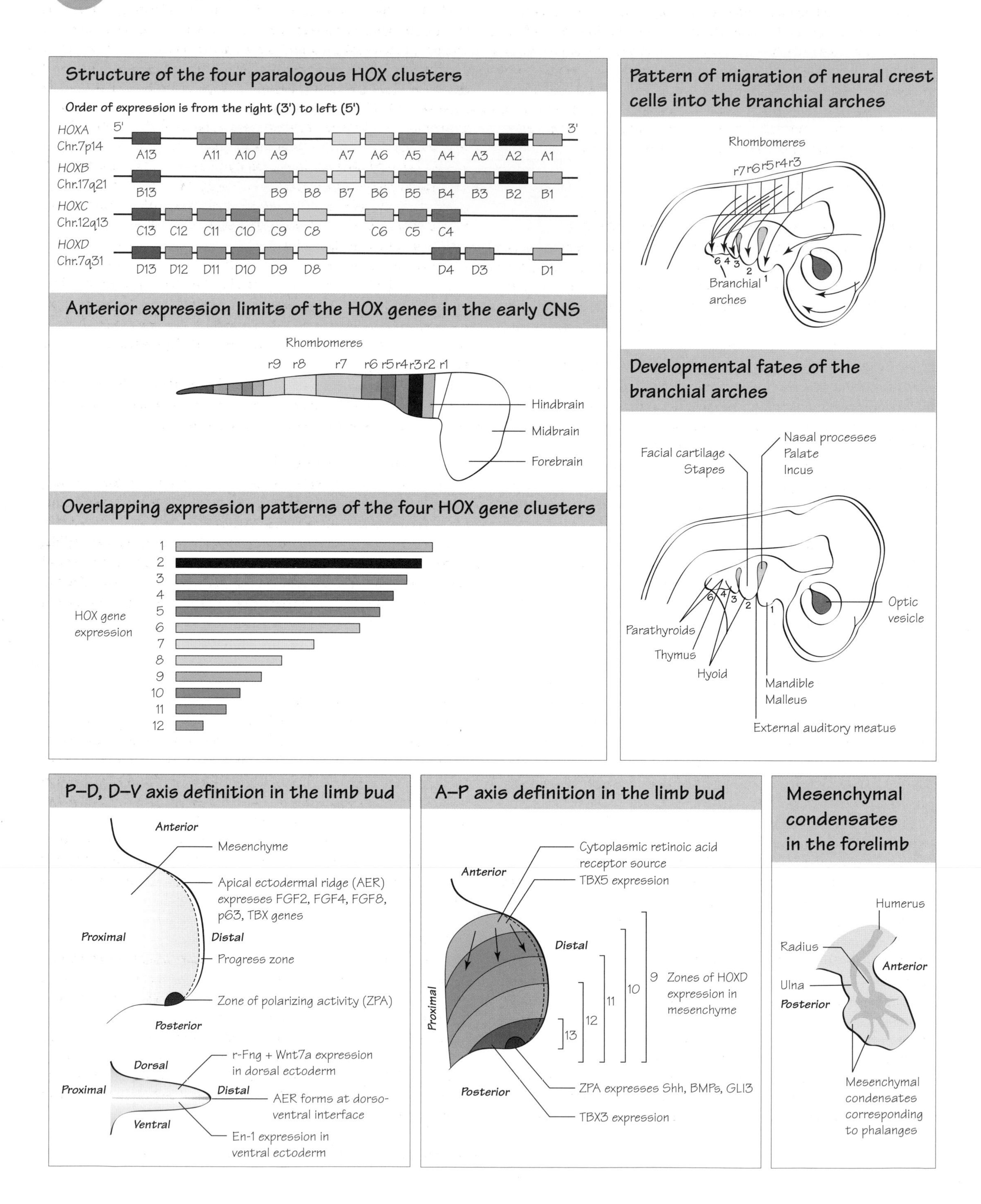

Overview

The human body shows regular features of anatomical organization that constitute what is known as 'body patterning'. Many of the important genes involved code for RNA transcription factors that bind to DNA, or protein morphogens that bind to cell surface receptors on target tissues.

Some of the gene names seem bizarre, as they are derived from research on other species.

Genes identified in non-human species are conventionally written in lower case, with an upper case capital if dominant (e.g. Shh), the equivalent human genes being written in upper case (e.g. SHH).

The main body

Differentiation along the antero-posterior axis

The antero-posterior axis is defined by the primitive streak, initiation and maintenance of which relates to the caudal movement of the primitive node and the sequential expression of members of four gene clusters, HOXA, B, C and D. Each cluster contains a very similar series of up to 13 genes encoding transcription factors, each containing the **homeobox** DNA binding domain.

Hox genes located at the 3′ (number 1) end are expressed earlier that those located 5′ and there is direct linear correlation between the position of each Hox gene in its cluster and its temporal and spatial expression. This derives from the graded sensitivity of gene expression controlling sequences to a common control molecule.

Primitive node function requires expression of the **Nodal** gene and its associated morphogen is believed to be **retinoic acid**, which it secretes increasingly abundantly as it moves in the caudal direction. More posterior target cells are thus exposed to larger concentrations of retinoic acid, with progressive activation of more Hox genes.

The fate of the neural crest (NC) cells is defined by the specific Hox genes that are active at their origin. NC cells from the fore- and midbrain migrate and differentiate into the mesenchyme of the first pharyngeal pouch, those of the anterior hindbrain to the mesenchyme of the second pharyngeal pouch. Cervical NC cells move into the third, fourth and sixth pharyngeal arches.

The fist embryonic pharyngeal arch forms the mandible and malleus, the first cleft the external auditory meatus and the mesenchyme of the first pharyngeal pouch, the nasal processes, palate and incus. The second arch forms part of the hyoid apparatus, the stapes and facial cartilage. The third arch also contributes to the hyoid cartilage. The third and fourth pouches become the thymus and parathyroids. The fourth and sixth arches form the laryngeal cartilages, the fifth arch degenerates.

The blood vessels within the arches form the aortic and pulmonary systems.

There is evidence that the gene **Tbx1** may be important specifically for the arteries of the fourth arch and **DiGeorge syndrome**, with partial absence of the thymus and facial malformation, etc. (see Chapter 50) is due to a Chromosome 22 microdeletion involving TBX1.

Differentiation of left from right

In the normal condition, **situs solitus**, the right (R) lung is trilobed, the left (L) bilobed, the apex of the heart points to the left, the spleen and stomach are on the left, the liver is on the right and the small bowel loops in a counter-clockwise direction. In **situs inversus** there is complete mirror-imaging, but usually no disease symptoms. **Situs ambiguous** involves randomization of the arrangement of heart, lung, liver, spleen and stomach about the midline and is often associated with congenital heart defects. Mirror image bilateral symmetry of the whole body is called **isomerism**, that of individual organs **heterotaxia**, and both are associated with a variety of pathologies.

The first observable sign of L/R asymmetry is looping of the heart tube to the right and the first relevant molecular signal detectable is of **sonic hedgehog (Shh)** protein from the notochord. Cilia at the primitive node, powered by the motor protein **dynein**, then cause asymmetrical flow of perinodal fluid, which activates the genes for **Nodal** protein and **Lefty-2 (LEFTB)**, specifically on the left side of the embryo. Both are members of the **transforming growth factor-β (TGF-β)** family of signalling proteins and Nodal is responsible for the rightward looping of the heart tube. These initiate signalling pathways that activate left-hand-specific transcription factors, including **Pitx2** and **eHAND**, which promotes differentiation of the left ventricle, while **dHAND** promotes differentiation of the right ventricle. **Lefty-1 (LEFTA)** prevents leakage of signals across the midline.

Situs inversus, isomerism and heterotaxia are produced by mutations in LEFTA, LEFTB and NODAL, while **Kartagener syndrome** involves random situs and other problems due to immotile cilia. Mutations in the zinc finger proteins, **ZIC3** and **GLI3** (see Chapter 7), cause rare abnormalities of asymmetry including **Grieg cephalopolysyndactyly** and **Pallister–Hall syndrome**.

Discrepancies in L/R asymmetry in MZ and conjoined twins indicate normal diffusion of lateralizing influence from the left, the twin arising on the R most commonly showing randomization.

Dorso-ventral differentiation

Bone morphogenetic protein-4 (BMP-4) is emitted by the primitive node and induces ventral characteristics, but on its dorsal side proteins **noggin** and **chordin** are also expressed and these bind directly to BMP-4 and prevent it activating its receptor dorsally. **Sonic hedgehog (Shh)** protein expressed in the notochord is responsible for dorso-ventral patterning of the neural tube. Mutations and duplications of SHH can cause **holoprosencephaly** (non-division of the forebrain) and **cyclopia** (a single, central eye).

The limbs

The proximo-distal axis

The limb bud grows by proliferation of mesenchyme cells in the **'progress zone'** less than a millimetre below the **apical ectodermal ridge (AER)** at its tip. At this stage the mesenchyme cells receive progressively changing instructions mediated by **fibroblast growth factors**, **FGF2**, **4** and **8** that define the extent of their proliferation, depending on which bony elements they are to form.

Limb abnormalities are a feature of **Apert syndrome**, in which there are mutations in the FGF2 receptor (**FGFR2**). Expression of **p63** is crucial for sustaining the AER and p63 mutations cause split hands and feet, called **ectrodactyly**.

The antero-posterior axis

At the posterior margin of the limb bud is the **ZPA**, or **zone of proliferating activity**, the source of morphogens that define the form, number and location of the digits. These diffuse anteriorly and generate a nested, overlapping pattern of HoxD and HoxA expression.

Mutations of HOXD13 cause **synpolydactyly** (fusion of the middle digits). Defects in the anterior and posterior elements of the upper limbs occur in **Holt-Oram** and **ulnar-mammary syndromes**, caused by mutations in **TBX5** and **TBX3** specifying thumb and little finger respectively.

13 Sexual differentiation

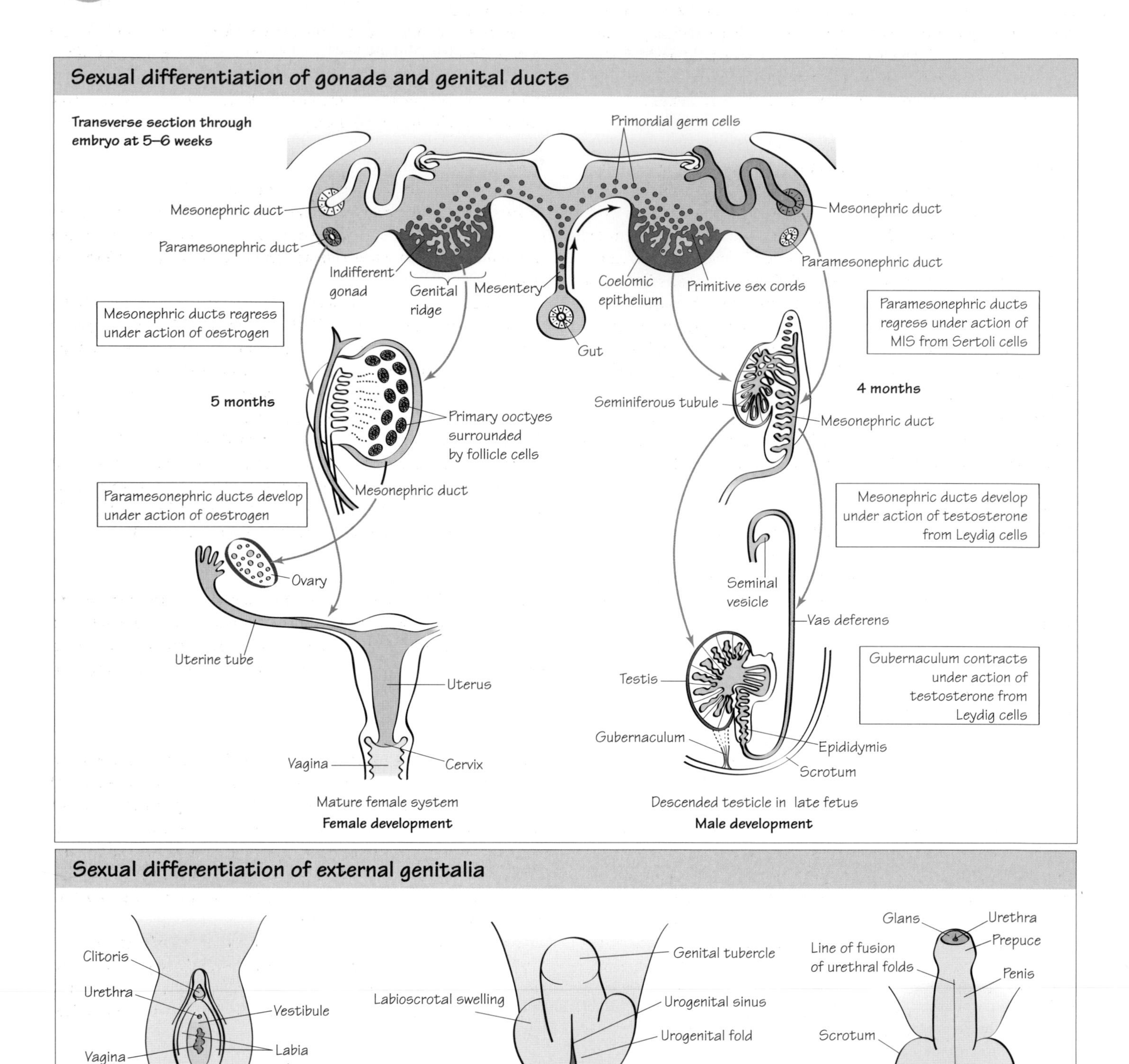

Overview

Sexual differentiation is initiated at fertilization, depending on whether the sperm carries an X or a Y chromosome. At the blastocyst stage in XX embryos, one X chromosome in every cell is permanently inactivated, otherwise development of the sexes is similar until the **SRY gene** on the Y chromosome comes into operation and certain structures, including the brain, become progressively more masculinized.

X chromosome inactivation

At the late blastocyst stage cells inactivate all but one of their X chromosomes. The nuclei of normal XX female cells therefore come to contain one inactive X, which can be seen at interphase as a **Barr body** in addition to their active X. Presence or absence of a Barr body is the basis of the original Olympic sex test (see Chapter 22). The choice of whether it is the paternal or maternal X which becomes inactive is random in each somatic cell, but in descendent cells it remains the same. Every woman therefore develops as a mosaic with respect to expression of her two X chromosomes. In the extra-embryonic trophoblast cells the paternal X is preferentially inactivated. In oogonia the inactive chromosome is reactivated.

Genes in the pairing (**pseudo-autosomal**) region and several other sites on the X are not subject to inactivation, accounting for the sexual abnormalities of XXY and XO individuals (see Chapter 25).

Early development

At the beginning of week 5, up to 2000 **primordial germ cells** migrate from the endoderm cells of the yolk sac and infiltrate the **primitive sex cords** within the mesodermal **genital ridges**, which are developments of the coelomic epithelium. The paired **indifferent gonad** is identical in males and females.

The ovary

In the early ovary the primitive sex cords break down, but the surface epithelium proliferates and gives rise to the **cortical cords**, which split into clusters, each surrounding one or more germ cells. The latter, now called **oogonia**, proliferate then enter meiosis as **primary oocytes**.

The testis

The SRY gene carried only on the Y chromosome is expressed in week 7 in the cells of the primitive sex cords. Its product is a zinc finger transcription factor that binds to DNA in those same cells, leading to a masculine gene expression pattern. These cells proliferate into the **testis cords**.

Leydig cells derived from the original mesenchyme of the gonadal ridge move in around the 8th week and until weeks 17–18 synthesize male sex hormones, or **androgens**, including **testosterone**, which initiate sexual differentiation of the genital ducts and external genitalia. By the 4th month the male gonads also contain **Sertoli cells** derived from the surface epithelium of the gonad (see Chapter 23).

Genital ducts

Initially both sexes have two pairs of genital ducts: **mesonephric** (or **Wolffian**) and **paramesonephric** (or **Mullerian**). In females the mesonephric ducts regress under the action of **oestrogens** produced by the maternal system, placenta and fetal ovaries, but the paramesonephric ducts remain and become the **uterine tubes** and **uterus** (see Chapter 23).

In males the Sertoli cells produce a growth factor called **Mullerian inhibiting substance (MIS)**, which causes the paramesonephric ducts to degenerate.

Testosterone binds to an intracellular receptor protein and the hormone-receptor complex then binds to specific control sites in the DNA and regulates transcription of tissue-specific genes. In male embryos testosterone converts the mesonephric ducts into the **vas deferens**, **seminal vesicle** and **epididymis**.

External genitalia

The external genitalia are derived from a complex of mesodermal tissue located around the **urogenital sinus**. At the end of the 6th week in both sexes this consists of the **genital tubercle** anteriorly, the paired **urogenital folds** on either side and lateral to these the **labioscrotal swellings**.

In females oestrogen stimulates slight elongation of the genital tubercle to form the **clitoris**, while the urogenital folds remain separate as the **labia minora**. The urogenital sinus remains open as the **vestibule** and the labioscrotal swellings become the **labia majora**.

The tissues around the **urogenital sinus** synthesize **5-α-reductase** which in males converts **testosterone** secreted by the Leydig cells to **dihydrotestosterone**. Under the action of this hormone the genital tubercle elongates into the **penis**, pulling the urethral folds forward to form the lateral walls of the **urethral groove**. At the end of the 3rd month the tops of the walls fuse to create the **penile urethra**, while the urogenital sinus becomes the **prostate** (see Chapter 23).

Descent of the testis

Usually in the 7th month the testes descend from the peritoneal cavity between the peritoneal epithelium and pubic bones and into the **scrotum**. This is mediated finally by the **gubernaculum** contracting under the influence of testosterone, but descent may not be completed until birth.

Puberty

Puberty is triggered by hormones secreted by the **pituitary gland** acting on ovaries, testes and adrenal glands. In girls, usually between ages 10 and 14 years, the ovaries respond by secreting oestrogen that stimulates breast growth. About a year later **menstruation** commences, accompanied by maturation of the uterus and vagina and broadening of the pelvis. Testosterone synthesis is stimulated in the adrenal glands and is responsible for growth of pubic and axillary hair in girls. Menstruation ceases at **menopause**, at around 50 years.

In boys, starting at about 11–12 years, the testes enlarge and synthesis of androgens is reactivated. The testis cords acquire a lumen, so forming the **seminiferous tubules**, which link up with the urethra. The androgens enhance growth of the penis and larynx and initiate spermatogenesis.

Medical issues

Disorders of sexual differentiation are dealt with in Chapter 23. Failure of testicular descent is called **cryptorchidism**. Tumours arising from primordial germ are known as **teratomas**; they can contain several well-differentiated tissues (e.g. hair, bone, sebaceous gland, thyroid tissue) and are usually benign (see Chapter 40).

14 The place of genetics in medicine

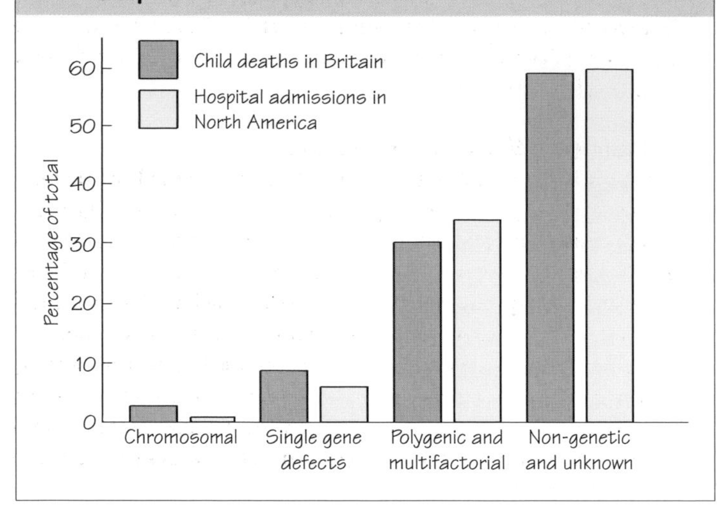

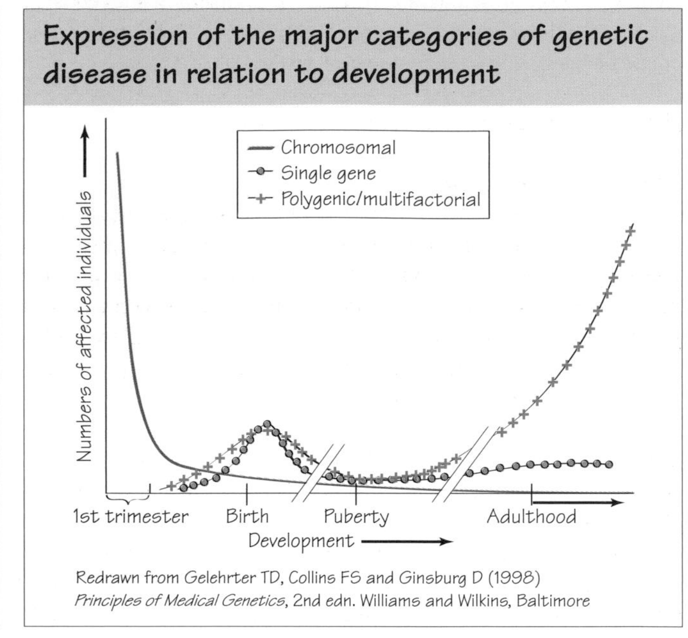

Redrawn from Gelehrter TD, Collins FS and Ginsburg D (1998) *Principles of Medical Genetics*, 2nd edn. Williams and Wilkins, Baltimore

Introduction

The true scale of genetic disease has only recently become appreciated. One survey of over a million consecutive births showed that at least one in 20 people under the age of 25 years develops a serious disease with a major genetic component. This, however, is probably an underestimate as it depends on how disease is defined and how strong the genetic component needs to be for it to be included.

Studies of the causes of death of more than 1200 British children suggest that about 40% died as a result of a genetic condition, while genetic factors are important in 50% of the admissions to paediatric hospitals in North America. Through variation in immune responsiveness and other host defences, genetic factors even play a role in infectious diseases.

Genetic diseases can be classed in three major categories: **chromosomal**, **single gene** and **multifactorial**. Chromosomal defects can create major physiological disruption and most are incompatible with even prenatal survival. These are responsible for more than 50% of deaths in the first trimester of pregnancy and about 2.5% of childhood deaths. Most single-gene defects reveal their presence after birth and are responsible for 6–9% of early **morbidity** and mortality. The multifactorial disorders account for about 30% of childhood illness and in middle-to-late adult life play a major role in the common illnesses from which most of us will die.

Overview of Part 2

Single gene defects (Chapters 15–21)

The foundation of the science of genetics is a set of principles of heredity discovered in the mid-19th century by an Augustinian monk called Gregor Mendel and described in Chapter 15. These give rise to characteristic patterns of inheritance, depending on whether the disease is dominant or recessive. Recognition of such patterns is central to prediction of the risk of producing an affected child, as described in Chapters 16 and 18. Chapter 18 also explains the risks associated with consanguineous mating. Chapter 20 deals with single-gene conditions that are neither strictly dominant nor recessive and introduces the concept of **pharmacogenetics**. Chapter 21 covers conditions that are progressive over the generations, or depend on which parent transmitted the disease allele.

Sex-related inheritance (Chapters 22 and 23)

There are many reasons why the sexes may express diseases differently. Of these the most important relates to the possession by males of only a single X-chromosome. Most sex-related inherited disease involves expression in males of recessive alleles carried on the X. The most common conditions in this category are defective colour vision and neurodevelopmental delay (mental retardation) in males. Mitochondrial disorders are uniquely transmitted by mothers to all their children, though expression may vary widely among family members. Chapter 23 also deals with conditions that cause failure of normal sexual differentiation.

Chromosomal defects (Chapters 24–27)

If chromosome segregation is incomplete or unequal at meiosis, chromosomally abnormal embryos can result. Since an average chromosome carries about 1000 genes, too many or too few chromosomes cause gross abnormalities of phenotype, most of which are incompatible with survival. Abnormal or unequal exchange of chromosomal material creates a variety of abnormalities, of varying severity. It is interesting to note that the three chromosomes associated with live birth of chromosomal trisomies (13, 18 and 21) (see Chapter 24) are the ones with the lowest gene density or of the smallest size.

Congenital and complex traits (Chapters 28–33)

Some conditions, including many congenital abnormalities, are due to the combined action of several genes and the adverse effects of environmental factors. These fall into the category of multifactorial inheritance. Genetic counselling in relation to this group is generally problematic as patterns of inheritance are usually not discernible. Multifactorial traits are of immense importance as they include most of the common disorders of adult life. Much current research is concentrated in this area, aimed at identification of the genes responsible.

Polymorphism (Chapters 34 and 35)

'Polymorphism' refers to genetic variants that occur commonly in the population. Polymorphic traits may be genetically silent, or can have phenotypic effect, including contribution to disease. The polymorphism concept is especially important in blood transfusion and organ transplantation and the practice of medicine on people of different ethnic backgrounds. The relative frequency of the different polymorphisms within populations is dealt with in Chapter 35.

Genetic linkage and gene mapping (Chapters 36 and 37)

If genes reside side-by-side on the same chromosome they are 'genetically linked'. If one is a disease gene, but cannot easily be detected whereas its neighbour can, then alleles of the latter can be used as markers for the disease allele. This allows prenatal assessment, informing decisions about pregnancy, selection of embryos fertilized *in vitro*, presymptomatic diagnosis and diagnosis of problematic conditions. The derivation of the complete human gene map is an outstanding recent achievement.

Mutation and its consequences (Chapters 38–41)

Mutation of DNA can involve chemical modification of bases, destruction, deletion or relocation of critical sequences. Repair mechanisms usually correct much of the damage, but new alleles are sometimes created that can be passed on to offspring. It is generally accepted that most mutational changes are either neutral in effect or deleterious, although very, very occasionally a new, apparently beneficial allele does appear. We therefore generally consider that exposures which increase the rate of mutation, such as to radiation or mutagenic chemicals, are best avoided.

Damage that occurs to the DNA of somatic cells can result in cancer, when a cell starts to proliferate out of control. This can give rise to a tumour which may break up, and its component cells migrate and establish secondary tumours. The molecular details of **carcinogenesis** are outlined in Chapter 40 and families with a tendency toward cancer are described in Chapter 41.

Immunogenetics (Chapters 42 and 43)

A healthy immune system may eliminate many thousands of potential cancer cells every day, in addition to disposing of infectious organisms. Maturation of the immune system is associated with rearrangements of genetic material that are believed to be unique to that system. These involve cutting, splicing and reassembly of alternative DNA sequences to create billions of new genes within individual B and T lymphocytes. An outline of these events and the cellular interactions that accompany them are given in Chapter 42. Chapter 43 outlines many ways in which the immune system can go wrong and investigates the still mysterious **genetic association** of certain alleles involved in the immune response with certain diseases.

Biochemical genetics (Chapters 44 and 45)

At the beginning of the 20th century, Sir Archibald Garrod coined the term 'inborn errors of metabolism' to describe inherited disorders of physiology. Although individually most are rare, the 350 known different inborn errors of metabolism account for 10% of all known monogenic disorders. The most important are detailed in these chapters.

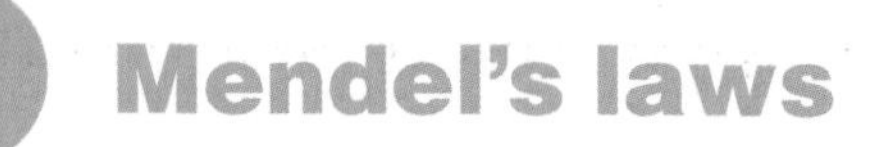

15 Mendel's laws

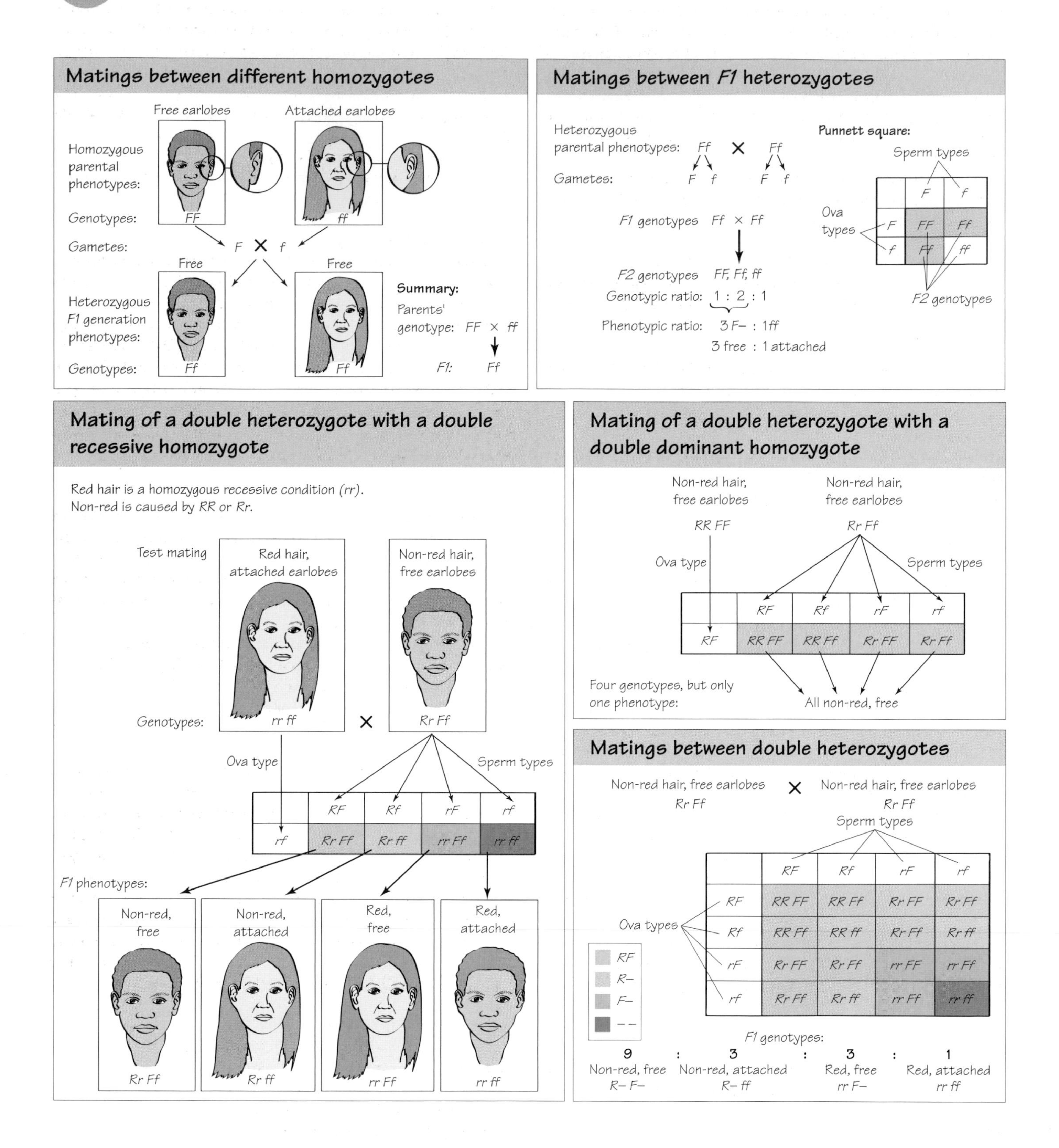

Overview

Gregor Mendel's laws of inheritance were derived from experiments with plants, but they form the cornerstone of the whole science of genetics. Previously heredity was considered in terms of the transmission and mixing of 'essences', as suggested by Hippocrates over 2000 years before. But, unlike fluid essences that should blend in the offspring in all proportions, Mendel showed that the instructions for contrasting characters segregate and recombine in simple mathematical proportions. He therefore suggested that the hereditary factors are particulate.

Mendel postulated four new principles concerning **unit inheritance**, **dominance**, **segregation** and **independent assortment** that apply to most genes of all diploid organisms.

The principle of unit inheritance

Hereditary characters are determined by indivisible units of information (which we now call genes). An allele is one version of a gene.

The principle of dominance

Alleles occur in pairs in each individual, but the effects of one allele may be masked by those of a dominant partner allele.

The principle of segregation

During formation of the gametes the members of each pair of alleles separate so that each gamete carries only one allele of each pair. Allele pairs are restored at fertilization.

Example

The earlobes of some people have an elongated attachment to the neck while others are free, a distinction determined by two alleles of the same gene, *f* for **attached**, *F* for **free**.

Consider a man carrying two copies of *F* (i.e. *FF*), with free earlobes, married to a woman with attached earlobes and two copies of *f* (i.e. *ff*). Both can produce only one kind of gamete, *F* for the man, *f* for the woman. All their children will have one copy of each allele, i.e. are *Ff*, and it is found that all such children have free earlobes because *F is dominant to f*. The children constitute the **first filial generation** or **F1 generation** (irrespective of the symbol for the gene under consideration). Individuals with identical alleles are **homozygotes**; those with different alleles are **heterozygotes**.

The **second filial**, or **F2, generation** is composed of the grandchildren of the original couple, resulting from mating of their offspring with partners of similar genotype. In each case both parents are heterozygotes, so both produce *F* and *f* gametes in equal numbers. This creates three genotypes in the F2: *FF*, *Ff* (identical to *fF*) and *ff*, **in the ratio: 1 : 2 : 1**.

Due to the dominance of *F* over *f*, dominant homozygotes are phenotypically the same as heterozygotes, and so there are three offspring with free earlobes to each one with attached. ***The phenotypic ratio 3 : 1 is characteristic of the offspring of two heterozygotes.***

The principle of independent assortment

Different genes control different phenotypic characters and the alleles of different genes re-assort independently of one another.

Example

Auburn and 'red' hair occur naturally only in individuals who are homozygous for a recessive allele ***r***. Non-red is dominant, with the symbol ***R***. All red-haired people are therefore *rr*, while non-red are either *RR* or *Rr*.

Consider the mating between an individual with red hair and attached earlobes (*rrff*) and a partner who is heterozygous at both genetic loci (*RrFf*). The recessive homozygote can produce only one kind of gamete, of genotype *rf*, but the double heterozygote can produce gametes of four genotypes: *RF*, *Rf*, *rF* and *rf*. Offspring of four genotypes are produced: *RrFf*, *Rrff*, *rrFf* and *rrff* and ***these are in the ratio 1 : 1 : 1 : 1***.

These offspring also have phenotypes that are all different: non-red with free earlobes, non-red with attached, red with free, and red with attached, respectively.

The test-mating

The mating described above, in which one partner is a double recessive homozygote (*rrff*), constitutes a **test-mating**, as his or her recessive alleles allow expression of all the alleles of their partner.

The value of such a test is revealed by comparison with matings in which the recessive partner is replaced by a double dominant homozygote (*RRFF*). The new partner can produce only one kind of gamete, of genotype *RF*, and four genotypically different offspring are produced, again in equal proportions: *RRFF*, *RRFf*, *RrFF* and *RrFf*. However, due to dominance all have non-red hair and free earlobes, so the genotype of the heterozygous parent remains obscure.

Matings between double heterozygotes

The triumphant mathematical proof of Mendel laws was provided by matings between pairs of double heterozygotes. Each can produce four kinds of gametes: *RF*, *Rf*, *rF* and *rf*, which combined at random produce nine different genotypic combinations. ***Due to dominance there are four phenotypes, in the ratio 9 : 3 : 3 : 1*** (total = 16). This allows us to predict the odds of producing:

1 a child with non red hair and free earlobes (*R-F-*) as 9/16;
2 a child with non-red hair and attached earlobes (*R-ff*) as 3/16;
3 a child with red hair and free earlobes (*rrF-*) as 3/16; and
4 a child with red hair and attached earlobes (*rrff*) as 1/16.

Biological support for Mendel's laws

When published in 1866 Mendel's deductions were ignored, but in 1900 they were rediscovered and rapidly found acceptance. The reason was that the chromosomes had by then been described and the postulated behaviour of Mendel's factors coincided with the observed properties and behaviour of the chromosomes: (i) both occur in homologous pairs; (ii) at meiosis both separate, but reunite at fertilization; and (iii) the homologues of both segregate and recombine independently of one another. This coincidence is because the genes are components of the chromosomes. Examples of simple dominant and recessive conditions of great medical significance are familial hypercholesterolaemia (see Chapter 17) and cystic fibrosis (see Chapter 18).

Exceptions to Mendel's laws

1 Sex-related effects (see Chapters 22, 23).
2 Mitochondrial inheritance (see Chapter 23).
3 Genetic linkage (see Chapter 36).
4 Polygenic conditions (see Chapters 29–32).
5 Incomplete penetrance (see Chapter 20).
6 Genomic imprinting (see Chapter 21).
7 Dynamic mutations (see Chapter 21).

16 Autosomal dominant inheritance, principles

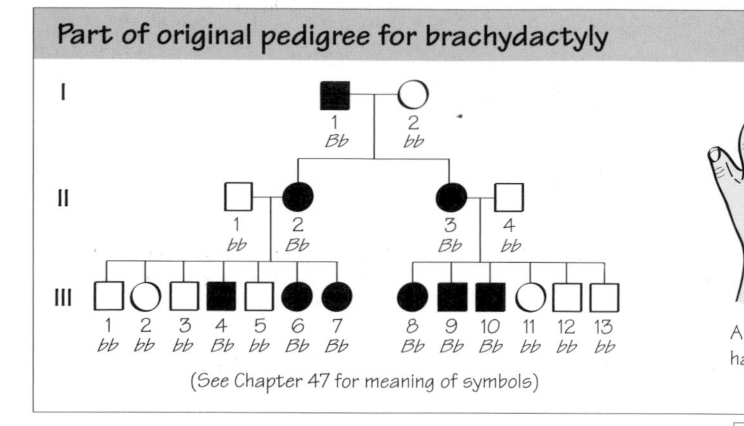

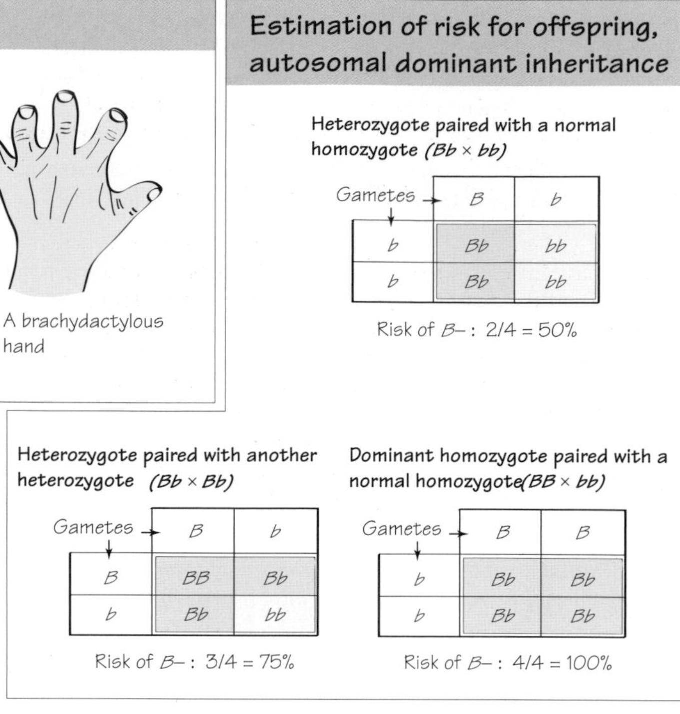

Overview

The best way to represent the distribution of affected individuals within a family is with a **pedigree diagram**, from which the mode of inheritance can often be easily deduced. The practical approach to drawing a real pedigree diagram is outlined in Chapter 47.

The pedigree diagram

Females are symbolized by circles (○), males by squares (□), persons of unknown sex by diamonds (◇). Individuals affected by the disorder are represented by solid symbols (■), those unaffected, by open symbols (□). In simple pedigrees, marriages or matings are indicated by horizontal lines linking male and female symbols. Offspring are shown beneath the parental symbols, in order of birth from left to right, linked to the mating line by a vertical, and numbered (1, 2, 3, etc.) from left to right in Arabic numerals. The generations are indicated in Roman numerals (I, II, III, etc.) from top to bottom on the left, with the earliest generation labelled I.

The patient who stimulated the investigation, the **propositus** (female: **proposita**), **proband**, or **index case**, is shown by an arrow (↑) with the letter P. The individual who sought genetic advice (the **consultand**) is shown by an arrow without the P. (NB. in older texts the proband is indicated by an arrow alone.) A diagonal line through the symbol indicates death.

Rules for autosomal dominant inheritance

The following are the basic rules for simple **autosomal dominant inheritance**. These rules apply only to conditions of complete penetrance (see Chapter 20) and when new mutations have not occurred.

1 *Both males and females express the allele and can transmit it equally to sons and daughters.*

2 ***Every affected person has an affected parent*** ('vertical' pattern of expression in the pedigree). *Direct transmission through three generations is practically diagnostic of a dominant.*

3 *In affected families, the ratio of affected to unaffected children is almost always 1 : 1.*

4 *If both parents are unaffected, all the children are unaffected.*

Example

The first condition in humans for which the mode of inheritance was elucidated was **brachydactyly**, characterized by abnormally short phalanges (distal joints of fingers and toes).

In Mendelian symbols, dominant allele ***B*** causes brachydactyly and every affected individual is either a homozygote (*BB*), or a heterozygote (*Bb*). In practice most are heterozygotes, because ***brachydactyly is a rare trait*** (i.e. < 1/5000 births), ***as are almost all dominant disease alleles***. Unrelated marriage partners are therefore usually recessive homozygotes (*bb*) and the mating can usually be safely represented:

$$Bb \times bb \;\rightarrow\; Bb, bb \quad 1:1.$$

Dominant disease alleles are kept at low frequency since their carriers are less fit than normal homozygotes.

Matings between heterozygotes are the only kind that can produce homozygous offspring:

$$Bb \times Bb \;\rightarrow\; \mathbf{BB}, Bb, bb \quad 1:2:1 \text{ (i.e. 3 affected: 1 unaffected).}$$

Dominant disease allele homozygotes are extremely rare and with many disease alleles homozygosity is lethal or causes a more pronounced or severe phenotype.

Matings between heterozygotes may involve inbreeding (see Chapter 18), or occur when patients have met as a consequence of their disability (e.g. at a clinic for the disorder).

Table 16.1 Some important autosomal dominant inherited diseases in order of approximate frequency in Caucasians.

Condition	Frequency	Map loc.	Gene product
Dominant otosclerosis	1/300		
Familial hypercholesterolaemia (see Chapter 17)	1/500	19p	LDL receptor
Dentinogenesis imperfecta	1/1000		
Adult polycystic kidney disease	1/1000		
Multiple exostosis	1/2000		
Hereditary motor and sensory neuropathy. Type I due to duplication of PMP22 gene. Slow nerve condition, exaggerated foot arch, clawing of toes.	1/3000	17p	
Neurofibromatosis Type 1. (see Chapter 20)			
Hereditary spherocytosis. Red blood cells appear spherical leading to haemolytic anaemia	1/5000	8p	ankrin -1
Osteogenesis imperfecta. Highly variable, with multiple fractures and lens deformity. There are recessive forms also. *Type I*: blue sclerae and deafness; *Type II*: lethal perinatally: *Type III*: severe progressive deformation; *Type IV*: mild bone breakage, short stature, dental abnormalities	1/5000–1/10 000	17q 7q	Collagen – COL 1A1 Collagen – COL 1A2
Myotonic dystrophy. Progressive muscle weakness with inability to relax muscle tone normally, cataracts, cardiac conduction defects, hypogonadism. (see Chapter 30)	1/8000	19q	DM kinase
Ehlers–Danlos syndrome. Numerous types and highly variable, genetic heterogeneity suspected; skin fragility and elasticity, joint hypermobility. Type IV has high risk of early death due to vascular rupture	1/10 000	2q, etc.	Collagen Type IV: COL 3A1
Marfan syndrome (see Chapter 17)	1/10 000	15q	
Achondroplasia (see Chapter 17)	1/10 000 – 1/50 000	4p	
Dominant blindness	1/10 000		
Dominant congenital deafness	1/10 000		
Familial adenomatous polyposis coli (see Chapter 30)	1/10 000	5q	APC t.s.
Tuberous sclerosis. Highly variable, cortical brain tubers, 'ash leaf spots' and raised lesions on skin, lung lesions, severe mental handicap, epilepsy (see Chapter 47)	1/15 000		
TSC 1		9q, etc.	Hamartin t.s.
TSC 2		16p	Tuberin t.s.
Adult onset cerebellar ataxia. Progressive cerebellar ataxia often associated with ophthalmoplegia and dementia.	1/20 000	6p, etc.	Spinal CA, type I; Ataxin
Huntington disease (see Chapters 20 and 21)	1/20 000	4p	Huntingtin
Neurofibromatosis Type 2. Bilateral acoustic neuromas and early cataracts	1/50 000	22q	schwannomin (merlin)t.s.
Facio-scapulo-humeral dystrophy. Progressive limb girdle and facial weakness particularly of the shoulder muscles	1/50 000	4q	

All offspring of affected homozygotes are affected, for example:

$$BB \times bb$$
$$\downarrow$$
$$Bb$$

Unaffected members of affected families are normal homozygotes, so do not transmit the condition: $bb \times bb \rightarrow bb$

Estimation of risk

In simply inherited autosomal dominant conditions where the diagnosis is secure, estimation of risk for the offspring of a family member can be based simply on the predictions of Mendel's laws. For example:

1 For the offspring of a heterozygote and a normal homozygote ($Bb \times bb \rightarrow 1\ Bb;\ 1\ bb$):
risk of $B- = 1/2$, or 50%.

2 For the offspring of two heterozygotes ($Bb \times Bb \rightarrow 1\ BB;\ 2\ Bb;\ 1\ bb$):
risk of $B- = 3/4$, or 75%.

3 For the offspring of a dominant homozygote with a normal partner ($BB \times bb \rightarrow Bb$):
risk of $B- = 1$, or 100%.

Calculations involving dominant conditions can however be problematical as we usually do not know whether an affected offspring is homozygous or heterozygous (see Chapter 48).

Estimation of mutation rate

The frequency of dominant diseases in families with no prior cases can be used to estimate the natural frequency of new point mutations (see Chapter 38). This varies widely between genes, but averages about one event in any specific gene per 500 000 zygotes. Almost all point mutations arise in sperm, each containing, at the latest estimates 20–25 000 genes (see Chapter 4). There are therefore perhaps 25 000 mutations per 500 000 sperm and we can expect around 5% of viable sperm (and babies) to carry a new genetic mutation. However, only a minority of these occurs within genes that produce clinically significant effects, or would behave as dominant traits.

17 Autosomal dominant inheritance, clinical examples

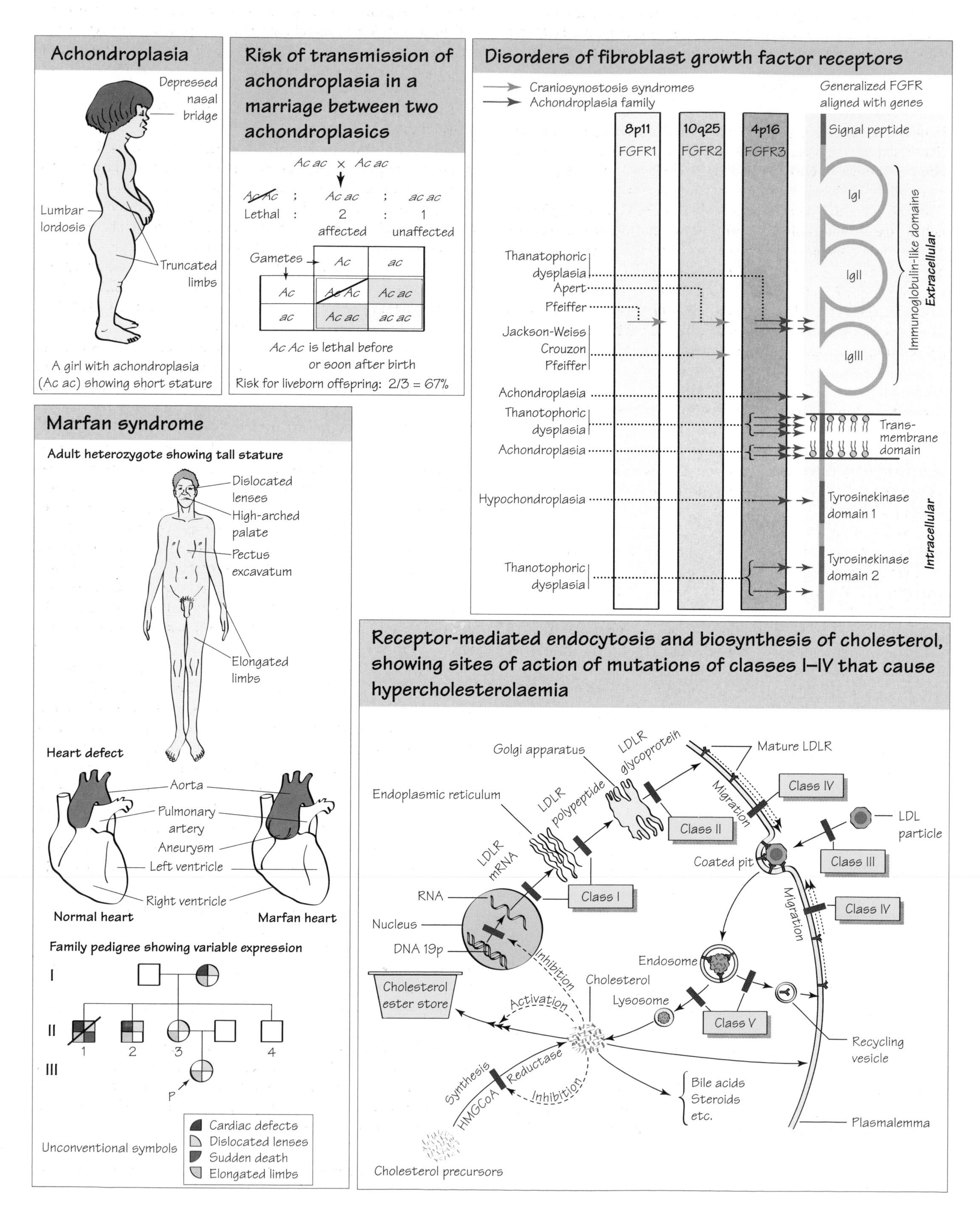

Overview

Over 4000 autosomal dominant (AD) diseases are known, although few are more frequent than 1/5000 and deemed 'common' (see Table 16.1). Typically the significant gene product in AD disease is a non-enzymic protein and this is the case with three of the most important detailed here: **achondroplasia**, **Marfan syndrome** and **familial hypocholesterolaemia**.

Diseases of the fibroblast growth factor receptors

Extracellular **fibroblast growth factor (FGF)** signals operate through a family of three transmembrane tyrosine kinases, the **fibroblast growth factor receptors (FGFRs)**. Binding of FGF by their extracellular domains activates intracellular tyrosine kinase activity.

Mutations in the genes that code for the FGFRs are implicated both in the **achondroplasia family** of skeletal dysplasias and the **craniosynostosis syndromes**. **Hypochondroplasia** is grossly similar to achondroplasia, but the head is normal; **thanatophoric dysplasia** is much more severe and invariably lethal. There is premature fusion of the cranial sutures in all the craniosynostoses, in **Apert syndrome** often associated with hand and foot abnormalities. In **Pfeiffer** the thumbs and big toes are abnormal; in **Crouzon** all limbs are normal.

Achondroplasia

Description Achondroplasia causes severe shortening of the proximal segments of the limbs, the average height of adults being only 49–51 inches (125–130 cm). The patient has a prominent forehead (**macrocephaly**), depressed nasal bridge and restricted foramen magnum that can cause cervical spinal cord compression, respiratory problems and sudden infant death. Middle ear infections are common and can lead to conductive deafness. Pelvic malformation causes a waddling gait. Lumbar **lordosis** can cause lower back pain and 'slipped disc'. Women usually deliver by Caesarean section.

Aetiology FGFR3 is expressed in chondrocytes, predominantly at the growth plates of developing long bones, where the normal allele inhibits excessive growth. The achondroplasia mutation causes premature differentiation of chondrocytes into bone, 80% of mutations being new (see Chapter 16).

Management issues Children are often hypotonic and late in sitting and walking. Spinal cord compression due to foramen magnum restriction can cause weakness and tingling in the limbs. Breathing patterns should be monitored during childhood. Frequent attacks of **otitis media** must be treated quickly, and there is orthopaedic treatment to lengthen limbs.

Affected individuals tend to marry and can conceive homozygotes that usually do not survive to term. Liveborn homozygotes have an extreme short-limbed, asphyxiating dysplasia causing neonatal death, so surviving offspring of achondroplasic partners have a 2/3 risk of being achondroplasic. Genetic status is determinable by DNA analysis during the first trimester (see Chapters 53 and 57).

Marfan syndrome (MFS)

Description MFS illustrates **pleiotropy**, as it affects several systems, notably the skeleton, heart and eyes. MFS can be confused with other conditions and if the family history is non-contributory, positive diagnosis requires a minimum of *three* of the major *Ghent criteria* plus involvement of a third organ system. If there is an affected close relative, *one* major criterion, plus involvement of a second organ system are deemed sufficient.

Skeleton Affected individuals have joint laxity, a *span : height ratio greater than 1.05 and reduced upper-to-lower segment body ratio.* Overgrowth of bone occurs due to stretching of the periosteum. There are unusually long, slender limbs and fingers, **pectus excavatum** (hollow chest), **pectus carinatum** (pigeon chest) and **scoliosis** that can cause cardiac and respiratory problems.

Heart Most patients develop prolapse of the mitral valve, its cusps protruding into the left atrium, allowing leakage back into the left ventricle, enlargement of which can result in congestive heart failure. More serious is **aneurysm** (widening) of the ascending aorta in 90% of patients, leading to rupture during exercise or pregnancy.

Eyes Most patients have myopia and about half **ectopia lentis** (lens displacement).

Aetiology The underlying defect is excessive elasticity of **fibrillin-1**. A dominant negative effect is created in heterozygotes by mutant protein binding to and disabling normal fibrillin. There are several hundred alleles.

Management issues Clinical management includes body measurement, echocardiography, ophthalmic evaluation and lumbar magnetic resonance imaging (MRI) scan. Aortic dilatation can be reduced by β-adrenergic blockade to decrease the strength of heart contractions. Surgical replacement should be undertaken if the aortic diameter reaches 50–55 mm. Heavy exercise and contact sports should be avoided. Pregnancy is a risk factor if the aorta is dilated.

Hormone treatment of prepubertal girls reduces final height and worsening of scoliosis. Squints may need correction. Antibiotics should be given prophylactically before minor operations, to obviate **endocarditis**.

Familial hypercholesterolaemia

Description Up to 50% of deaths in many developed countries are caused by **coronary artery disease (CAD)**. This results from **atherosclerosis**, following deposition of low density lipid (LDL; including cholesterol) in the intima of the coronary arteries. FH heterozygotes account for 1/20 of those presenting with early CAD and approximately 5% of **myocardial infarctions** (MIs) in persons under 60 years of age. FH heterozygote plasma cholesterol levels are twice as high as normal, resulting in distinctive cholesterol deposits (**xanthomas**) in tendons and skin. Approximately 75% of male FH heterozygotes develop CAD and 50% have a fatal MI by the age of 60 years. In women the equivalent figures are 45% and 15%.

Aetiology All cells require cholesterol as a component of their plasma membranes, which can be derived either by endogenous intracellular synthesis, or by uptake via LDL receptors (LDLRs) on their external surfaces.

Newly synthesized receptor protein is normally glycosylated in the Golgi apparatus before passing to the plasma membrane, where it becomes localized in **coated pits** lined with the protein **clathrin**. LDL-bound cholesterol attaches to the receptor and the coated pit sinks inwards, internalizing the LDL particle. There the lipid separates from the receptor and inhibits *de novo* cholesterol synthesis. The receptor then returns to the surface to bind another LDL. Each LDLR repeats this cycle every 10 minutes. High cholesterol levels in the circulation of FH heterozygotes arise from defective LDLRs.

There are over 900 FH alleles in five classes (see figure):

- **Class I**: no LDLR protein is produced;
- **Class II**: LDLR synthesis fails before glycosylation;
- **Class III**: glycosylated LDLR reaches the coated pits, but cannot bind LDL;
- **Class IV**: receptors reach the cell surface, but fail to congregate in coated pits;
- **Class V**: the receptor cannot release bound LDL.

Management issues Dietary cholesterol should be restricted and bile acid absorbing resins can be used to sequester cholesterol from the enterohepatic circulation. Other drugs ('**statins**') block endogenous synthesis by inhibiting **HMGCoA reductase**.

18 Autosomal recessive inheritance, principles

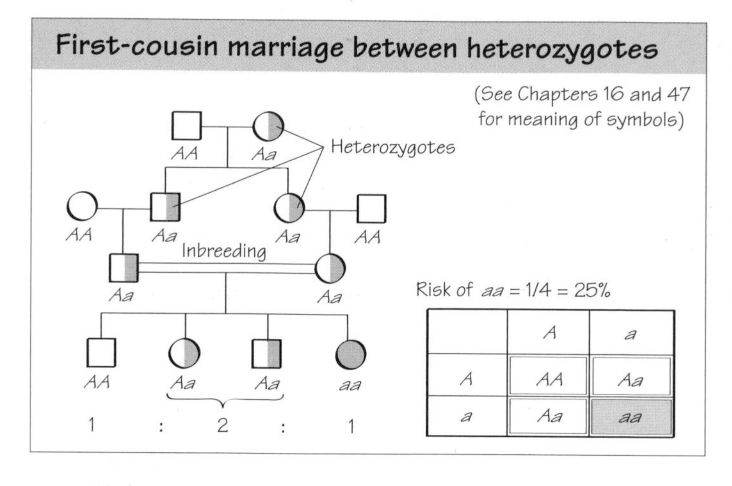

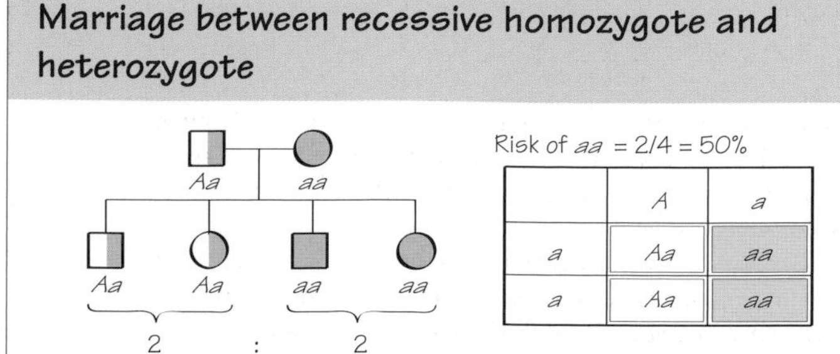

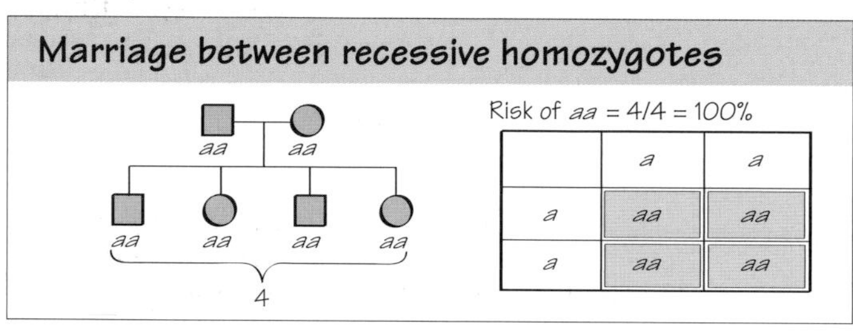

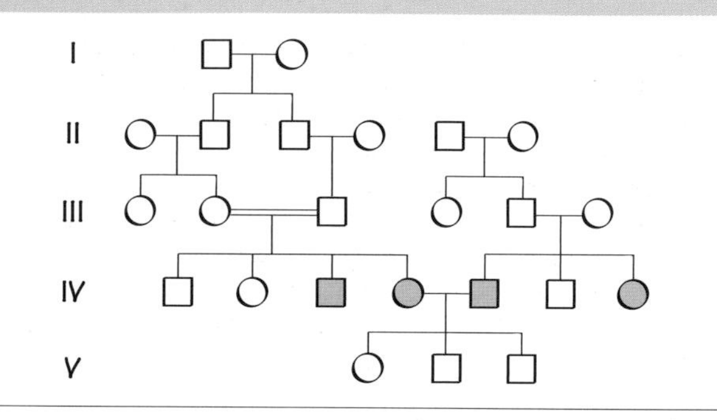

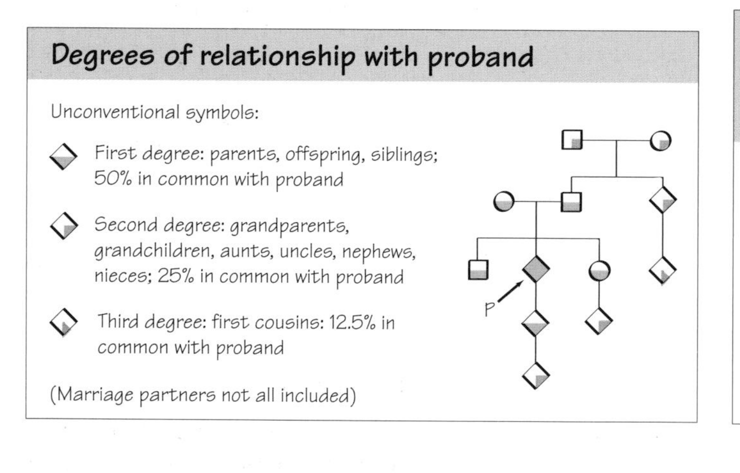

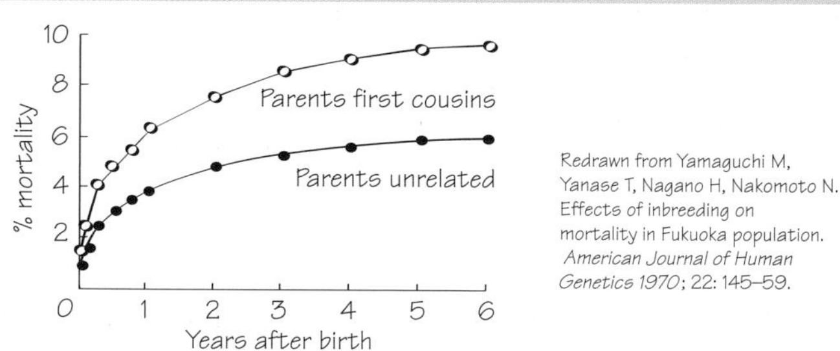

Overview

The pedigree diagram for a family in which autosomal recessive disease is present differs markedly from those with other forms of inheritance. Recessive diseases can be relatively common, as heterozygous carriers can preserve and transmit disease alleles without adverse selection.

Rules for autosomal recessive inheritance

The following are the rules for simple **autosomal recessive inheritance**:

1 ***Both males and females are affected.***

2 ***There are breaks in the pedigree and typically the pattern of expression is 'horizontal'*** (i.e. sibs are affected when parents are not).

3 ***Affected children can be born to normal parents***, usually in the ratio of one affected to three unaffected.

4 ***When both parents are affected all the children are affected***, unless mimic genes are involved (see 'congenital deafness', below.)

5 ***Affected individuals with normal partners usually have only normal children.***

Example: albinism

Homozygotes for **oculocutaneous albinism** (**OCA**) represent around 1 in 10 000 births. They have very pale hair and skin, blue or pink irises and red pupils. They suffer from **photophobia** (avoidance of light) and involuntary eye movements called **nystagmus**, related to faults in the neural connections between eye and brain, and poor vision. The biochemical defect (in OCA1) is in the enzyme **tyrosinase**, which normally converts tyrosine, through DOPA (dihydroxy-phenylalanine),

Table 18.1 Some important autosomal recessive inherited diseases in order of approximate frequency in Caucasians.

Condition	Freq.	Carrier freq.	Map locn.	Gene prod.
Primary haemochromatosis. Iron accumulation especially in the liver, with cirrhosis, cardiomyopathy, diabetes mellitus	1/400	1/10	6p	HLA-H
Recessive mental retardation	1/2000		Many	
Cystic fibrosis (see Chapter 19)	1/2500	1/25 (in white people)	7q31	CFTR
Retinitis pigmentosa. 50% of type AR, 15% AD, 5% X-linked. Night blindness, tunnel vision, pigmented areas in retina	1/4000		Several	
Spinal muscular atrophy (see Chapter 19)	1/10 000	1/50	5q13	SMN factor
Recessive blindness	1/10 000			
Congenital adrenal hyperplasia. Masculinization of female genitalia, precocious puberty in males, salt deficiency	1/10 000	1/50	6	21-hydroxylase
Medium chain acyl CoA dehydrogenase deficiency. Presents in early years with low blood glucose in response to infection or starvation, inability to produce ketones	1/10 000	1/50	1p	MCAD
Phenylketonuria (see Chapters 19, 51, 60)	1/10 000–1/15 000	1/50–1/60	12	PA hydroxylase
Gaucher disease (see Chapter 50)	1/25 000	1/15 (in Ashkenazi Jews)	1	β-glucosidase
Smith–Lemil–Opitz syndrome. Type 2 is lethal neonatally, with microcephaly, heart defect, renal dysplasia, cleft palate and polydactyly; Type 1 is less severe with mental handicap, ptosis and genito-urinary malformations	1/30 000			7-dehydrocholesterol reductase (7 DHCR)
Zellweger syndrome. Peroxisome function disrupted, raised plasma levels of long chain fatty acids, severe developmental delay, hypotonia, renal and hepatic failure	1/50 000		Several	
Classical galactosaemia. Vomiting, hepatomegaly, jaundice and oedema. In later life, cataracts and mental handicap (see Chapter 60)	1/55 000		9	Galactose-1-phosphate uridyl transferase
Sickle cell disease (see Chapters 34, 60)	1/600	1/12 (in African Americans)	11p	β-globin
Alpha-thalassaemia (see Chapters 34, 60)	1/2500	1/25 (in Southeast Asians, Chinese)	16p	α-globin
Beta-thalassaemia (see Chapters 34, 60)	1/3600	1/30 (in Greeks, Italians)	11p	β-globin
Friedreich ataxia. Ataxia, pigeon chest, loss of muscle function in legs			7q	Frataxin
Adenosine deaminase deficiency. Severe immunodeficiency, recurrent infections	1/100 000		20q	Adenosine deaminase
Ceroid lupofuscinosis. Presents in infancy or middle childhood with rapid loss of vision and dementia; early death	1/150 000		1p 16p	PPT CLNS

into DOPA quinone, a precursor of the dark pigment, **melanin** (see Chapter 51).

Every person with OCA1 is a recessive homozygote (***aa***) and most are born to phenotypically normal parents, who can also produce normal homozygotes and heterozygotes in the ratio of one dominant homozygote to two pigmented heterozygotes to every one with albinism:

$Aa \times Aa \rightarrow 1\,AA : 2\,Aa : 1\,\mathbf{aa}$;   3 pigmented : 1 albino.

The babies produced by OCA partners all have OCA:

$aa \times aa \rightarrow aa$

People with OCA who have normally pigmented partners usually produce only pigmented offspring as the albinism allele is relatively rare:

$\mathbf{aa} \times AA \rightarrow Aa$

On rare occasions, however, a normally pigmented partner is a heterozygote and a half of the children of such matings are recessive homozygotes:

$\mathbf{aa} \times Aa \rightarrow Aa, \mathbf{aa}$;   1 pigmented : 1 albino.

Superficially the latter pattern resembles that due to dominant heterozygotes with normal partners (see Chapter 16) and is referred to as '**pseudodominance**'.

Recessive diseases can be common in reproductively closed populations and molecular tests, if available, can be used to identify unaffected carriers. The frequency of heterozygotes can be calculated from that of homozygotes by the **Hardy–Weinberg law** (see Chapter 35).

Estimation of risk

Recessive homozygotes are produced by three kinds of mating, although the first of these is by far the most common.

1 Two heterozygotes:

$Aa \times Aa \rightarrow 1\,AA : 2\,Aa : 1\,\mathbf{aa}$;   risk = 1/4, 0.25, or 25%.

2 Recessive homozygote and heterozygote:

$aa \times Aa \rightarrow 1\,Aa : 1\,aa$;   risk = 1/2, 0.5, or 50%.

3 Two recessive homozygotes:

$aa \times aa \rightarrow aa$; risk = 1.0, or 100%.

Example: congenital deafness

There are many (> 30) non-syndromic, autosomal recessive forms of congenital deafness that mimic one another at the gross phenotypic level in that all homozygotes are deaf. Such a situation is known as '**locus heterogeneity**'. The frequency of heterozygotes is about 10%.

Deaf individuals frequently choose marriage partners who are also deaf and often produce offspring with normal hearing. This can occur *if the marriage partners are homozygous for mutant recessive alleles at different loci.*

If alleles *d* and *e* both cause deafness in the homozygous state, a mating between two deaf homozygotes could be represented:

dd*EE* × *DD***ee**
deaf deaf
↓
DdEe

all offspring have normal hearing.

Consanguineous matings

Consanguinity means that partners share at least one ancestor. **Inbreeding** between consanguineous partners is potentially harmful as it brings recessive alleles 'identical by descent' into the homozygous state in the offspring. **Incestuous** matings, for example between parent and child, or sibs (brother and sister) involve the greatest risk. The probability that a particular allele present in one individual is present also in an incestuous partner is 0.5.

If each of us on average were heterozygous for *one* harmful (but non-lethal) recessive allele, the probability of a homozygous recessive offspring resulting from incestuous mating would be:

$0.5 \times 0.25 = 0.125$, or 1/8.

For marriages between first cousins, the equivalent figures are 1/8 that an allele is shared and 1/32 (3%) that a homozygous baby would be produced. This accords with the observed frequency of recessive disease among offspring of first-cousin marriages, although excluding early miscarriages and other possible complications. The observation supports the hypothesis that on average we each carry at least one harmful recessive allele in the heterozygous state.

Recessive disease occurs in outbred marriages at one quarter of the square of the heterozygote frequency (see Chapter 35) and averages about 2% overall. In general, the rarer the disease and the greater the frequency of consanguineous marriages, the higher the proportion of recessive homozygotes produced by such marriages.

The offspring of first-cousin marriages have 2.5 times as many congenital malformations and 70% higher postnatal mortality than those of outbred matings, both features of decreased vigour, known as **inbreeding depression**. In the UK double first cousins (i.e. both sets of parents are full siblings) are the closest relatives permitted to marry.

Problems

1 A man asks what is the probability he is a carrier of cystic fibrosis, as his unaffected sister has had a baby with cystic fibrosis. What would you tell him?

Answer His sister is an '**obligate heterozygote**' (i.e. she *must* be a heterozygote) and he has a 50% chance of also being heterozygous. You could point out that the frequency of carriers is as high as 1/25 among Caucasians, but that screening for the most common alleles that cause cystic fibrosis is available both for him and any intended partner. The affected child could also be tested to compare their disease alleles.

2 A young woman has received a proposal of marriage from her father's brother's son. She has a sister who suffers from oculocutaneous albinism (OCA) and is concerned that if she married him their children would have the same health problem. What would you advise her?

Answer The mating that produced the affected sister would be $Aa \times Aa$, which can also produce normal homozygotes (AA) and heterozygotes (Aa) in the ratio 1 : 2. The normally pigmented woman therefore has a 2/3 chance of being a carrier. Her father is an obligate heterozygote and the chance his brother is also a carrier is 1/2. The risk her cousin is a carrier is therefore $1/2 \times 1/2 = 1/4$ and the risk that the proposed marriage would produce offspring with OCA is: $2/3 \times 1/4 \times 1/4 = 1/24$ for each child.

19 Autosomal recessive inheritance, clinical examples

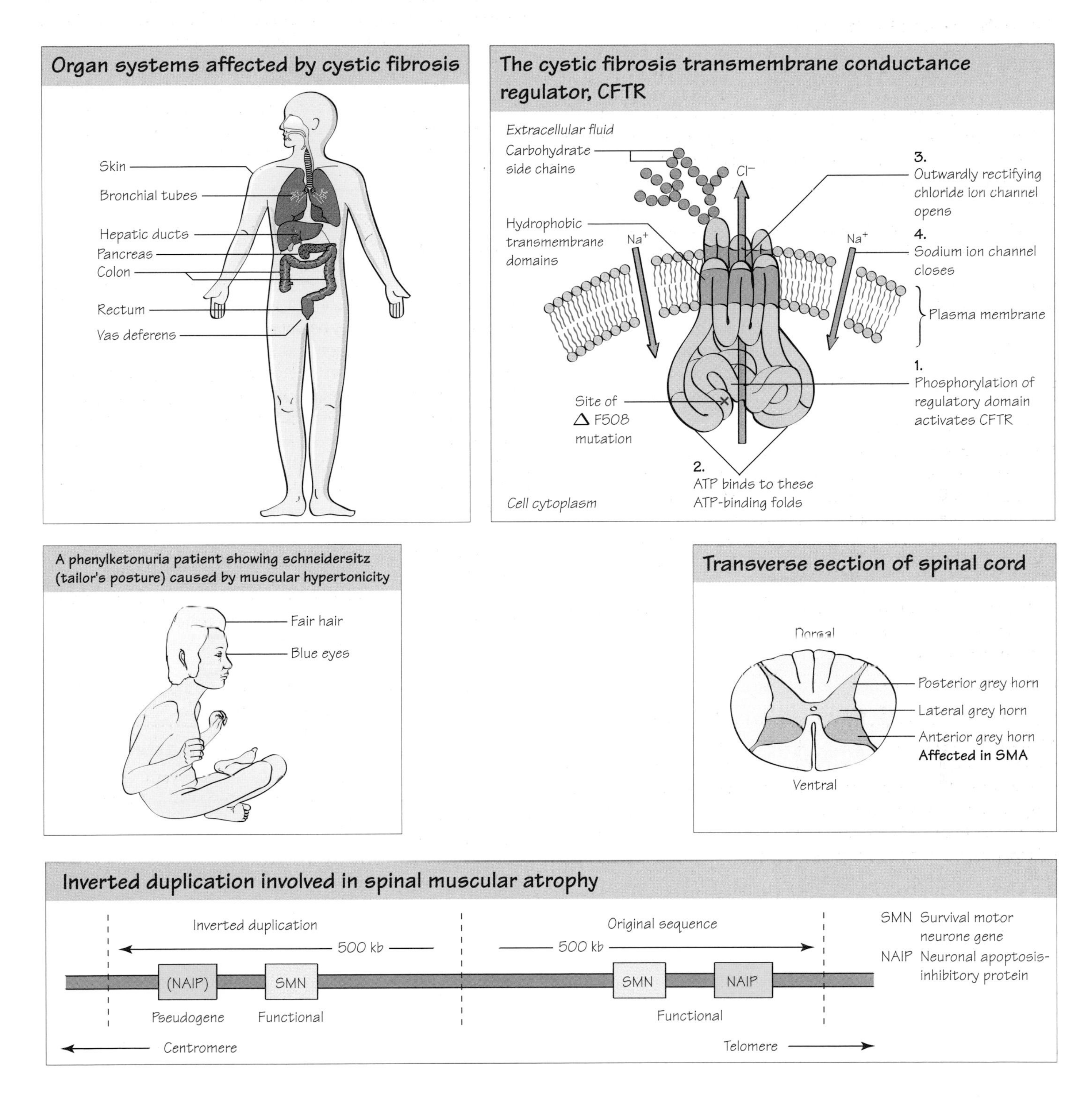

Overview

We are still unable to explain the high frequencies of most common recessive diseases. High allele frequencies may arise by random 'drift', or by the 'founder effect', i.e. by expansion of isolated small populations. An allele could have been advantageous in the past, but now cause disease because lifestyles have changed, an example being those that promote efficient food utilization which in wealthier times predispose to diabetes mellitus (see Chapters 32, 46). A disadvantageous allele may perhaps 'hitch-hike' along with another that is selectively advantageous, as the latter increases in frequency by natural selection. For G6PD deficiency and sickle cell disease there is good evidence for **heterozygote advantage** in resistance to malaria (see Chapter 34). In the case of cystic fibrosis perhaps the best explanation is reproductive advantage for heterozygotes, as in highly fertile partnerships where the ΔF508 allele is present almost every baby born at high parities is a girl. This situation would preferentially promote the mutant allele and if continued over 5000 years would account for its present high frequency.

Cystic fibrosis (CF)

Frequency 1/~2500 Caucasians; 1/15 000 African-Americans; 1/30 000 Asian-Americans.

Genetics AR, 7q31; more than 1300 alleles, but **ΔF508** accounts for 70%.

Features Cystic fibrosis is one of the commonest serious autosomal recessive diseases in northern Europeans, in whom about one in 25 are unaffected heterozygous carriers (see Chapter 35). Among newborns 10–20% have a thick plug that blocks the colon called **meconium ileus**. Most patients have pancreatic insufficiency, there is intestinal malabsorption, anaemia and failure to thrive, rectal prolapse and blockage of liver ducts. The sweat is very salty. Almost all males have **congenital bilateral absence of the vas deferens (CBAVD)**. The most serious problem is chronic obstructive airway disease due to thick mucus, accompanied by bacterial infection which causes destruction of lung tissue and death in 90% patients by 25–30 years of age. Death can also result from heat prostration.

Aetiology The basic defect is in the **cystic fibrosis transmembrane conductance regulator (CFTR)** protein responsible for controlled passage of chloride ions through cell membranes. CFTR forms cyclic AMP-regulated Cl^- ion channels that span the plasma membranes of specialized epithelial cells. Normally, activation of the CFTR by phosphorylation of the regulatory domain, followed by binding of ATP opens the outwardly rectifying Cl^- ion channel and closes adjacent Na^+ channels. Defective ion transport creates salt imbalance and water depletion.

CFTR structural gene modifications include missense, frameshift, splice site, nonsense and deletion mutations (see Chapter 39). They either block or reduce CFTR synthesis, prevent it reaching the epithelial membrane (e.g. ΔF508), or cause its malfunction.

Patients with CFTR activity of below 3% of normal have severe 'classic' CF with pancreatic insufficiency (PI); those with 3–8% have respiratory disease but pancreatic sufficiency (PS); at 8–12% male patients have CBAVD only.

Management The mainstay of treatment for lung problems is thrice-daily percussive physiotherapy and antibiotics. Inhalers and nebulizers are helpful and heart-lung transplants have been successful in very severe cases. Nutritional therapy includes pancreatic enzymes and special diets. Exercise including swimming is beneficial. Gene replacement therapy is still at the experimental stage.

Prenatal diagnosis is based on microvillar enzymes in amniotic fluid, or DNA analysis of amniotic fluid cells. Neonatal diagnosis includes measurement of NaCl in sweat and of immunoreactive trypsin (IRT) in the blood, a consequence of pancreatic duct blockage *in utero* (see Chapter 60). Population screening at birth is routine in some populations and for carriers in CF-affected families (known as 'cascade screening').

Problems requiring immediate attention

- Breathing tube obstruction and lung infection; sodium balance.

Tay–Sachs disease, GM2 gangliosidosis

Frequency 1/3600 in Ashkenazi Jews (carrier frequency, 1/30), but now reduced to 5/360 000 by genetic intervention; 1/360 000 in American non-Jews (carrier frequency 1/300).

Genetics AR; 15q

Features Tay–Sachs disease is of two overlapping main types, '**infantile**' and '**late infantile**' (**Sandhoff disease**). In the infantile form affected infants usually present with poor feeding, lethargy and hypotonia and in 90% of patients there is a cherry-red spot in the macula of the retina. In the second half of the first year there may be developmental regression, feeding becomes increasingly difficult, with progressive loss of skills. Deafness develops, or hypersensitivity to sound. Visual impairment leads to complete blindness by 1 year. In the 2nd year head size can increase, there may be outbursts of inappropriate laughter and seizures. Hypotonia leads to spasticity, then paralysis. Death due to respiratory infection usually occurs by the age of 3 years, or in the late infantile form at 5–10 years.

Aetiology The most common mutation for Tay–Sachs disease is a four-base insertion in the gene for the α-subunit of **hexosaminidase A**. Hexosaminidase A is responsible for converting the glycosylated membrane phospholipid, or **ganglioside**, GM2 to GM3, the deficiency causing build-up of GM2 in the lysosomes (see Chapters 45, 51). It has α and β subunits while its isozyme **hexosaminidase B** has two β subunits. In Sandhoff disease there is a defect in the β subunit and both hexosaminidases A and B are affected.

Management Management is supportive. Prenatal or pre-implantation DNA-based diagnosis is possible if both parents are known to be carriers (see Chapter 51). Diagnosis in newborns is routine, on the basis of hexosaminidase A deficiency and heterozygotes are identified by intermediate levels (see Chapter 60).

Problems requiring immediate attention

- Confirmatory diagnosis and feeding.

Phenylketonuria (PKU)

Frequency 1/10 000–1/15 000 Caucasians; carriers 1/50–1/60.

Genetics AR; 12q24; > 450 alleles.

Features Typically PKU homozygotes are fair-haired with blue eyes. Children have convulsions and become severely mentally retarded, phenylalanine (PA) accumulates in the blood and related metabolites are excreted in the urine.

Aetiology The basic cause is deficiency in **phenylalanine hydroxylase (PAH)** necessary for conversion of PA into tyrosine (see Chapter 51 for details and diagnostic tests). In the early days there is severe vomiting and occasionally convulsions. There is learning disability and the baby's skin can become dry and eczematous. Untreated patients have a 'mousy' smell due to phenylacetic acid in the sweat and urine and muscular hypertonicity. Life expectancy is reduced.

Management Physiological independence of a baby from its mother is acquired at birth and only thereafter does the homozygous infant risk trauma from PA build-up, untreated babies losing 1–2 IQ points per week. PA is essential for growth, but a PA-low diet must be introduced well before 1 month and continued for at least 10 years. Special care must be taken during pregnancy in affected females to prevent mental damage, microcephaly and congenital heart defects in offspring.

Problems requiring immediate attention

- Diet and convulsions.

Spinal muscular atrophy (SMA)

Frequency 1/10 000; carrier frequency 1/50.

Genetics AR, 5q13

Features SMA includes a biochemically and genetically heterogeneous group of disorders that are among the commonest genetic causes of death in childhood.

- **Type 1 SMA (Werdnig–Hoffmann disease).** This is the most severe and most common form. Children present within the first 6 months with severe hypotonia and lack of spontaneous movement. They may have poor swallowing and respiratory function leading to death before the age of 3 years.
- **Type 2 SMA.** Muscle weakness and hypotonia are again the main features, but are less severe and onset is at 6–18 months. Children can sit unaided, but cannot achieve independent locomotion. Most survive into early adulthood.
- **Type 3 SMA (Kugelberg–Welander disease).** This form is relatively mild, with age of onset after 18 months and all patients able to walk without support. Muscle weakness is slowly progressive. There can be recurrent respiratory infection and scoliosis.

Aetiology Disability is due to degeneration of the anterior horn cells of the spinal cord which leads to progressive muscle weakness and ultimately death.

Two relevant genes on Chromosome 5q are involved in a 500 kb inverted duplication. These are **SMN**, the **survival motor neuron gene** and **NAIP**, which codes for **neuronal apoptosis inhibitor protein**. The duplicated section carries an alternative version of SMN and a non-functional pseudogene of NAIP. In 95% of Type 1 patients there is homozygous deletion of exons 7 and 8 of the telomeric copy of SMN. The adjacent NAIP gene is also deleted in 45% of Type 1 patients and up to 20% of those with Types 2 and 3, but additional genes are probably also involved.

Management Because of the complex genetic situation, prenatal diagnosis and carrier detection by DNA analysis is difficult, but diagnosis of patients can be confirmed by electromyography. Type 3 patients need wheelchairs in early adult life. There is no effective treatment, but up-regulation of the centromeric SMN gene is an attractive future possibility.

Problems requiring immediate attention

- Respiration and feeding.

20 Aspects of dominance

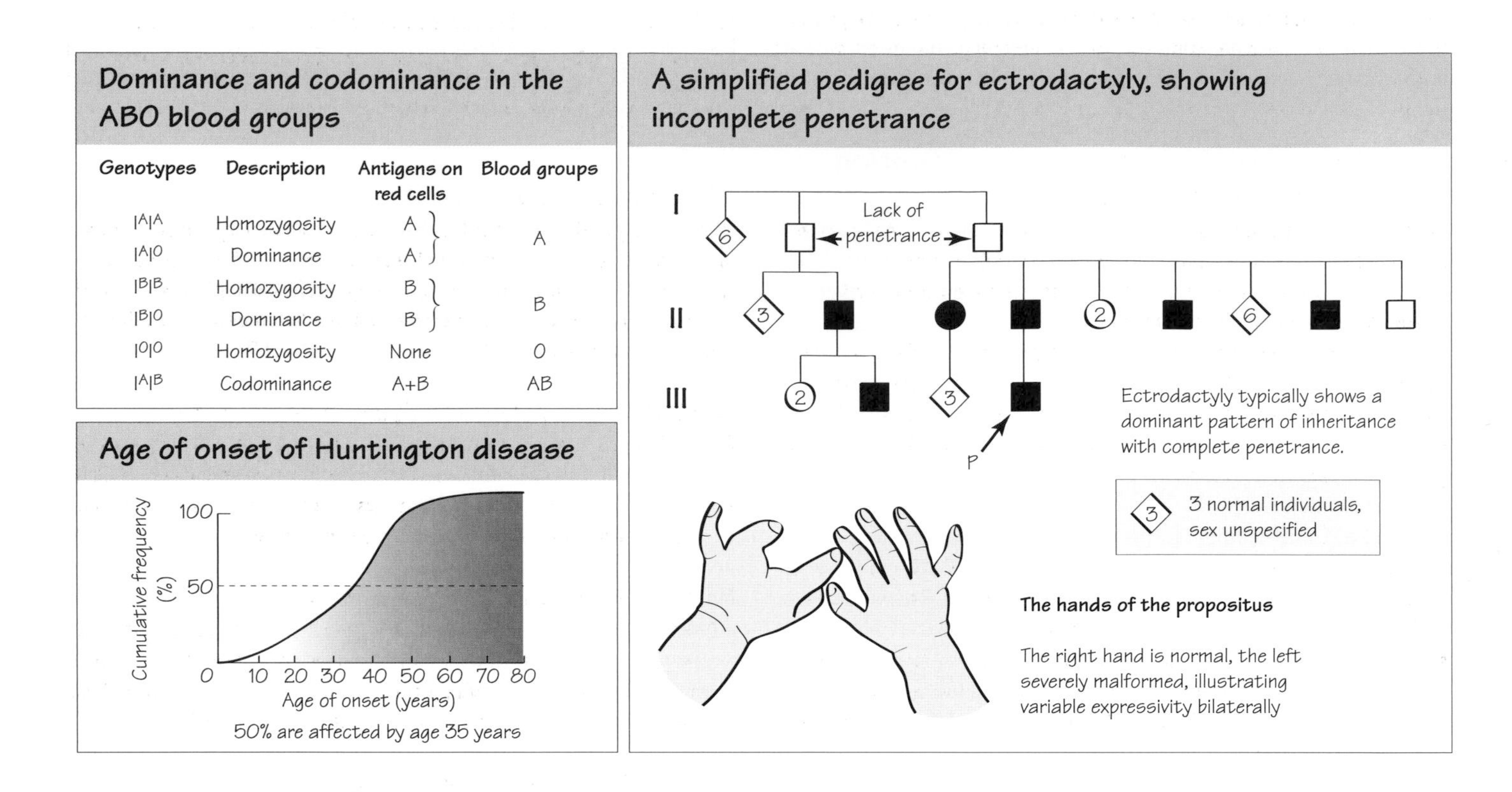

Dominance and codominance in the ABO blood groups

Genotypes	Description	Antigens on red cells	Blood groups
I^AI^A	Homozygosity	A	A
I^AI^O	Dominance	A	
I^BI^B	Homozygosity	B	B
I^BI^O	Dominance	B	
I^OI^O	Homozygosity	None	O
I^AI^B	Codominance	A+B	AB

Overview

If a child is born with what is known to be a genetic disease, but there is no family history of that disease, it could be due to a new mutation in a germ cell that led to that individual. Close to 90% of achondroplasia and 50% of NF1 cases (see below) seem to be new mutations. If there are several new cases in one sibship it could be due to gonadal mosaicism arising from a mutation during development of a parent.

Different mutations of the same gene can show different patterns of inheritance. A mutation would be considered recessive if it only slightly reduces enzyme activity in single dose, but cause significant deficiency in double dose, while a more serious mutation of the same gene that causes disease in the heterozygous state would be classed as dominant. A useful rule is: ***a dominant disease allele can produce disease in a heterozygote, whereas a recessive allele cannot***. Like achondroplasia, most 'dominant' diseases are probably more severe in the affected homozygote than in the heterozygote.

Mutations that cause gain of function at the protein level are requently expressed as dominant (e.g. HD; see Chapter 21). Mutations that cause loss of function typically result in recessive disease (e.g. FH; see Chapter 17). 'Dominant negative' conditions often involve protein multimers in which an abnormal polypeptide interferes with functioning of a normal homologue with which it interacts (e.g. MFS; see Chapter 17).

Codominance (Co-D), the ABO blood groups

If neither of two alternative alleles is dominant to the other, the situation is called **codominance**. In the ABO blood group system groups A, B, AB and O are distinguished by whether the red blood cells are agglutinated by anti-A or anti-B antibody (see Chapter 35). Group O cells have a precursor glycosphingolipid embedded in their surfaces which is elaborated differentially in A, B and AB, by the products of alleles I^A and I^B.

The erythrocytes of both I^B homozygotes and I^B/I^O heterozygotes are agglutinated by anti-B antibody, so both are considered Group B. Similarly Group A includes both I^A homozygotes and I^A/I^O heterozygotes. *Alleles I^A and I^B are both dominant to I^O.*

The red cells of I^O homozygotes are not agglutinated by antibodies directed against A or B. They are placed in Group O.

The red cells of Group AB individuals carry both A and B antigens. They are agglutinated by *both* anti-A and anti-B, and are therefore of Group AB. *Since both are expressed together, alleles IA and IB are **codominant**.*

The alleles of several other blood groups, the tissue antigens of the HLA system, the electrophoretic variants of many proteins and the DNA markers (see Part III) can also be considered codominant, as their properties are assessed directly, irrespective of their derivative properties.

Incomplete dominance (ID), sickle cell disease

Alpha- and β-globin, together with haem and iron, make up the **haemoglobin** of our red blood cells. The normal allele for β-globin is called HbA and the **sickle cell allele,** HbS, differs from it by one base (see Chapter 39). In HbS homozygotes the abnormal haemoglobin aggregates, causing the red cells to collapse into the shape of a sickle and to clog small blood vessels. **Sickle cell disease** is characterized by anaemia, intense pain, and vulnerability to infection.

Heterozygotes have both normal (A) and abnormal (S) haemoglobin molecules in their erythrocytes, which stay undistorted most of the time, allowing them to live a normal life. At this level HbA is dominant to HbS. However, under conditions of severe oxygen stress, a proportion of cells undergoes sickling and this causes transient symptoms similar to those of homozygotes. On this basis the HbS allele is classified as **incompletely dominant**. HbS/HbA heterozygotes are said to possess '**sickle cell trait**'.

Incomplete penetrance

Some apparently dominant alleles sometimes 'skip a generation'. **Ectrodactyly**, in which formation of the middle elements of hands and feet is variably disrupted, is caused by such a **dominant allele of reduced penetrance** (see Chapter 12).

'**Degree of penetrance**' relates to the percentage of carriers of a specific 'dominant' allele that show the relevant phenotype. For example, about 75% of women with certain mutations in the BRCA1 gene develop breast or ovarian cancer (see Chapter 41). The joint penetrance of those mutations is 75%.

Delayed onset

Huntington disease can remain unexpressed for 30–50 years and is an example of **age-related penetrance** or a **disease of late onset**. Patients eventually undergo progressive degeneration of the nervous system, with uncontrolled movements and mental deterioration (see Chapter 21). Other examples are **haemochromatosis** (a disorder of iron storage), **familial Alzheimer disease** (see Chapter 32) and many inherited cancers (see Chapter 41).

Variable expressivity

Sometimes a disease allele is expressed in every individual who carries it (i.e. it is dominant and fully penetrant), although its severity and expression vary considerably. This is called **variable expressivity**. The causes of variable expressivity are largely unknown, but include '**modifier genes**'. For example, a gene on Chromosome 19 seems to influence whether or not a patient with CF will develop meconium ileus (see Chapter 19). A well studied example is neurofibromatosis type 1.

Neurofibromatosis type 1 (NF1), Von Recklinghausen disease

Frequency 1/3000–1/5000

Genetics AD; penetrance virtually 100% by the age of 5 years, variable expressivity. 80% are new mutations.

Features NF1 is highly variable in expression. In mild form it generally includes **café-au-lait spots** (pale brown spots) and axial or inguinal freckling, sometimes benign '**Lisch nodules**' on the retina and a few non-malignant peripheral nerve tumours called **neurofibromas**. When severely expressed there may be thousands of neurofibromas, **optic gliomas** (benign tumours of the optic nerve), epilepsy, learning disabilities, hypertension, scoliosis and malignant tumours of peripheral nerve sheaths.

Identical twins with NF1 have similar symptoms, suggesting influence of modifier genes (see Chapter 33).

Problems requiring immediate attention

- Sometimes high blood pressure.

Pharmacogenetics

Pharmacogenetic traits are a special case of incomplete penetrance and variable expression in which the presence of deficient alleles is revealed by specific chemicals, including drugs. Genes known to be of especial importance in drug deactivation are those of the **Cytochrome P450** group (see Chapter 34).

G6PD deficiency (X-linked R) (see Chapters 22 and 35)

G6PD deficiency causes sensitivity to certain drugs, notably ***primaquine*** (used for treatment of malaria), ***phenacetin***, ***sulphonamides*** and **fava beans** (broad beans), hence the name '**favism**' for the haemolytic crisis that occurs when they are eaten by male hemizygotes.

N-acetyl transferase deficiency (AR)

Fifty per cent of members of Western populations are homozygous for a recessive allele that confers a dangerously slow rate of elimination of certain drugs, notably ***isoniazid*** prescribed against tuberculosis. The Japanese are predominantly rapid inactivators.

Pseudocholinesterase deficiency (AR)

One European in 3000 and 1.5% of Inuit (Eskimo) are homozygous for an enzyme deficiency that causes lethal paralysis of the diaphragm when given ***succinylcholine*** as a muscle relaxant during surgery.

Halothane sensitivity, malignant hyperthermia (genetically heterogeneous)

One in 10 000 patients can die in high fever when given the anaesthetic, ***halothane***, especially in combination with succinylcholine.

Thiopurine methyltransferase deficiency (ACo-D)

Certain drugs prescribed for leukaemia and suppression of the immune response cause serious side-effects in about 0.3% of the population with deficiency of ***thiopurine methyltransferase.***

Debrisoquine hydroxylase deficiency (AR)

This enzyme is one of the P450 group. Five to 10 per cent of Europeans show serious adverse reactions when given ***debrisoquine*** for hypertension. The enzyme is involved in the metabolism of many other drugs.

Porphyria variegata (AD)

Skin lesions, abdominal pain, paralysis, dementia and psychosis are brought on by sulphonamides, barbiturates, etc., in about one in 500 South Africans. Death can result from concentration of haem in the liver, following induction of haem-containing Cytochrome P450 proteins.

21 Genomic imprinting and dynamic mutation

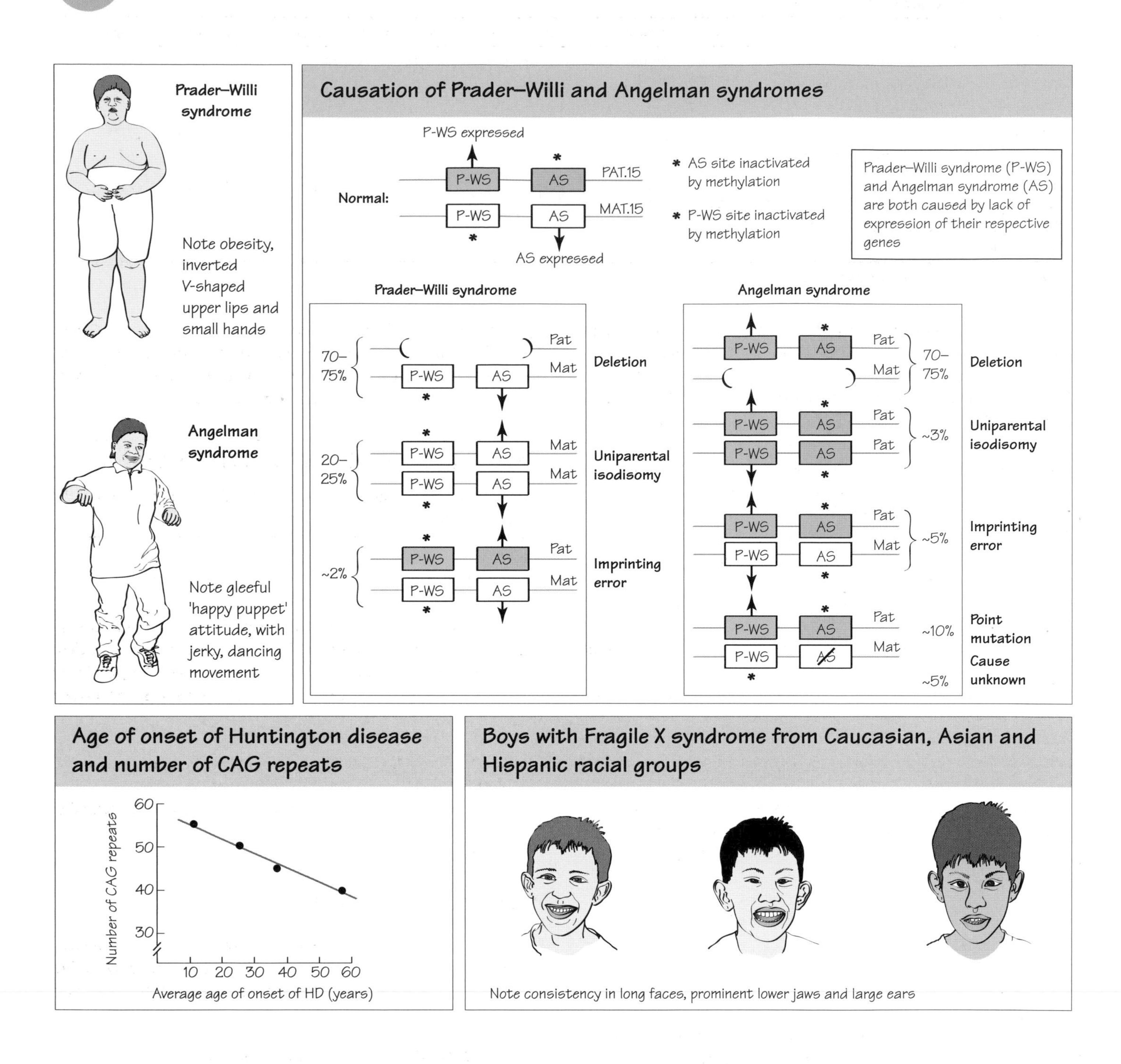

Overview

During gametogenesis possibly as many as 40 genes receive '**genomic imprinting**' that normally ensures later expression of *only one* of the two inherited alleles. In contradiction of Mendel's laws, mutations of such genes can cause dramatically different disorders depending on whether they come from the mother or the father. Genomic imprinting is a factor in **assisted reproduction** as the incidence of imprinting disorders increases after use of ***in vitro* fertilization** and **intracytoplasmic sperm injection** (**ICSI**; see Chapter 52).

Dynamic mutation refers notably to the progressive expansion of '**triplet repeats**'. There are close to 20 diseases of this type falling into three categories (Table 21.1). Symptoms in later generations often become more severe or appear at progressively younger ages, a phenomenon called **anticipation**.

Genomic imprinting

Within the '**critical region**' on Chromosome 15q, which includes the **Prader-Willi** and **Agelman** sites, several genes are transcriptionally active only on the paternal homologue, others only on the maternal. The main mechanism of this differential activation/deactivation is methylation

Table 21.1 Diseases caused by expansion of repeat sequences. Categories 1 and 2 involve trinucleotide repeats; in Category 3 units of other numbers of nucleotides are also involved.

Disorder	Repeat unit	Normal range	Disease range	Anticipation	Parent*	Sequence
Category 1 Neurological, e.g. Huntington disease and most of the **cerebellar ataxias**, etc.	CAG	6–35	21–220	Yes	Father	Coding
Category 2 Musculoskeletal, e.g. **cleidocranial dysplasia**, etc.	G--	5–15	6–25	No	Unknown	Coding
Category 3 Neurological and muscular, e.g. MD1, MD2, FRAX A, **FRAX E**, **Friedreich ataxia**, two of the cerebellar ataxias, etc.	Various	5–75	30–11 000	Yes	Mother	Non-coding

* Parent in which repeat expansion occurs.

of the DNA. Imprinting is affected by mutations in imprinting control elements, deletions, duplications and epigenetic modification.

Prader–Willi and Angelman syndromes (P-WS and AS)

Frequency 1/25 000. Prader–Willi syndrome is characterized by short stature, hypotonia, compulsive eating, obesity, small hands and feet, hypogonadism and *mild-to-moderate* neurodevelopmental delay. Fifty to sixty per cent of patients have a visible deletion and 15% a submicroscopic deletion at 15q11-12. *In P-WS it is always the paternal homologue that is deleted*, while most of the remaining 25% have *maternal* 15q isodisomy (see Chapters 24 and 27).

Angelman syndrome is characterized by epilepsy, *severe* neurodevelopmental delay, uncoordinated movements and compulsive laughter. Some 70% of AS patients also have a deletion of 15q11-12, but *on the maternal homologue*. In a further 2–3% there is *paternal* uniparental isodisomy of 15q.

These conditions seem to involve two adjacent genes that normally are differentially inactivated by methylation during the production of sperm and oocytes, the imprinting pattern in oocytes being the opposite of that in sperm. Normal development requires just *one* active copy of *both* the AS and P-WS sites in the brain, the paternal P-WS site and the maternal AS site being preferentially expressed. In up to 10% of AS patients there are mutations in the maternal AS site and a small percentage of both classes of patient have a deletion in the **imprinting centre** that controls the imprinting process.

Beckwith–Wiedemann syndrome (B-WS)

Frequency 1/4000

Genetics AD; 11p15

Features Fetuses are large for gestational age, with excess amniotic fluid (**polyhydramnios**), protrusion of the umbilicus (**omphalocoele**), asymmetrical limb length, prominent eyes, enlarged internal organs, facial haemangioma, and a predisposition to embryonal tumours. A large, protruding tongue can cause orthodontic, breathing and speech problems.

The **insulin-like growth factor 2** (**IGF2**) gene is normally active only on the paternally derived Chromosome 11 and disease can arise from defective imprinting of the maternal copy. High levels of IGF2 are believed to cause the overgrowth features of B-WS.

About 20% of B-WS patients have childhood tumours, uniparental 11p isodisomy and abnormal methylation of a 1 megabase (Mb) region of Chromosome 11. There are three imprinting centres here and about 50% of patients are defective in the second of these, but have no predisposition to tumours. Embryonal tumours are associated with methylation of a non-coding region designated H19.

Problems requiring immediate attention

- Umbilical abnormalities, neonatal hypoglycaemia, breathing and feeding problems due to large tongue.

Dynamic mutation: the triplet repeat disorders

Two of the best examples of dynamic mutation are **Huntington disease** (**HD**) and **myotonic dystrophy** (**MD**), both of which show anticipation. MD provides examples of three additional genetic principles: **pleiotropy** (see also MFS, Chapter 17), **locus heterogeneity** and **meiotic drive**.

Huntington disease (HD); Huntington's chorea

(Table 21.2)

Genetics AD; 4p16.3; shows anticipation when transmitted paternally.

Gene product Huntingtin

Frequency 1/10–20 000 Caucasians

Features Slowly progressive neuronal death, characteristic 'choreic' movements (facial grimacing, twitching, folding of arms and crossing of legs); gait becomes unsteady and speech unclear. There is insidious

Table 21.2 Huntington disease (HD) phenotypes.

Phenotype	No. of CAG repeats	Features
Normal	< 26	Stable throughout meiosis
Normal	27–35	'Premutation' unstable in paternal meiosis
Mild HD	36–39	Late onset or non-penetrance
Adult-onset HD	> 40	Symptoms from average age 41 years
Juvenile-onset HD	> 55	Symptoms before age 20 years

impairment of intellectual function and psychiatric disturbance culminating in dementia. Advanced patients have difficulty swallowing, and generally die of pneumonia, cardiorespiratory failure, subdural haematoma after head trauma, or suicide. The average age of onset is 41 years and the mean duration of illness 15 years. Up to 5% of cases present before 20 years with rigidity, slow clumsiness and early progressive dementia, often with epileptic seizures. Eighty per cent of juvenile-onset HD cases show paternal transmission and these have especially long repeat series.

Aetiology The huntingtin gene normally contains a highly polymorphic **CAG** trinucleotide repeat series in an exon near the 5′ end. In most patients this is abnormally expanded, possibly due to slippage of DNA polymerase during spermatogenesis. Cleavage of huntingtin by the proteinase **caspase** creates a toxic product that kills cells. The CAG repeats result in a polyglutamine series that promotes abnormal aggregation of huntingtin within and near neuronal nuclei, especially in the corpus striatum, and probably promoting their early loss.

Management Development of HD can be monitored by magnetic resonance imaging (MRI). Treatment is with benzodiazepines to control choreic movements, anti-psychotic drugs and antidepressants. Caspase-specific inhibitors may be beneficial.

Myotonic dystrophy type 1 (MD1) (Table 21.3)

Frequency 1/8000

Genetics AD, 19q13.3

Gene product **Dystrophia myotonica protein kinase (DMPK)**

Features Tonic muscle spasm with prolonged relaxation, cardiac conduction defects and arrhythmia, testicular atrophy, cataracts, disturbed gastro-intestinal peristalsis, weak sphincters, increased risk of diabetes mellitus and gallstones, somnolence and frontal balding.

Aetiology The disease mutation is an expanded **CTG** trinucleotide repeat in the 3′ untranslated region of the DMPK gene. The number of repeats often increases maternally in succeeding generations, the age of onset recedes, clinical symptoms increase in severity and more body systems become involved.

In the congenital form, newborns present with hypotonia, talipes (club foot) and respiratory distress, which can be life-threatening. Survivors tend to show lack of facial expression (**myopathic facies**), delayed motor development and learning difficulties.

Management Diagnosis is usually by DNA analysis. Regular surveillance for cardiac conduction defects is advised and education on the risks of anaesthesia.

Problems requiring immediate attention

- Respiratory problems in some newborn offspring of affected females.

Pleiotropic expression In a mouse model of MD1 the CTG expansion reduces production of DMPK, causing cardiac arrhythmia; cataract, possibly by interfering with a downstream transcription factor gene, and myotonic myopathy due to the RNA transcript blocking RNA binding proteins.

Meiotic drive The relatively high population frequency of MD 'premutation' alleles may be due to healthy heterozygotes preferentially transmitting alleles with greater than 19 CTG repeats.

Locus heterogeneity: MD1 and MD2 MD2 is phenotypically similar to MD1, but associated with expansion of a different part of the genome, the 4-base sequence **CCTG** at 3q21.

Table 21.3 Myotonic dystrophy type 1 (MD1) phenotypes.

Phenotype	No. of CTG repeats	Features
Normal	5–37	
Mild MD1	38–100	Cataracts in older people
Full MD1	100–1000	Moderate adult-onset disease
Congenital MD1	1000–2000	Severe congenital disease

Fragile X disease A (FRAX-A) (Table 21.4)

FRAX-A involves repeats of **CGG** at Xq27.3. Methylation of the extended **FMR-1** gene blocks transcription and leads to mental retardation, etc. (see Chapter 22). With > 200 repeats the X chromosome tends to break when cells are cultured in folic acid-deficient medium.

Table 21.4 Fragile X disease A (FRAX-A) phenotypes.

	No. of repeats	Fragile site	IQ, etc.
Male phenotype			
Normal	10–50	Absent	Normal
Normal	50–200	Absent	'Normal transmitting male' with 'premutation'
Full disease	200–2000	In < 50% of cells	Moderate learning difficulties
Female phenotype			
Normal	50–200	Absent	Normal, but 'premutation' unstable
Mild disease	200–2000	In < 10% of cells	50% have mild learning difficulties

X-linked inheritance

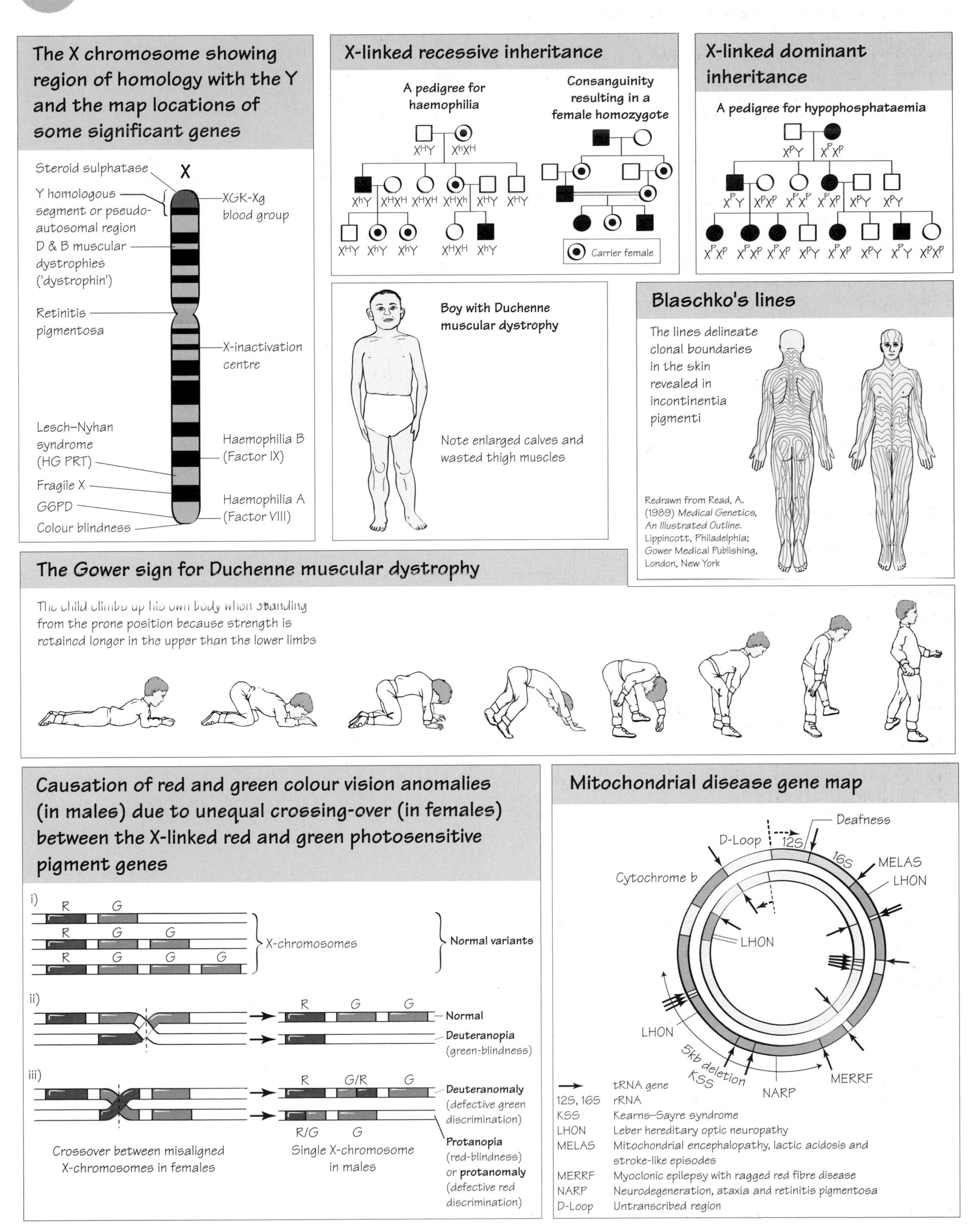

Overview

Most so-called '**sex-linked disorders**' are caused by X-linked recessive alleles in males. For example, since **haemophilia** is recessive, heterozygous females are normal, but males, being **hemizygous** for X-linked genes, are affected. ***X-chromosome inactivation*** (see Chapter 13), however, ***can create mosaic patterns of expression in female heterozygotes, some seriously affected when the inactivation is skewed***. Female homozygotes for X-linked recessive alleles generally occur at a frequency equal to the square of that of affected males.

A man (XY) receives his X chromosome from his mother (XX) and passes that X to every daughter. Both mother and daughter are therefore **obligate carriers** of any X-linked recessive expressed by the man.

Rules of X-linked recessive inheritance

1 ***The incidence of disease is very much higher in males than in females.***
2 ***The mutant allele is passed from an affected man to all of his daughters, but they do not express it.***
3 ***A heterozygous 'carrier' woman passes the allele to half of her sons, who express it, and half her daughters who do not.***
4 ***The mutant allele is NEVER passed from father to son.***

Table 22.1 Sex-related diseases: ***X-linked recessive diseases.***

	Frequency per 10 000 caucasian male births
G6PD deficiency (geographically very variable)	0–6500
Red and green colour blindness (rhodopsin)	~800
Non-specific X-linked mental retardation	5
Duchenne muscular dystrophy (dystrophin)	3.5
Fragile X syndrome	2.5
Haemophilia A (Factor VIII)	2
Becker muscular dystrophy (dystrophin)	0.5
Haemophilia B (Factor IX)	0.3
Agammaglobulinaemia (X-linked)	0.1
Ocular albinism	< 0.1
Hunter syndrome (Mucopolysaccharidosis II)	< 0.1
Retinitis pigmentosa	< 0.1
Fabry disease (angiokeratoma)	< 0.1
Anhidrotic ectodermal dysplasia	< 0.1
Menkes syndrome	< 0.1
Adrenoleukodystrophy	< 0.1
Lesch–Nyhan syndrome (HGPRT deficiency)	< 0.1
Ornithine transcarbamylase deficiency	< 0.1
Chronic granulomatous disease	< 0.1

Table 22.2 Sex-related diseases: ***X-linked dominant diseases.***

Hypophosphataemia (vitamin D resistant rickets)
Hereditary motor and sensory neuropathy
Incontinentia pigmenti (lethal in males)
Rett syndrome (can be lethal in males)
Oro-facio-digital syndrome

Estimation of risk for offspring

Haemophiliac man and unaffected woman

$X^{h}Y$ (**affected man**) × $X^{H}X^{H}$ (unaffected woman)

↓

$X^{H}Y$ (unaffected son) ; $X^{H}X^{h}$ (carrier daughter)

There is no risk of haemophilia in these children.

Carrier woman and unaffected man

Four kinds of offspring can be produced: half the sons are affected and half the daughters are carriers

$X^{H}X^{h}$ (carrier woman) × $X^{H}Y$ (unaffected man)

↓

$X^{H}X^{H}$	$X^{H}X^{h}$	$X^{H}Y$	$X^{h}Y$
unaffected daughter	carrier daughter	unaffected son	**affected son**
1	1	1	**1**

The risk of haemophilia in the offspring is 1/4 or for males 1/2.

Haemophiliac man and carrier woman

Half of the children are affected irrespective of sex.

$X^{h}Y$ (**affected man**) × $X^{H}X^{h}$ (carrier woman)

↓

$X^{H}X^{h}$	$X^{h}X^{h}$	$X^{H}Y$	$X^{h}Y$
carrier daughter	**affected daughter**	unaffected son	**affected son**
1	1	1	**1**

The overall risk is 2/4, or 1/2.

Unaffected man and homozygous haemophiliac woman

All the sons are affected, and all the daughters are carriers.

$X^{h}X^{h}$ (**affected woman**) × $X^{H}Y$ (unaffected man)

↓

$X^{H}X^{h}$	$X^{h}Y$
carrier daughter	**affected son**
1	1

The overall risk is 1/2.

Haemophilia A (HbA), classic haemophilia

Frequency 1/5000 males

Genetics XR; Xq28 (see also Chapter 39)

Gene product Blood clotting Factor VIII

Features Visible bruising, severe bleeding from large wounds. Haemorrhage into the joints causes painful inflammation and diminished joint function (**haemarthrosis**).

Fifty per cent of patients have several bleeding episodes per month and Factor VIII levels below 1% of normal. Those with levels at 5–25%, have coagulation problems only after surgery or severe trauma.

Aetiology Mutations in Factor VIII that disrupt conversion of prothrombin into thrombin include inversions, major deletions and nonsense mutations.

Management Prenatal diagnosis is by DNA testing (see Chapter 57). Perinatal diagnostic criteria include excessive bleeding from the umbilical cord.

Without treatment haemophilia is often fatal by the age of 20 years. Factor VIII for prophylactic use can be isolated from plasma, heat treated and screened to eliminate infection, or produced by recombinant DNA technology. It has a half-life of only 8 hours, so repeated infusions may be necessary. Ten to fifteen per cent of patients develop immunity to administered Factor VIII and require immunosuppression.

Problems requiring immediate attention

- Bleeding from the umbilicus.

Red and green colour blindness

Frequency in males Caucasians 8% (1/12); Asians 4.5%; Africans 2.5%.

Frequency in females The square of that in males, e.g. 0.64% in Caucasians.

Features A quarter of colour vision defective males are **dichromatic**, unable to perceive either red (**protanopia**) or green (**deuteranopia**) light. Most of the remainder perceive reds and greens abnormally and are termed **protanomalous** and **deuteranomalous**. (Absence of both red- and green-sensitive cones is rare and causes **blue cone monochromacy**.)

Aetiology On each X chromosome is a gene for red-sensitive **opsin** immediately adjacent to one or several green opsin genes. Their sequences are very similar, promoting a tendency for crossover errors (see Chapter 26). Protanomaly and deuteranomaly arise when crossover creates 'hybrid' genes.

The X-linked muscular dystrophies

Duchenne muscular dystrophy (DMD)

Frequency in males 1/3500

Genetics XR; Xp21

Features Before 5 years of age, boys show clumsiness, muscle weakness and pseudo-hypertrophy of the calves caused by replacement of degenerate muscle with fat and connective tissue. Patients are confined to wheelchairs by the age of 11 years. Subsequent deterioration leads to lumbar lordosis, joint contractures and cardiorespiratory failure, death ensuing at a mean age of 18 years. Creatine kinase (CK) leaks into the bloodstream and can increase to over 20 times the normal levels. A third of boys have mild-to-moderate intellectual impairment. Female heterozygotes can be mildly affected.

Becker muscular dystrophy (BMD)

Frequency in males 1/18 000

Features Onset around 11 years and slower progression than DMD.

Aetiology The DMD/BMD gene codes for the protein **dystrophin**, with 79 exons, by far the largest gene known in humans. Dystrophin is localized on the cytoplasmic side of the muscle fibre membrane and links the internal cytoskeleton to extracellular material via glycoproteins that span the plasma membrane. Most DMD patients have serious mutations and lack dystrophin, whereas BMD have the protein in reduced quantity or abbreviated form.

Management Assay of dystrophin enables distinction between DMD, BMD and other limb girdle muscular dystrophies. Deletions are usually detected by multiplex polymerase chain reaction (PCR; see Chapter 57), other mutations by sequencing. Carrier females may be identified by mutation testing or by linkage to intragenic markers (allowing for an intragenic recombination rate of 12%). Diagnosis is assisted by electromyography and muscle biopsy. Physiotherapy and treatment with steroids are beneficial.

Fragile X syndrome (FRAX-A [and FRAX-E])

Frequency 1/4000 males; 1/8000 females (FRAX-E: ~1/16 000 and ~1/32 000)

Genetics The FMR-1 gene contains a CGG triplet repeat at Xq27.3 which expands only in females, although is occasionally transmitted as a 'premutation' by '**normal transmitting males**' (see Chapter 21).

Features FRAX-A accounts for 40% of all males with learning difficulties. They have a high forehead and prominent lower jaw, large ears, excess joint mobility and after puberty, **macroorchidism**. There can also be mitral valve prolapse, autistic features and/or hyperactive behaviour. Speech may be halting and repetitive. Normal transmitting males sometimes suffer tremor and ataxia.

Aetiology The FRAX-A full mutation leads to methylation of the promoter and lack of expression of the gene product.

Management Diagnosis involves measurement of the length of the repeat series and its degree of methylation, by enzyme digestion, PCR and Southern blotting (see Chapters 56 and 57).

Other examples

G6PD deficiency See Chapter 35.

Lesch–Nyhan syndrome Disorder of purine metabolism with mental retardation, spasticity and self-mutilation (see Chapter 44).

Adreno-leucodystrophy A peroxisome abnormality causing behavioural, visual and neurological problems.

Fabry disease A variety of vascular defects caused by deficiency in galactosidase A.

X-linked dominant disorders

Rules

1 The condition is expressed and transmitted by BOTH sexes.
2 The condition occurs twice as frequently in females as in males.
3 An affected man passes the condition to every daughter, but never to a son.
4 An affected woman passes the condition to half her sons and half her daughters.
5 Females are usually less seriously affected than males.

Examples

Vitamin D-resistant rickets, hypophosphataemic rickets

Genetics XD
Features Hereditary rickets when there is adequate dietary intake of vitamin D. The kidneys have impaired ability to reabsorb phosphate, resulting in abnormal ossification.

Problems requiring immediate attention

- Correction of serum phosphate level.

Hereditary motor and sensory neuropathy (HMSN), Charcot–Marie–Tooth disease

Frequency of all forms 1/2500

Genetics XD, AD (the most common) and AR; classified as forms I, II, III, etc., by nerve conduction velocity (see also Chapter 39).

Gene product of X-linked form Gap junction protein connexin 32 (see Chapter 2).

Features Heterogeneous, with slowly progressive distal wasting of the legs (between the ages of 10 and 30 years in HMSN I) and often later of the arms, often with ataxia and tremor. The feet develop an exaggerated arch (**pes cavus**). There is often demyelination and thickening of peripheral nerves and progressive hearing loss.

Management Monitoring of hearing and provision of hearing aids. Can be diagnosed pre-implantationally by PCR.

Incontinentia pigmenti (IP)

Frequency Rare, perhaps 1/40 000

Genetics XD, Xq28

Features Diagnosis in infants is based on reddening of a skin rash to blisters, and eventually to pigmented lesions. These follow **Blaschko's lines** (see figure), fading during adolescence. There are conical or missing teeth, ocular and neurological abnormalities.

Aetiology The abbreviated product fails to block apoptosis by tumour necrosis factor. Since IP is lethal in male embryos, offspring are in the ratio 33% affected females : 33% unaffected females : 33% unaffected males.

Problems requiring immediate attention

- Management of seizures in infancy.

Rett syndrome

Genetics XD

Frequency 1/10 000–1/15 000 females; fewer males due to embryonic lethality.

Features Autistic behaviour, deterioration in cognition, epileptic seizures breathing irregularities, gait ataxia and stereotyped hand movements, reduced life expectancy.

Aetiology Most cases have a mutation in MECP2, the protein product of which fails to regulate transcription of genes concerned with brain development.

Management Monitoring of special educational needs.

Problems requiring immediate attention

- Breathing irregularity, seizures.

23 Sex-related disorders other than X-linked

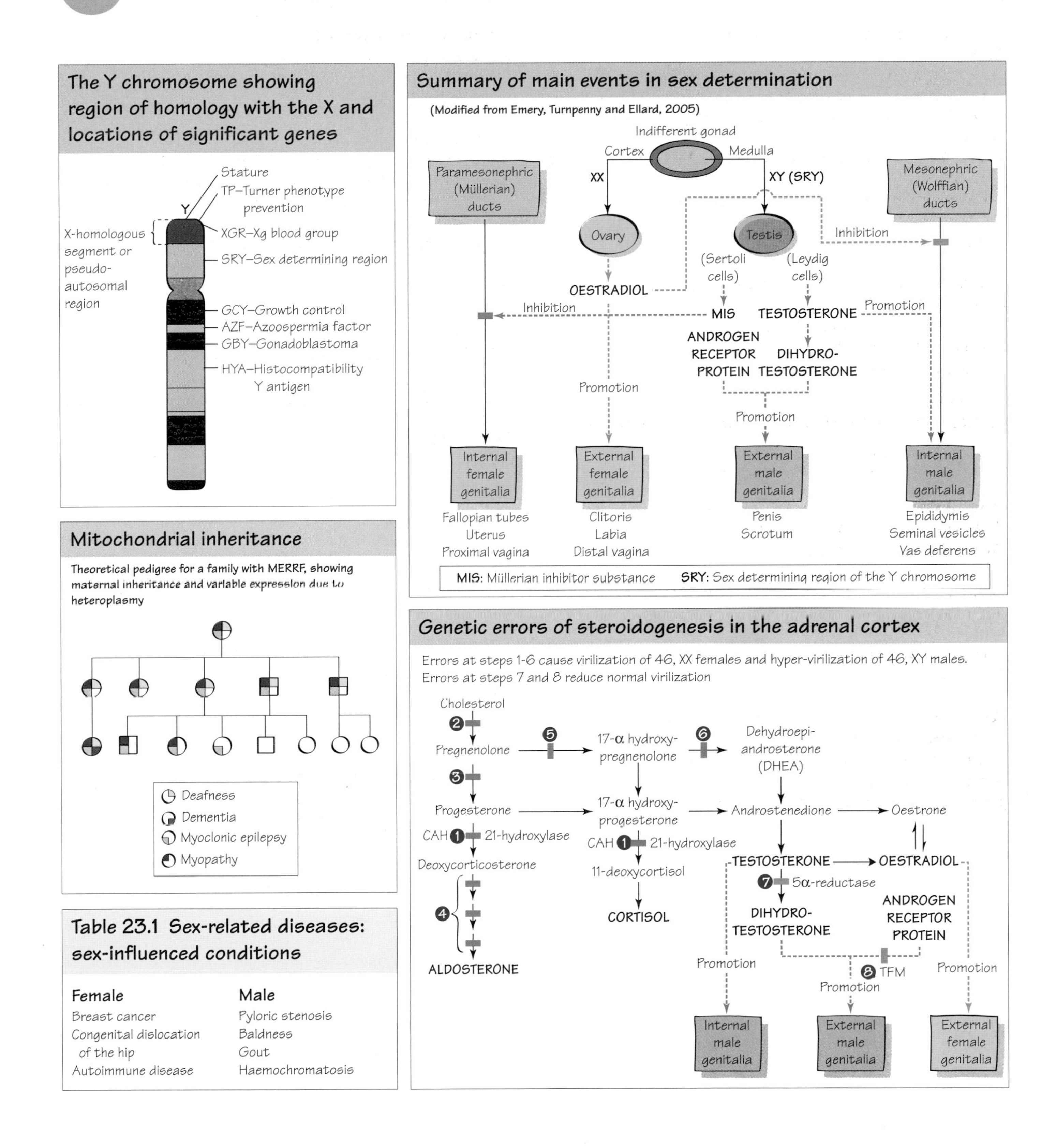

Table 23.1 Sex-related diseases: sex-influenced conditions

Female	Male
Breast cancer	Pyloric stenosis
Congenital dislocation of the hip	Baldness
Autoimmune disease	Gout
	Haemochromatosis

Overview

This chapter includes Y-linked, pseudoautosomal and mitochondrial traits, sex-limited and sex-influenced conditions and disorders of sexual definition.

Y-linked or holandric inheritance

DNA sequencing indicates at least 20 genes on the Y chromosome, including **SRY** that initiates male differentiation through the '**testis determining factor**' (**TDF**) and the normal allele for **azoospermia** (**AZT**) which ensures production of sperm. There is a gene for the male-specific tissue transplantation antigen **HYA** and **GCY,** concerned with male stature.

Rules for Y-linked inheritance

Y-linked genes are expressed in and transmitted only by males, to all their sons.

Possible example Hypertrichosis (hairiness) of ear rims.

Pseudoautosomal inheritance or 'partial sex linkage'

Crossing-over between the X and Y occurs in the **pseudoautosomal region** during male meiosis. Here are several housekeeping genes, one that ensures non-development of **Turner syndrome** in males (see Chapter 25), others for stature and the **Xg blood group**.

Rules of pseudoautosomal inheritance

Genes in the X/Y homologous segment are transmitted by women equally to both sexes, but by a man predominantly to offspring of one sex, although that sex varies between men.

Example **Steroid sulphatase deficient X-linked ichthyosis**, scaly skin.

Mitochondrial inheritance

Mitochondria are acquired solely from the cytoplasm of the ovum, so mitochondrial inheritance is strictly maternal. (See mitochondrial gene maps in Chapters 6 and 22.)

Rules of mitochondrial inheritance

1 Typically the condition is passed from a mother to ALL her children.
2 The condition is NEVER transmitted by men.

MtDNA occurs in several copies per mitochondrion, each encoding two rRNAs, 22 tRNAs and 13 polypeptides involved in oxidative phosphorylation. (Another 90+ mitochondrial polypeptides are encoded in the nucleus.)

Altogether more than 50 mutations and over 100 mitochondrial deletions and duplications are known. Further accumulation of mutations throughout life probably contributes to the ageing process.

Apart from the red blood cells and lens fibres, almost every cell in the body contains thousands of mitochondria and since they play a critical role in ATP production, they are especially numerous in tissues of high energy requirement, such as muscle and brain. The mitochondria do not have DNA repair enzymes, so mtDNA has a high rate of spontaneous mutation. In most individuals the DNA is the same in all mitochondria (**homoplasmy**), but mutations can create more than one mitochondrial type in one individual, called **heteroplasmy**. When representation of the two mitochondrial populations varies between tissues and individuals.

Typically mitochondrial defects show a combination of neurological and myopathic features. Duplications and deletions give rise to **Kearns–Sayre syndrome** (**KSS**; muscle weakness, cerebellar damage and heart failure) and **Pearson syndrome** (infantile pancreatic insufficiency, pancytopaenia, lactic acidosis and chronic progressive external ophthalmoplegia).

Myoclonic epilepsy with ragged red fibre disease (MERRF)

Features Progressive myoclonic epilepsy, widespread degeneration in the brain with slowly progressive dementia and optic atrophy.

Aetiology There is a point mutation in the gene for tRNA lysine.

Mitochondrial encephalopathy, lactic acidosis and stroke-like episodes (MELAS)

Features Short stature, stroke-like episodes with vomiting, headache or visual disturbance, sometimes hemiplegia and hemianopia. Type 2 diabetes often coincides with deafness.

Aetiology Eighty per cent of patients have two substitutions in a leucine tRNA.

Neurodegeneration, ataxia and retinitis pigmentosa (NARP)

Features Night blindness, developmental delay, seizures and dementia.

Aetiology The mutation is a substitution in the ATPase gene.

Leigh disease

Genetics There are both mitochondrial and AR forms.

Features Typical spongiform brain lesions, slow recovery from anaesthesia, sometimes death in infancy. Some patients have cytochrome-C deficiency.

Leber hereditary optic neuropathy (LHON)

Genetics There are about a dozen known mutations in the mitochondrial ND4 gene.

Features Sudden loss of central vision at age 12–30 years, especially in males.

Barth syndrome, X-linked cardioskeletal myopathy, endocardial fibroelastosis

Features Congenital generalized myopathy, cardiomyopathy and growth retardation. Tissues are deficient in cardiolipin and skeletal muscle shows a raised lipid content.

Aetiology There are mutations in the X-linked TAZ gene that codes for a protein in the cytochrome-C system.

Management Diagnosis requires measurement of 3-methyl glutaconic acid in urine.

Sex limitation and sex influence

Some genes are carried on the autosomes, but are limited or influenced by sex. Sex limited traits occur in only one sex due, for instance, to anatomical differences. Penetrance and expressivity of mutant alleles may differ for recognized physiological reasons; for example, **pattern baldness** acts as AD in entire, but not castrated, males, but weakly AR in females. Gout is largely confined to males and post-menopausal women. **Breast cancer**, **autoimmune disease** and **depressive illness** are most common in women, **haemochromatosis** (a disorder of iron accumulation) in men, women probably being protected by menstrual bleeding.

Congenital dislocation of the hip and **cleft palate** are most commonly found in girls and **pyloric stenosis**, **talipes** (clubfoot), **cleft lip and palate** and **Hirschprung disease**, involving intestinal obstruction due to failure of innervation of the large bowel, are most commonly found in boys (see Chapter 28).

Abnormalities of sexual differentiation

Sexual differentiation begins in the early 'indifferent' gonads with secretion of oestrogen or androgen, depending on whether the Y-chromosome is absent or present. Subsequently steroidogenesis is triggered in the adrenal cortex and this becomes responsible for much of later sexual differentiation and maturation.

Disorders of sexual differentiation have been divided into five categories:

1 ***Congenital development of ambiguous genitalia*** – e.g. virilization of a 46,XX individual by exposure to androgens, due to congenital adrenal hyperplasia.
2 ***Congenital disjunction of internal and external sex anatomy*** – e.g. female external anatomy in a 46,XY individual with testes, due to androgen insensitivity.
3 ***Incomplete development of sex anatomy*** – e.g. failure of gonadal development.
4 ***Sex chromosome anomalies*** – e.g. Turner or Klinefelter syndrome (see Chapter 25).
5 ***Disorders of gonadal development*** e.g. individuals with an ovary on one side and a testis on the other, or a mixture of ovarian and testicular tissue.

Problems in girls

Virilization influences in females create ambiguous genitalia arising from defects at six or more steps in the biosynthesis of **aldosterone** and/or **cortisol** (**hydrocortisone**). All are inherited as autosomal recessives. By far the most significant is **congenital adrenal hyperplasia** (**CAH**; or **adrenogenital syndrome**); due to deficiency in **21-hydroxylase** (Step 1 in the figure 'Genetic errors of steroidogenesis in the adrenal cortex'). This so-called '**classic OHD**' causes deficiency of aldosterone and cortisol and build-up of adrenocortical steroids proximal to the block, many of which have androgenic properties. About 25% suffer excessive salt excretion and circulatory collapse at 2–3 weeks. Reduced cortisol production stimulates **adrenocorticotrophic hormone** (**ACTH**) secretion and overgrowth of the adrenal glands.

An estimated 1% of the inhabitants of New York, of Jewish, Hispanic, Slavic and Italian origin, have '**non-classic OHD**', with defects in one of five or so enzymes of related function (Steps 2–6 in the figure 'Genetic errors of steroidogenesis in the adrenal cortex').

Other causes of ambiguous sexuality in females are maternal androgen ingestion and androgen secreting tumours. There can also be abnormal representation of SRY on the X in an XX individual, due to illegitimate crossover between the X and Y in the father.

Problems in boys

Androgen insensitivity syndrome (**testicular feminization**, or **TFM**) allows development of female external genitalia in XY individuals due to lack of the receptor for dihydrotestosterone (Step 8 in the figure 'Genetic errors of steroidogenesis in the adrenal cortex'). Classically they present with a convincing external female phenotype, but lack of onset of menstrual periods, or inguinal hernia containing a testis, which can develop malignant cancer.

Males with deficiency in **5α-reductase**, responsible for converting testosterone into dihydrotestosterone, may initially be classified as girls, but require reclassification at puberty when the deficiency is corrected by a surge of androgen from late developing testes (Step 7 in the figure 'Genetic errors of steroidogenesis in the adrenal cortex').

Other causes of ambiguous sexuality are Klinefelter syndrome (e.g. 47,XXY; see Chapter 25) and 45,X/46,XY mosaicism due to loss of the Y from a progenitor cell during embryogenesis. There can also be absence of the SRY allele from the Y due to previous illegitimate crossover between the X and Y.

One target of TDF is the **SOX 9** gene, mutation of which can cause **campomelic dysplasia**, with female phenotype development and bowing of the long bones. Production of cholesterol is deficient in **Smith–Lemli–Opitz syndrome** and involves hypovirilization of boys (see Chapter 44).

Males with 'non-classic OHD' may have hypervirilization, with increased penis size.

24 Autosomal aneuploidies

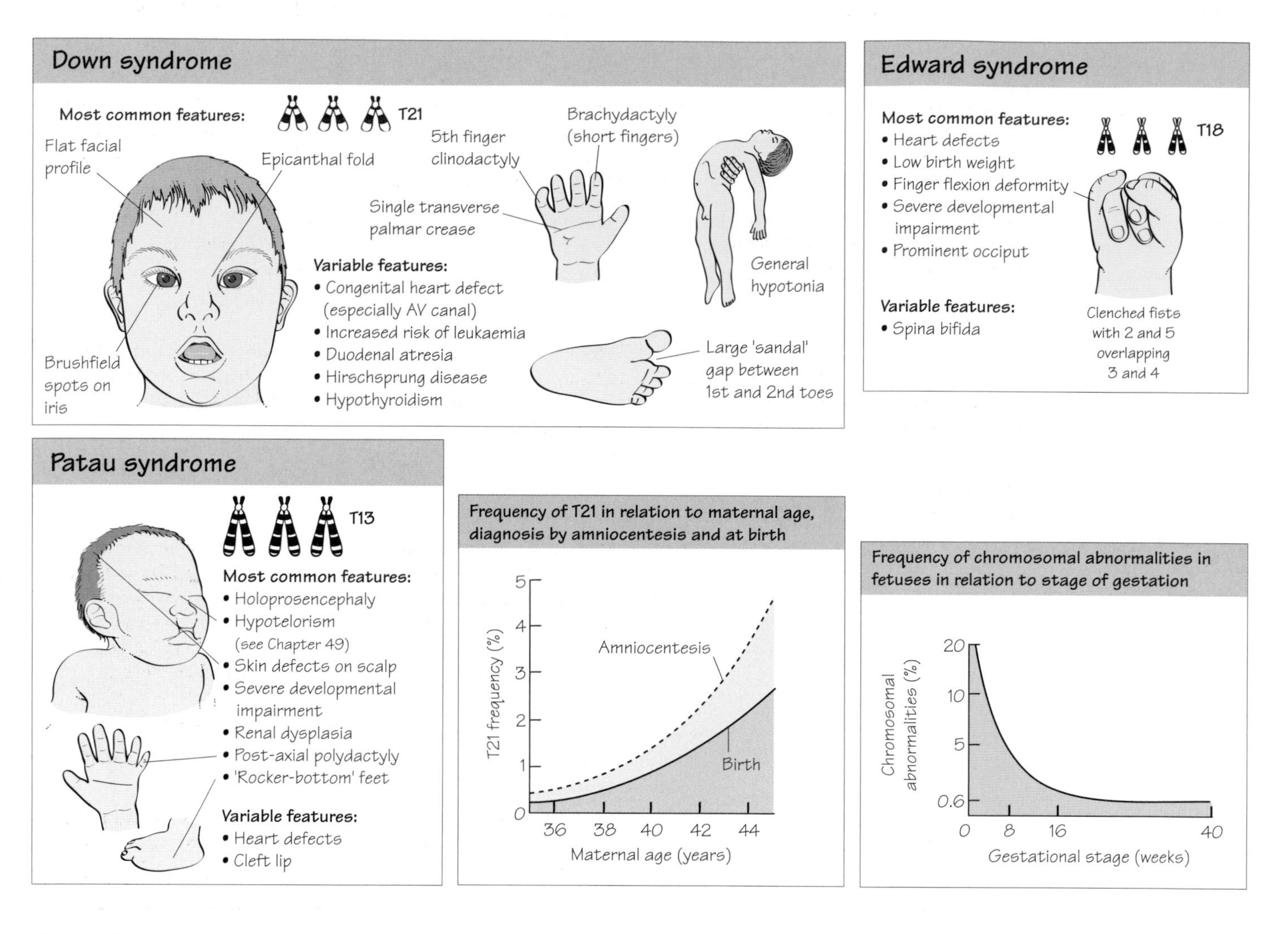

Overview

Chromosomal disorders involve both abnormal numbers of chromosomes and aberrations in their structure (see Chapter 26). **Euploidy** means that the chromosome number per body cell is an integral multiple of the haploid number, N = 23, a**neuploidy** that it is other than an integral multiple. Aneuploidy is usually ascribed to **failure of conjugation**, or **non-disjunction** (non-separation) of chromosomes in Meiosis I; or non-disjunction, **premature disjunction,** or **anaphase lag** (delayed separation) in Meiosis II.

Diploidy describes the normal situation, a typical body cell in humans having 2N = 46 chromosomes. Women have 23 similar pairs, including a pair of X chromosomes, their **karyotype** formula being **46,XX**. In normal men there is an X and a Y chromosome, their karyotype being **46,XY**. The non-sex chromosomes are called **autosomes**. **Polyploidy** refers to multiples of the haploid number (e.g. **triploidy**, 3N = 69).

Trisomy (2N + 1) is presence of three copies of one chromosome. Possession of only a single copy of an autosome (2N–1) is called **monosomy**. Autosomal monosomies are nearly always incompatible with survival.

Chromosomal abnormalities are present in at least 10% of spermatozoa and 25% of oocytes. Approximately 50% of spontaneous first trimester miscarriages have a chromosome abnormality, including probably 95% of Trisomy 13 (T13) and T18 fetuses. The most common is T16, not seen in livebirths.

Aetiology

Trisomy 21, causing **Down syndrome** (**DS**), T18, causing **Edward syndrome** (**ES**) and T13, causing **Patau syndrome** (**PS**), are the only autosomal trisomies compatible with survival to birth and all three syndromes can also be caused by translocations (see Chapter 26) or as somatic mosaics.

The majority (95% of DS and ES, 80% of PS) have complete trisomy and a severe clinical phenotype. The birth frequency of this class increases with maternal age, especially after 35 years of age. Nevertheless 75% of DS babies are born to women under 35, since most babies are born to younger mothers.

Around 4% of DS and ES and close to 20% of PS have major translocations involving the relevant chromosomes. Translocation DS almost always involves another acrocentric chromosome, i.e. 13, 14, 15, or 22; t14,21 is the most common. Translocations that lead to partial trisomy are associated with milder manifestation and longer survival.

Table 24.1 Newborn and diagnostic features of the autosomal trisomies.

	Down syndrome	Edward syndrome	Patau syndrome
Trisomic karyotype	47,XX,+21 or 47,XY,+21	47,XX,+18 or 47,XY,+18	47,XX,+13 or 47,XY,+13
Frequency	Overall corrected incidence ~1/700 (assuming 50% termination)	1/3000–1/6000 live births	1/5000–1/8000 live births
Head and face	Small, flattened head, short neck with excess nuchal skin. Face broad. Tongue without a central fissure. Low nasal root, ears small	Microcephaly, fine features, elongated skull with prominent occiput, small, low-set ears with unravelled helices and large lobes, small mouth, micrognathia	Microcephaly with sloping forehead; facial features coarse and 'pugilistic'; cleft lip and palate; micrognathia
Eyes	Eyes slanting upwards, with marked epicanthic folds; cataracts, squint and nystagmus (involuntary eye movements). Most have white speckles on the iris		Microphthalmia, anophthalmia, cyclopia or hypotelorism (closely spaced eyes)
Hands and feet	Half have a single palmar flexion crease. Limbs and fingers short, little finger in-turned, with single crease. Large 'sandal gap'. Webbing of toes 2 and 3	'Rocker bottom' feet with prominent heels; a distinctive way of clenching the fists with index and little fingers overlapping the middle ones; often a single palmar crease	'Rocker-bottom' feet; frequently a single palmar crease, post-axial polydactyly (6th finger present)
Muscle tone	Babies are always 'floppy' (hypotonic) and tend to be sleepy		
General	See text	Prenatal growth deficiency; hypotonia; major malformations of the renal and CN systems. Severe learning difficulty; most require complete care and can never walk or feed themselves	Midline malformations include failure of separation of the cerebral ventricles, and cardiac abnormalities. Frequently malformations of the CN and renal systems. Seizures common. Skills limited to those of a child of 2 years. All boys have undescended testes
Life expectancy	50–60 years	50% die in the first few weeks, 95% in the first year	50% die within the first month, 95% by 3 years
Problems requiring immediate attention	Congenital heart disease; oesophageal, anal or duodenal **atresia** (closure)	Pneumonia, **apnoea**, diaphragmatic hernia; **omphalocoele**, infection, heart defects, **spina bifida**	Special care with feeding; repair of oral/facial clefts; investigation of heart and renal systems; learning disability

Around 1–4% of patients with each syndrome show mosaic expression.

Recurrence risk for T21 is 0.5–1.0%, depending on maternal age; for translocation cases: 1–3% for male carriers; 10–15% for female.

Maternal serum screening in the second trimester detects 75–80% of DS pregnancies. This is based on 'triple' or 'quadruple testing' (see Chapter 60), followed by chromosomal analysis or FISH (see Chapter 50).

Down syndrome (DS)

Problems in infancy and childhood

Hearing deficit is a problem in 60–80% and epilepsy in 5–10%. About 20% have either an overactive or underactive thyroid gland. There is risk of obesity, sleep apnoea and skeletal problems including dislocation of cervical vertebrae.

Acute lymphocytic leukaemia accounts for 5% of deaths in childhood. Upper respiratory tract infections are common.

Congenital heart disease affects around 40% of DS babies. The most common anomalies are failure of fusion of the inter-atrial and inter-ventricular septa (AV canal) and/or retention of the (i.e. '**patent**') **ductus arteriosus**. 'Failure to thrive' is among the first signs.

There is usually significant intellectual delay, with specific deficits in speech and auditory short-term memory.

Problems in adolescence and adulthood

More than 80% of DS patients survive beyond 10 years. Average adult height is ~ 150 cm, average IQ of young adults 40–45. Males are nearly always sterile and about 40% of females fail to ovulate.

Life expectancy is reduced and there are Alzheimer-like features in half those over 40 years of age.

25 Sex chromosome aneuploidies

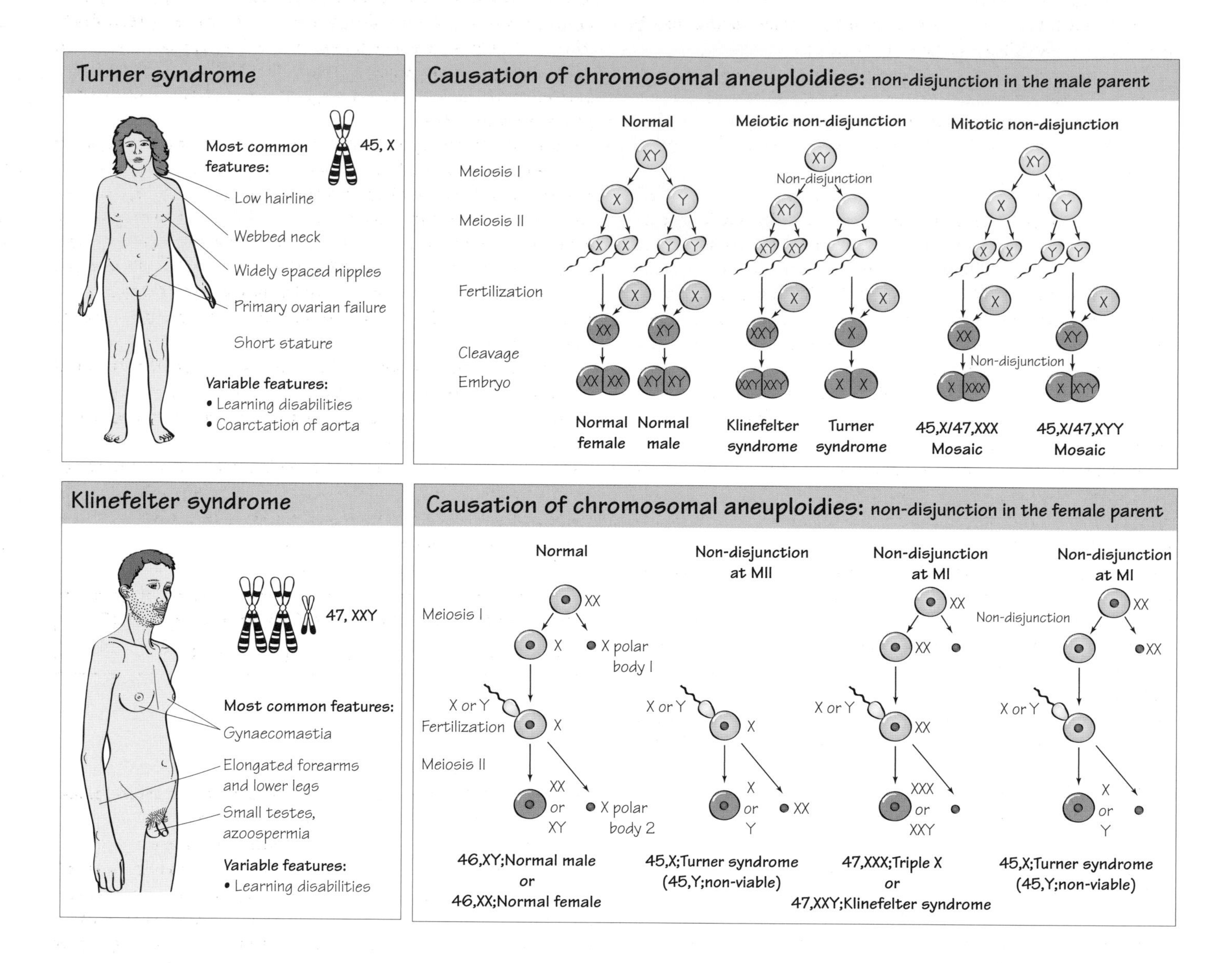

Overview

Monosomy of the X chromosome is the only whole body monosomy compatible with postnatal life, but the associated Turner syndrome demonstrates the requirement in both sexes for two active copies of the pseudoautosomal region, as well as several other X-linked genes. Monosomy X probably occurs in 1–2% of conceptions, but almost all are lost prenatally.

Karyotype formulae indicate the ***total*** number of chromosomes, together with the sex chromosome constitution.

Klinefelter syndrome

Genotype Karyotype **47,XXY**; or **48,XXXY**; **49,XXXXY**, etc.; abnormal presence of Barr bodies, one less than the number of X chromosomes (see Chapter 13).

Frequency 1/500–1/1000 male births

Life expectancy Normal, but 50% die before birth.

Body form Phenotype is basically male, tall with elongated lower legs and forearms, but with a feminine body shape and low muscle mass. There is **gynaecomastia** in one third and risk of **osteoporosis** and breast cancer.

Fertility Small, soft testes (<10 mL, 2 cm); most are sterile or produce few sperm, as a result of atrophy of the seminiferous tubules. Testicles and penis remain small; there is low libido and impotence. Blood tests show high gonadotrophin and low testosterone levels. Pubic, axillary and chest hair are sparse and daily facial shaving is rarely necessary.

IQ 10–15 points reduced, representing around 1% of men in institutions for the learning disabled.

Other features There may be **scoliosis**, **emphysema**, varicose veins and leg ulcers, diabetes mellitus in 8% and thyroid problems are common.

Aetiology Around 15% show 46,XY / 47,XXY mosaicism. Mental deficiency and physical abnormality increase with the number of supernumerary X chromosomes.

Management Klinefelter syndrome presents in childhood with clumsiness, learning difficulties, and poor verbal skills.

Testosterone therapy by long-term implants should be initiated at the beginning of puberty. Fertility has been achieved using testicular sperm aspiration and **intra-cytoplasmic sperm injection (ICSI)**.

Turner syndrome, X chromosome monosomy

Genetics Karyotype **45,X**; body cells abnormal for females in containing no Barr bodies. They can show X-linked recessive disease as in males.

Frequency 1/2000–1/3000 female births

Body form Phenotype basically female, but patients fail to mature; short stature from age of 3 years, no adolescent growth spurt. Mature height averages 145 cm (4ft 9in; 20 cm below average); shield-shaped chest with widely spaced nipples.

Head and face Heart-shaped face with micrognathia and low posterior hairline; excess skin forms a web between neck and shoulders; high arched palate with overcrowding of teeth.

Eyes High incidence of long or short sight, **strabismus**, **epicanthic folds**, **ptosis** of eyelids.

Ears Ears are low-set and posteriorly rotated, **otitis media** is frequent and can lead to conductive deafness.

Hands and feet Short fingers and toes, especially 4th metacarpals (in 50%), frail nails; increased carrying angle at elbow (**cubitus valgus**). There is often **lymphoedema** in the hands and feet of newborns.

Fertility Breasts, pubic hair and menstruation are usually absent. Ovaries may appear normal at birth, but atrophy progressively, some have borne children.

Heart Twenty per cent have heart defects, most commonly obstructive lesions of the left side (50% have a bicuspid aortic valve, 15–30% **coarctation** of the aorta) leading to hypertension in 30% and peripheral vascular problems. Life expectancy is reduced.

IQ Patients may have difficulty with specific visual–spatial coordination tasks and mathematics.

Thyroid Hypothyroidism due to lymphocytic thyroiditis.

Other features Half have structural kidney defects; there is occult aneurysm of cerebral arteries, many **naevi** (moles).

Aetiology Sixty to 80% are caused by loss of the paternal derived sex chromosome during paternal meiosis or early cell division in the embryo.

In 45,X fetuses the lymphatic system sometimes becomes obstructed, the common thoracic duct fails to empty and the posterior cervical area develops as a large, fluid-filled sack (**cystic hygroma**). Coarctation of the aorta may result from compression and the fluid imbalance may result in **hydrops** (heart failure and widespread swelling), culminating in collapse of the circulation, the primary cause of fetal death. Alternatively the cystic hygroma can recede, leaving a short neck with redundant skin, low posterior hairline and low-set ears.

Management Adolescents usually present with decreased growth or **primary amenorrhoea**.

Ultrasound scanning in the second trimester can reveal generalized oedema (**hydrops fetalis**), or swelling localized to the neck.

- ***Sexual development.*** Oestrogen administration at 12–13 years can ensure breast development, growth of pubic hair and maturation of the uterus and vaginal epithelium. Cyclic treatment with oestrogen and progesterone maintains female phenotype and prevents osteoporosis. Pregnancy can be achieved by *in vitro* fertilization with donor eggs.
- ***Short stature.*** Height can be increased by growth hormone administration.
- ***Aorta.*** Coarctation is indicated by a diminished femoral pulse, when surgical correction is recommended.
- ***Eyes.*** Optical checks and provision of spectacles, correction of strabismus.
- ***Ears.*** Regular hearing checks after otitis media bouts; treatment of 'glue ear'.
- ***Hypothyroidism.*** Thyroxine administration if necessary.
- ***Hand–eye coordination.*** Physical therapy.

Problems requiring immediate attention

- Possible heart surgery; treatment of hypothyroidism.

Table 25.1 Chromosomal errors in Turner patients.

Proportion of Turner patients (%)	Chromosomal error
50	Monosomy: 45,X
30–40	Mosaicism: mostly 45,X / 46,XX; a few 45X / 45,XY
10–20	Isochromosomes, ring chromosomes, deletions, etc.

47,XYY syndrome

Genotype Karyotype 47,XYY

Frequency 1/1000 male births; 2–3% of males institutionalized because of learning problems or anti-social criminal behaviour.

Features Very tall stature, large teeth. Fertility is normal.

IQ Ten to twenty points below controls. Minor behavioural disorders such as attention deficit, hyperactivity, learning disabilities, sometimes problems in motor coordination. They can show aggression in childhood, emotional immaturity and impulsive behaviour. A slightly higher than normal proportion become involved in criminal activity.

Triple-X syndrome

Genotype Karyotype, **47,XXX** (and **48,XXXX**, **49,XXXXX**, etc.); each body cell contains one fewer Barr bodies than the number of X chromosomes.

Frequency 1/1000–1/1500 female births

Features Generally tall with slender body shape. They have a mild reduction in intellectual skills and sometimes 'oppositional behaviour' and difficulty in interpersonal relationships. Abnormalities are in proportion to the number of X chromosomes they possess. The additional X is of maternal origin in 95% of cases.

Twenty five percent are infertile, sometimes ascribed to 45,X oocytes in 45,X / 47,XXX mosaics.

26 Chromosome structural abnormalities

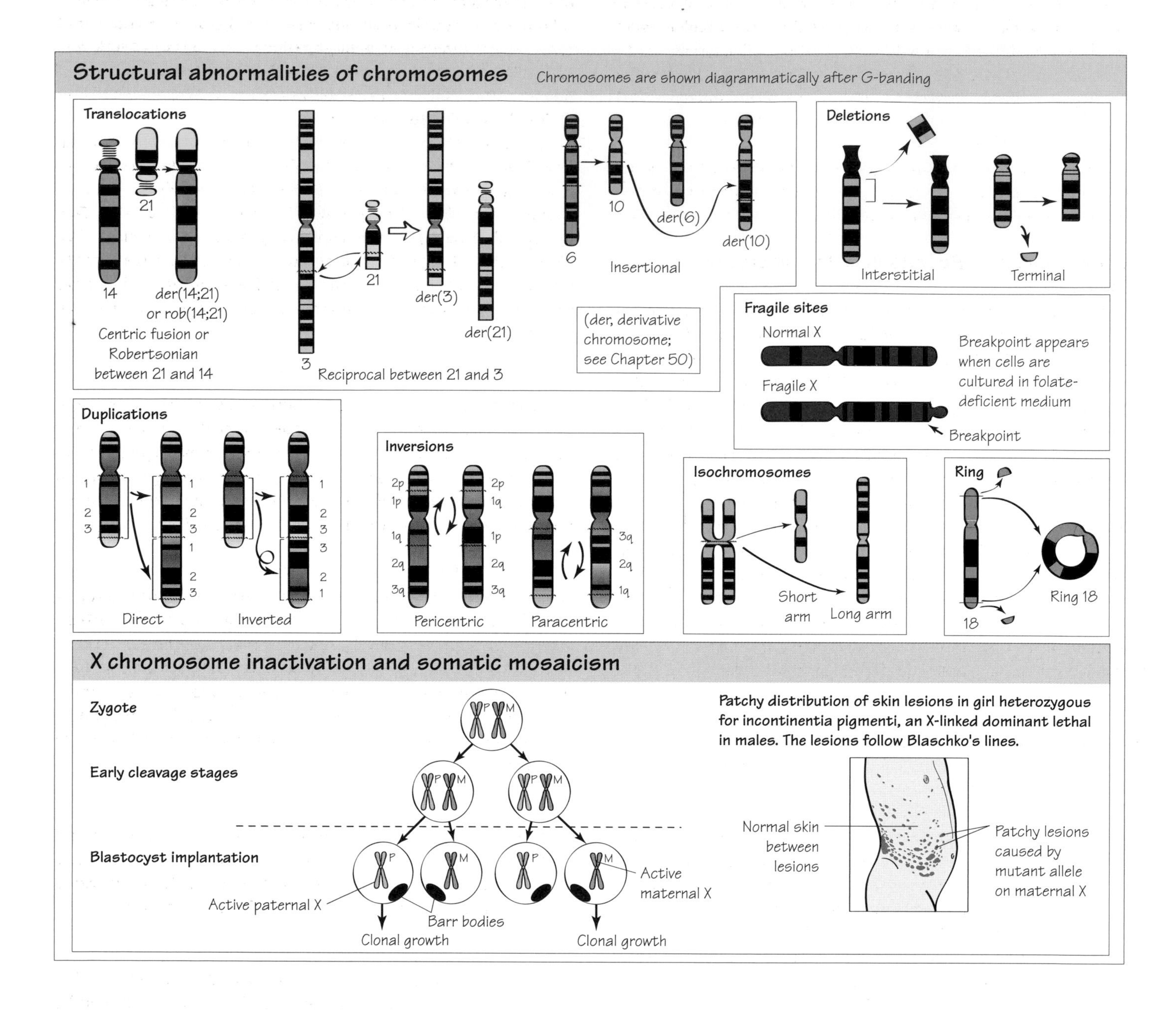

Overview

Chromosome abnormalities are a principal cause of pregnancy loss, an estimated 10–15% of conceptions having a chromosome abnormality of which 95% are lost before term. Close to 90% of the abnormalities are aneuploidies, the remainder being chromosome structural abnormalities. Around two-thirds of the structural abnormalities arise in oocytes, one-third in sperm, the latter increasing with paternal age.

Structural aberrations include **translocations**, **deletions**, **ring chromosomes**, **duplications**, **inversions**, **isochromosomes**, **centric fragments** and **fragile sites**. Most of these result from unequal exchange between homologous repeated sequences on the same or different chromosomes, or when two chromosome breaks occur close together and enzymic repair mechanisms link the wrong ends.

Somatic mosaicism

Mosaicism refers to the existence in the body of more than one genetically distinct cell line following a single fertilization event (c.f. **chimaerism**, in which different cell lines result from multiple fertilizations). Both yield incidence patterns that depart from general rules.

If an abnormal birth occurs in a family with no previous history of that disorder, it could be caused by a new mutation in a single germ cell, in which case the risk of recurrence would be negligible. If the mutation occurs throughout a mosaic patch of tissue that includes germ cells, the recurrence rate is usually estimated as around 1% or up to 6% for highly mutable genes such as **osteogenesis imperfecta** and **Duchenne muscular dystrophy** (see Chapter 21).

X chromosome inactivation (see Chapter 13) creates a mosaic for expression of the two X chromosomes in normal women, which in heterozygotes can allow pathological expression of X-linked recessive alleles. For example, a woman heterozygous for recessive colour blindness is colour blind if the normal X is inactivated in all her photoreceptor cones (see Chapter 22). Her genetic status as a heterozygote would be revealed, however, if she produced both normal and colour-blind sons.

Translocations

A translocation involves transposition of chromosome material usually between chromosomes. Three types are recognized: **centric fusion** or '**Robertsonian**', **reciprocal** and **insertional**.

Centric fusion or 'Robertsonian translocations' (code: 'rob')

Centric fusion arises from breaks at or near the centromeres of two chromosomes, followed by their fusion. The long arms of Chromosomes 13, 14, 15, 21 and 22 only are involved, especially 13 with 14 (rob13;14), and 14 with 21 (rob 14;21). These are all **acrocentric** chromosomes with very small short arms (see Chapter 50), the latter carrying multiple copies of the ribosomal RNA genes (see Chapter 6). Their tendency to undergo centric fusion possibly relates to their joint contribution to the function of the nucleolus (see Chapter 2).

Although centric fusion involves loss of rRNA genes sufficient intact copies remain on other chromosomes for no serious consequence to result. The carrier of a pair of centrically fused chromosomes may therefore have only 45 chromosomes, but be quite healthy as the overall loss is insignificant. This is a **balanced translocation**. However, such balanced translocation carriers run into problems at meiosis, with the result that a woman could have many miscarriages and individuals of either sex can have offspring with effective T21 and Down syndrome (see Chapter 27).

Reciprocal translocations (code: 't')

Reciprocal translocation involves inter-chromosomal exchange. Either arm of any chromosome can be involved and carriers are usually healthy. The medical significance is therefore usually for *future* generations, as carriers can produce chromosomally unbalanced fetuses.

X-linked recessive disease can arise in heterozygous females as a consequence of X-autosome translocation. For example, the reciprocal translocation between chromosomes X and 1, formulated as 46,X,t(X;1)(p21;q31) (see Chapter 50) interferes with X inactivation, as the translocation breakpoint occurs between that gene and the inactivation centre.

Reciprocal translocation can also activate genes in cancer (see Chapters 27, 41).

Insertional translocations (code: 'ins')

Insertional translocation involves insertion of a deleted segment interstitially at another location. It is extremely rare and balanced carriers are usually healthy, but may produce chromosomally unbalanced offspring with either a duplication or a deletion.

Deletions (code: 'del')

Deletion of part of a chromosome can be **interstitial** or **terminal**. Interstitial deletions can arise from two breaks, followed by faulty repair, from unequal crossing-over in a previous meiosis, or as a consequence of a translocation in a parent. The error is described using the code 'del' followed by a description of the missing region in a separate set of brackets. For example, DiGeorge syndrome, caused by a deletion at 22q11.22, is formulated: del(22)(q11.22). A terminal deletion of the long arm of Chromosome 1 from band 21 would be formulated: 46,XX,del(1)(q21;qter) (see Chapter 50).

The smallest deletions detectable by **high resolution banding** (see Chapter 50) are of about 3 megabases (i.e. 3 million base pairs). Since a gene may be as short as 1 kb (1000 bases), visible deletions tend to indicate loss of many genes. They are generally characterized by mental handicap and multiple congenital malformations (see Chapter 28). Several syndromes are ascribed to microscopically invisible **microdeletions** and when several genes are deleted together the term **contiguous gene syndrome** is applied to the corresponding phenotype.

Ring chromosomes (code: 'r')

If two breaks occur in the same chromosome the broken ends can fuse as a ring. Acentric rings are lost, but if the ring contains a centromere it can survive subsequent cell division. Clinically a ring represents two deletions. They can double by sister chromatid exchange, leading to effective trisomy, or be lost, resulting in monosomy. They are sometimes associated with growth failure and mental handicap.

Duplications (code: 'dup')

Duplication is the presence of two adjacent copies of a chromosomal segment and can be either '**direct**' (or '**tandem**'), or '**inverted**'. Duplications may originate by unequal crossing-over in a previous meiosis, or as a consequence of translocation, inversion, or presence of an isochromosome (see below) in a parent. Duplications are more common, but generally less harmful than deletions. An example is **cat eye syndrome** involving **iris coloboma** formulated: dup(22)(p13;q11).

Inversions (code: 'inv')

Inversions arise from two chromosomal breaks with end-to-end switching of the intervening segment. If this includes the centromere it is **pericentric**, if not, the inversion is **paracentric**. They can lead to chromosomally unbalanced gametes following crossing-over.

Isochromes (code: 'iso')

An isochromosome has one chromosome arm deleted and the other duplicated. In live births the commonest involves the long arm of the X, resulting in Turner syndrome due to short arm monosomy. Most cause spontaneous abortion.

Fragile sites (code: 'fra')

A fragile site is an apparent gap in a chromosome. Some are common (or 'universal'), others are rare and sensitive to folate levels in the medium in which the cells under examination are cultured. These are inherited in a Mendelian fashion, a well known example being the defect associated with fragile X syndrome (see Chapter 22).

27 Chromosome structural abnormalities, clinical examples

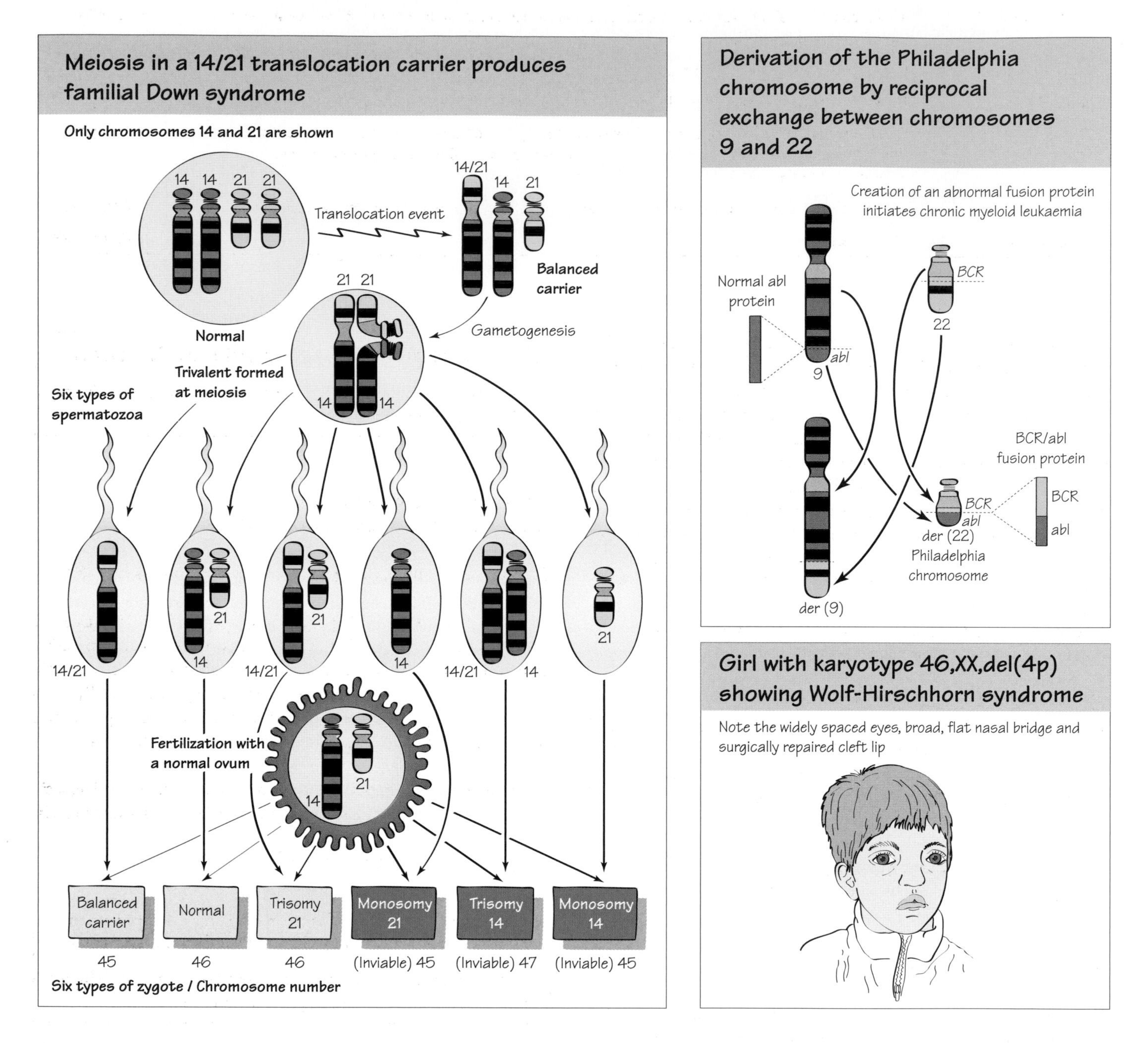

Overview

Congenital abnormalities are increasingly being ascribed to very small deletions rendered visible by applications such as **fluorescence *in situ* hybridization (FISH)** (see Chapter 50). Even smaller 'microdeletions' are detectable by **array comparative genome hybridization (CGH)** and pathological microduplications are now also recognized. Loss of several closely adjacent genes can result in a **contiguous gene syndrome**, such as **WAGR** and **DiGeorge syndrome**. In such cases the contiguous gene series is usually flanked by identical series of repeats that promote unequal crossover and variable deletion.

Although chromosomal syndromes are typically quite variable, several generalizations are nevertheless possible:

- Most chromosomal abnormalities are associated with developmental delay in childhood and mental retardation in teenagers and adults.
- Most produce characteristic facial appearances.
- Most are associated with retardation in growth.
- Many include congenital malformation of the heart.

See Chapter 49 for explanation of dysmorphic terms.

Translocations

Translocation Down syndrome

About 4% of Down syndrome cases involve a Robertsonian translocation between the long arm of Chromosome 21 and another acrocentric, usually 14 (see Chapter 26).

Table 27.1 Additional microdeletion syndromes.

Syndrome	Clinical features	Karyotype
'1p36 syndrome'	Microcephaly, straight eyebrows, sunken eyes, midface hypoplasia; hypotonia, growth delay, severe learning difficulties, epilepsy	del(1)(p36)
Langer–Giedion	Characteristic facies, sparse hair, bone overgrowth, mental retardation	del(8)(q24.11)
Miller–Dieker	Characteristic facies, **lissencephaly** (smooth brain surface)	del(17)(p13.3)
Rubinstein–Taybi	Broad thumbs and great toes, large convex nose, long eyelashes, strabismus, vertebral and sternal abnormalities, pulmonary stenosis, microcephaly, mental retardation, developmental delay, undescended testes	del(16)(p13.3)
Alagille	Characteristic facies, neonatal jaundice, 'butterfly' vertebrae, pulmonary valvular stenosis	del(20)(p12)
Azoospermia	Male infertility	del(Y)(q11.23)

Consider an individual defined as 45,XX,der(14;21)(q10;q10). This woman lacks one normal 14 and one normal 21 and instead has a chromosome derived by reciprocal translocation between the entire long arms of 14 and 21. Since there is little genetic information in either short arm her phenotype is normal. However, during meiosis the abnormal derivative chromosome may segregate in either of several ways to yield an ovum which, if fertilized by a normal sperm, could create a fetus with either translocation Down syndrome, with effective T21, monosomy 21 (M21); effective T14, or M14. Embryos with the latter three karyotypes fail to survive to term, but additional prenatal losses reduce the frequency of live born Down syndrome babies to 10–15%. The equivalent figure for fathers with the balanced 14;21 translocation is 1–2%.

By comparison, the recurrence risk for a Down syndrome pregnancy with a karyotypically normal woman under 30 years is around 1%.

The Philadelphia chromosome

The 'Philadelphia chromosome' is a derivative of Chromosomes 22 and 9, created by reciprocal translocation. The modified 22 carries the coding for an abnormal 'fusion protein' with increased enzymic activity that initiates chronic myeloid leukaemia (see Chapter 41).

Deletions and microdeletions

Cri-du-chat; Lejeune syndrome

Frequency 1/20 000–1/50 000; possibly 1% of profoundly learning disabled.

Genetics 46,XX,del(5)(p15.2)

Features The newborn baby has a low birthweight and makes a distinctive cry similar to that of a kitten (French: '*cri du chat*': 'cry of the cat'), due to underdevelopment of the larynx. Typically there are microcephaly, hypertelorism, epicanthic folds, divergent strabismus, low-set ears, hypotonia, severe breathing problems and often failure to thrive. Patent ductus arteriosus is present in 30%. The face is round in children, elongated in adults; severe mental retardation (IQ ~35).

Management Antenatal diagnosis is possible by chorionic villus sampling at 10–12 weeks, or amniocentesis at 16 weeks. A structured exercise regime is recommended, plus verbal stimulation and correction of squints.

Lifespan Survival into adulthood sometimes occurs.

Problems requiring immediate attention

- Surgical correction of congenital heart disease; severe respiratory and feeding difficulties.

Wolf–Hirschhorn syndrome

Frequency 1/50 000; male : female ratio 3 : 4.

Genetics e.g. 46,XY,del(4)(p16.1); balanced translocation in 10%.

Features Microcephaly, hypertelorism, epicanthic folds; lack of indentation of the nasal bridge is described as resembling the protective nosepiece of an ancient Greek helmet. Hypotonic at birth and muscle tone remains poor; cleft lip with or without cleft palate (CL ± P); low-set ears, short upper lip, heart defects, convulsions, hypospadias and undescended testes, severe learning difficulties, failure to thrive.

Management Developmental checks are necessary; antenatal diagnosis is possible by chorionic villus sampling at 10–12 weeks (see Chapter 53).

Lifespan Sometimes into the teens.

Problems requiring immediate attention

- Nasogastric feeding; heart surgery; correction of facial clefts and hypospadias; selection of appropriate anticonvulsant.

Prader–Willi (P-WS) and Angelman (AS) syndromes (see also Chapter 21)

Frequency 1/25 000

Genetics Seventy per cent have the deletion or microdeletion del(15)(q11-12), others have uniparental isodisomy, or mutation of a neighbouring gene or imprinting centre.

Aetiology If the deletion occurs *de novo* on the *paternal* 15 this leads to P-WS; if the *maternal*, to AS. Most non-deletion cases of P-WS are caused by uniparental isodisomy with both maternal chromosomes 15.

Non-deletion cases of AS are due to uniparental disomy of both paternal chromosomes 15 or mutation in the gene UBE3A.

WAGR syndrome (Wilms tumour, Aniridia, Genitourinary abnormalities and mental Retardation)

Frequency 1/10 000

Genetics Contiguous gene deletion del(11)(p13).

Features Embryonal renal tumours (Wilms tumour), gonadal tumours, failure of iris development in each eye, general retardation of growth and development.

Aetiology Loss of gene PAX6 is responsible for aniridia; loss of WT1 causes Wilms tumour (see Chapter 41).

Management A WT1 DNA probe can be used for antenatal diagnosis.

Williams syndrome; infantile hypercalcaemia

Frequency 1/10,000

Genetics Microdeletion del(7)(q11.23); possibly inherited as AD.

Features Broad forehead, short palpebral fissures, tip-tilted nose with low bridge and outward facing nostrils, long philtrum, full cheeks, large mouth with full lips; excessive vomiting; sleeplessness; slow growth rate. Children have a 'cocktail party manner', with outgoing attitude, hyperactivity and advanced facility in language, but become withdrawn as adults and sensitive especially to loud noise. There are mental retardation, supravalvular aortic stenosis (SVAS), multiple peripheral pulmonary arterial stenoses, dental malformations and short stature, with sloping shoulders.

Aetiology Deletion of elastase locus and contiguous genes.

Management Dietetic advice, energetic play. Mental retardation prevents independency. May be dignosed prenatally by FISH (see Chapter 50).

Problems requiring immediate attention

- Special care with feeding; regulation of serum calcium; possible cardiac surgery.

DiGeorge or Velocardiofacial syndrome (VCFS)

Frequency 1/4000 live births; one of the commonest microdeletion syndromes.

Genetics Three megabases (3 million base pairs) deletion: del(22)(q11.2), sometimes related to unbalanced translocation of 22q; can be inherited as AD.

Features Recognizable facial appearance with micrognathia and congenital short or cleft palate; thymic hypoplasia causing T-cell deficiency and parathyroid hypoplasia depressing serum calcium levels; heart malformations particularly of the cardiac outflow tract. About half have partial growth hormone deficiency and 40% of adults have schizophrenia-like episodes.

Aetiology Deletion of multiple contiguous genes with primary effect on migration of neural crest cells to the cervical region (see Chapters 12, 43)

Lifespan Many die in the 1st year.

Management Investigation for cardiac abnormality, calcium and parathyroid status and renal anomalies, prevention of infection.

Problems requiring immediate attention

- Surgery of cardiac abnormality and cleft palate; serum calcium and growth hormone regulation.

Smith–Magenis syndrome

Frequency Rare, affecting more girls than boys.

Genetics del(17)(p11.2)

Features Small head, mid-face hypoplasia, small nose; ears low-set and of unusual shape. Initially delayed growth, but excessive weight gain in older children, despite unexceptional appetite (c.f. P-WS; see Chapter 21). Seizures, learning difficulties and speech delay. Most often recognized by aggressive or hyperactive, self-harming behaviour, persistent disturbed sleep and characteristic 'self-hugging'. Congenital heart disease in a third, scoliosis develops in late childhood in more than half, middle ear infections and hearing impairment in two-thirds.

Aetiology Contiguous gene deletion.

Management Speech and hearing therapy; dietetic advice.

Problems requiring immediate attention

- Cardiac surgery; treatment of ear infection; use of melatonin to control sleep pattern.

Sotos syndrome, cerebral gigantism

Frequency Rare

Genetics Mutations in NSD1 gene on chromosome 5q35.

Features Large head with prominent forehead, hypertelorism with outwardly down-slanting palpebral fissures, characteristic nose in childhood and prominent chin. Usually high birthweight, hypotonia, feeding difficulties, often motor delay and ataxia. Cerebral ventricles may appear dilated on MRI or CT scan. Children are tall with long arms, large hands and feet, and advanced bone age.

Management Psychological problems related to stature. Scoliosis can develop in adolescence.

28 Congenital abnormalities, pre-embryonic, embryonic and of intrinsic causation

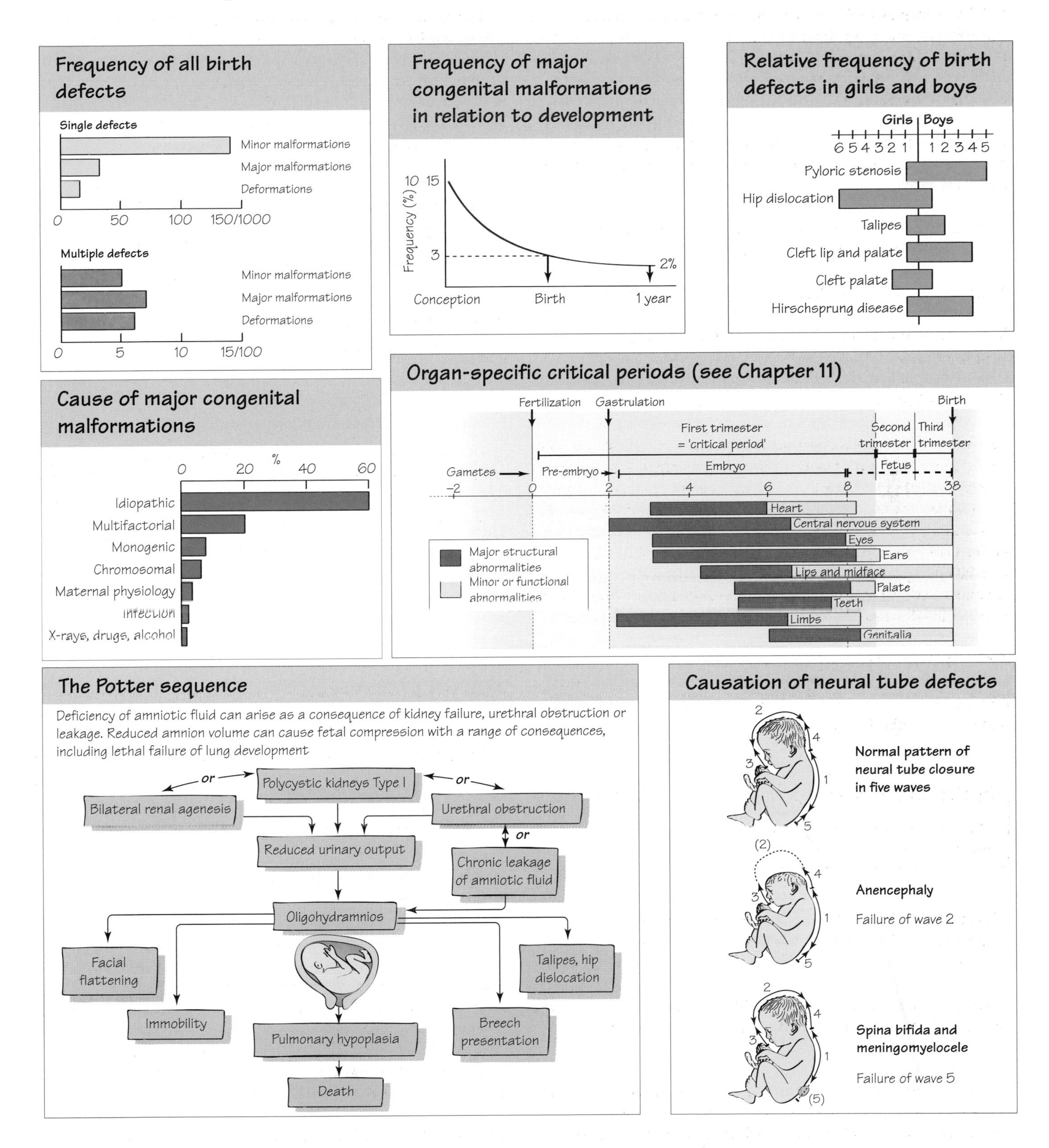

Overview

The word '**congenital**' means 'existing at birth' and includes all 'birth defects' regardless of causation. Congenital abnormalities are apparent in 1/40 newborn babies and account for 20–25% of infant deaths. At birth 0.7% of babies have *multiple major* abnormalities, 2–3% a *single major* defect and 14% a *single minor* defect (Table 52.1). Probably 15–25% of congenital abnormalities have a recognized genetic, 10% an environmental and 20–25% a multifactorial basis. Twinning accounts for 0.5–1.0% (see Chapter 33) and 40–60% are **idiopathic**, i.e. of unknown causation.

For medico-legal purposes malformations are regarded as 'congenital' only if recognized within the first 2 weeks after birth.

Classification of defects

Single abnormalities

1 **Malformations** are due to errors occurring in the initial formation of structures, e.g. cleft lip with or without palate (CL ± P), polydactyly; most are multifactorial (see Chapters 31 and 32).

2 **Disruptions** are due to disturbances after an organ has been formed, e.g. **phocomelia** resulting from a vascular problem.

3 **Deformations** are mechanical distortions, e.g. clubfoot (**talipes**). They frequently resolve completely soon after birth.

4 **Dysplasias** are abnormalities in tissue organization, e.g. in the differentiation of blood cells from vessels; most are monogenic.

Multiple abnormalities

1 **Sequences** are cascades of effects, e.g. **Pierre–Robin sequence**, in which a primary defect in mandibular development produces secondary **glossoptosis** (drooping tongue) and cleft palate.

2 **Syndromes** are groups of anomalies that consistently occur together due to a single underlying cause, e.g. Down syndrome due to trisomy 21.

3 **Associations** are where traits coincide more often than expected by chance.

The overall frequency of **multiple malformations** is 7/1000, the most frequently diagnosed being Beckwith–Wiedeman (see Chapter 21), DiGeorge, Noonan and Williams syndromes (see Chapter 27, **CHARGE** syndrome and **VATER** associations).

Noonan syndrome

Frequency 1/2000 births.

Genetics Defect in tyrosine phosphatase, non-receptor-type 11 (PTPN 11) at 12q22 in most but not all patients.

Features Similar to Turner syndrome (Chapter 25), but affecting both sexes: short stature, neck webbing, increased carrying angle at the elbow, also learning difficulties, hypertelorism, down-slanting palpebral fissures, low-set ears and congenital heart disease. Pulmonary stenosis is the most common heart lesion, but there are also aventricular (ASD) and ventricular septal defect (VSD) and hypertrophic cardiomyopathy (see below). Some have bleeding problems and a quarter have chest deformity.

CHARGE syndrome

CHARGE involves the co-occurrence of **C**oloboma, **H**eart defects, cho**A**nal atresia, **R**etarded growth, **G**enital abnormalities and abnormal **E**ars. Mutation in either CHD 7 or SEMA3E genes.

VATER/VACTERL association

VATER involves **V**ertebral defects, **A**nal atresia, **T**racheo-o**E**sophageal fistula (i.e. abnormal fusion) and **R**enal defects. **VACTERL** also includes **C**ardiac and **L**imb defects.

Timing and aetiology

Pre-embryo

Damage to the pre-embryo generally results in spontaneous abortion or regulative repair, so few errors in newborns are ascribable to pre-implantation damage. The following are exceptions:

1 **Monozygotic twinning** (see Chapter 33).

2 **Germ layer defects**, e.g. **ectodermal dysplasia** affecting skin, nails, hair, teeth and stature.

Embryo

The **first trimester**, especially between weeks 2 and 8, is the **critical period**. The palate and lips, eyes, ears, brain, neural tube and heart are all particularly susceptible at this stage and the CNS, eyes, lips and mid-face, teeth and genitalia remain especially vulnerable throughout gestation.

The following errors are most important during the first trimester:

1 **Failure of cell migration**, e.g. neural crest cells; DiGeorge syndrome.

2 **Failure of embryonic induction**, e.g. **anophthalmia**.

3 **Failure of tube closure**, e.g. the **neural tube defects** (see Chapter 31).

4 **Developmental arrest**, e.g. **cleft lip** (see Chapter 30).

5 **Failure of tissue fusion**, e.g. **cleft palate** (see Chapter 31).

6 **Defective morphogenetic fields**, e.g. **sirenomelia**.

The foundations of **consequent disturbances** are laid at this stage, e.g. the **Potter sequence**.

The Potter/oligohydramnios sequence

Babies are sometimes born with the combination of squashed facial features, severe talipes, dislocated hips, growth deficiency and lethal pulmonary hypoplasia. Such babies typically adopted breech presentation. The features arise from the 'Potter sequence', involving prolonged deficiency of amniotic fluid, called **oligohydramnios**.

Oligohydramnios develops due to defective urinary output by the baby, or chronic leakage. This leads to fetal compression and immobility, with the consequences described. The primary causes of reduced urinary output are bilateral **renal agenesis** (1/3000 births), **polycystic kidney disease type 1** and obstruction of the urethra. The recurrence risk for subsequent pregnancies is 1/33.

Renal agenesis classes as a *malformation*, which through oligohydramnios causes secondary *deformations*, the combination constituting a *syndrome* and the series of events, a *sequence*.

Defects of the CNS

Neural tube defects (NTDs)

NTDs arise from failure of closure of the neural tube at the end of Week 3 (see Chapter 11). An anterior defect results in either **anencephaly** or **encephalocele** (absence or protrusion of the brain). A posterior defect can lead to lumbosacral **myelocele** or **meningomyelocele** (protruding spinal cord exposed, or covered by meninges), **spina bifida** and leg deformity (see Chapter 31).

Holoprosencephaly

Holoprosencephaly is failure of cleavage of the embryonic forebrain, resulting in severe mental impairment and abnormal facies, in severe cases cyclopia. Survival is usually less than 1 month.

It can be associated with Triploidy 13 (see Chapter 24) and Smith–Lemli–Opitz syndromes (see Table 18.1), maternal diabetes mellitus (see Chapter 29) and several deletions and mutatations in various genes.

Isolated hydrocephalus

This is enlargement of the brain ventricles without NTD. It can arise from intracranial haemorrhage, infection or genetic defect, or be idiopathic.

Management involves insertion of a cerebrospinal fluid (CSF) drain, usually to the peritoneum.

Prenatal diagnosis is by serial ultrasound in the second trimester.

Lissencephaly (smooth brain)

This is caused by defective neuronal migration at 3–5 months. It can be associated with epilepsy and mental retardation and is a feature of Miller–Dieker syndrome and other disorders (see Chapter 27). As an isolated condition it has an empiric recurrence risk of 10% (see Chapter 48).

Macrocephaly and microcephaly

These terms apply to head circumferences greater than the 97th and less than the 3rd percentile (see Chapter 49). **Microcephaly vera** (i.e. without other abnormalities) is usually AR, but there is a variety of causes of each.

Congenital heart defects

Heart development occurs at 3–8 weeks and developmental defects occur in 7/1000 live births. Congenital heart defects can result in inadequate oxygenation of blood and/or poor perfusion of tissues (see Chapter 31).

Gastro-intestinal (GI) tract defects

Oesophageal atresia

This arises from an error in the formation of the oesophagus and can lead to **polyhydramnios** (excessive amniotic fluid because of failure to swallow). There may be associated tracheo-oesophageal fistulae. It occurs in 1/2500 live births, is multifactorial, associated with tetralogy of Fallot, ano-rectal agenesis and NTD and requires urgent surgical correction.

Pyloric stenosis

See Chapters 29 and 30.

Duodenal atresia

At Week 7 the midgut is solid; **duodenal atresia** occurs when the lumen fails to open. The frequency is 1/330, 35% of cases being associated with T21.

Surgical correction is required urgently.

Hirschsprung disease (HSCR); congenital intestinal aganglionosis

This is a defect in peristaltic activity of the hindgut, due to failure of migration of neural crest cells (see Chapter 12). Typically there is no passage of meconium in the first 48 hours. The frequency is 1/5000 live births, (3 ♂ : 1 ♀). Inheritance is due to mutation in single genes or may be multifactorial. The recurrence risk is 3–4% in the absence of monogenic causation. Management requires surgical removal of affected tissue.

Imperforate anus

This has a frequency of 1/5000. It is multifactorially inherited and corrective surgery is urgent.

29 Congenital abnormalities arising at the fetal stage

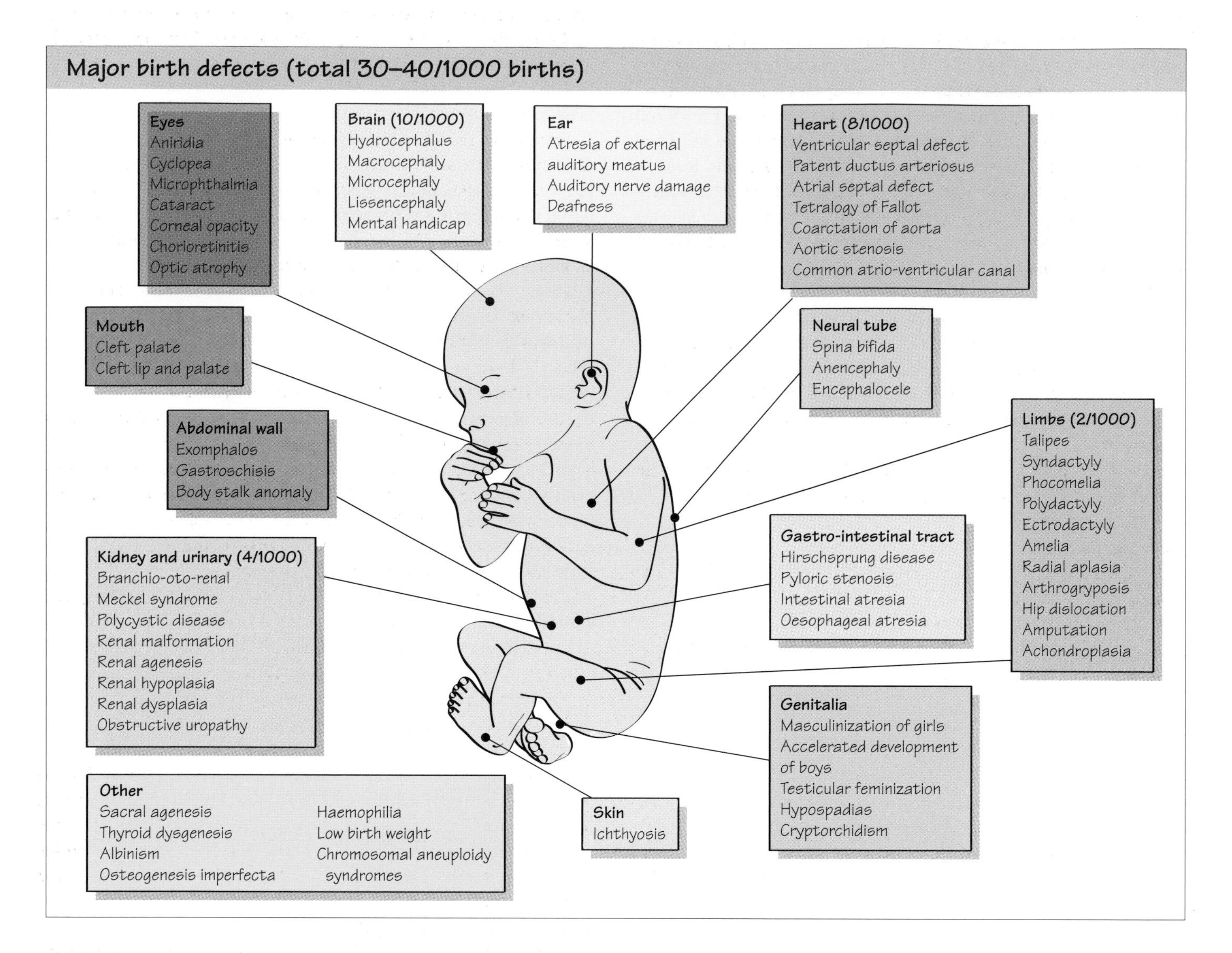

Overview

The 'embryonic' period ends at about 9 weeks, when the rudiments of all the major organs have been formed. In the subsequent 'fetal' period the main processes are growth and morphogenesis and there is extensive **programmed cell death**, or **apoptosis**.

Partial chromosomal duplication or deficiency may cause postnatal **neurodevelopmental delay**, pre- or postnatal **growth delay**, **dysmorphism** or death. The aetiology of two-thirds of congenital defects is unknown or multifactorial, but a genetic component is suspected in about a third. Other pathogenic influences include abnormal maternal physiology and infection, exposure to medicines and non-prescription drugs, environmental chemicals and external physical influences. Extrinsic agents, especially chemicals, that cause birth defects are called **teratogens**.

The practical application of **dysmorphology** is outlined in Chapter 49. For genital defects, see Chapters 13 and 23.

Pathogenic mechanisms

1 **Absence of normal apoptosis**, e.g. finger webbing.
2 **Disturbances in tissue resorption**, e.g. **anal atresia**.
3 **Failure of organ movement**, e.g. **cryptorchidism** .
4 **Destruction of formed structures**, e.g. **phocomelia** due to interference in blood supply.
5 **Hypoplasia** (reduced proliferation), e.g. **achondroplasia** (see Chapter 16).
6 **Hyperplasia** (enhanced proliferation), e.g. **macrosomia**.
7 **Constriction by amniotic bands** (strands of broken amnion), e.g. limb amputation.
8 **Restriction of movement**, e.g. talipes.

Maternal illness

Diabetes mellitus (see Chapter 32)

High maternal blood glucose levels in early pregnancy due to Type 1 diabetes mellitus is associated with a 2–3 fold increase in congenital abnormalities, including heart disease, neural tube defects, sacral agenesis, femoral hypoplasia, holoprosencephaly and **sirenomelia**. The causative influence is high maternal blood glucose levels in early pregnancy.

Phenylketonuria (see Chapter 19)

Uncorrected high maternal blood levels of phenylalanine can cause severe mental retardation, microcephaly and congenital heart disease.

Epilepsy

There is a 2–4 times increased incidence (to 5–10%) of birth defects in babies exposed prenatally to anti-epileptic drugs, and the number increases if more than one drug is used. They include NTDs (in about 10%), oral clefting, genitourinary abnormalities, and heart and limb defects. Learning difficulties and behaviour problems are increased. Sodium valproate exposure is associated with the highest incidence, NTDs and characteristic facies. The recommended maternal medication is single drug treatment avoiding sodium valproate.

Other predisposing conditions are **systemic lupus erythematosis** and **Graves disease** (see Chapter 43).

Maternal infection

Microorganisms that cause multiple malformations are summarized by the acronym, **TORCH**, for *Toxoplasma*, **O**ther (e.g. syphilis, *Treponema pallidum*), ***R**ubella*, ***C**ytomegalovirus* and ***H**erpes varicella zoster* (chickenpox). The most important are *Toxoplasma*, *Rubella* and *Cytomegalovirus*.

Toxoplasmosis

Maternal infection with the Protozoan, *Toxoplasma gondii*, confers a 20% risk to the fetus during the first trimester, rising to 75% in the second and third trimesters.

Rubella (German measles)

Rubella virus causes cardiovascular malformations in 15–20% of all babies infected in the first trimester.

Cytomegalovirus (CMV)

Risk is greatest if infection occurs during the first trimester. About 5% of infected pregnancies result in fetal damage.

Congenital deformations

Congenital dislocation of the hip

Incidence is 1/1000 (6 ♀ : 1 ♂). It is multifactorial, positively associated with breech birth and neuromuscular disorder and commonest in populations in which babies are swaddled.

Talipes equinovarus (club foot)

The feet are **plantar-flexed** and inverted (i.e. soles facing inwards). The incidence is 1/1000 live births; (3 ♂ : 1 ♀) (see Table 31.2).

Amputations

In 1/5000 live births there is limb amputation due to constriction by 'amniotic bands' formed by premature rupture of the amnion. It is frequently associated with oligohydramnios (see Chapter 28).

Congenital myotonic dystrophy

This can occur in association with hypotonia, respiratory insufficiency, mental retardation and can be lethal (see also Chapter 21).

Anterior abdominal wall defect

The overall incidence is 1/6000 live pregnancies.

- **Omphalocele** is a persistent midgut hernia into the umbilical cord; associated with T13 (30%) and congenital heart disease (10%).
- **Gastroschisis** is extrusion of the bowel through the abdominal wall.

Pyloric stenosis

Hypertrophy and hyperplasia of the pyloric sphincter muscles lead to projectile vomiting, constipation and dehydration in early infancy (see Chapter 30).

Limb malformations

Overall frequency: 2/1000.

Polydactyly is a feature of many syndromes, including T13, but can be inherited as AD or be of unknown aetiology.

Arthrogryposis is a heterogeneous group of malformations characterized by stiffness and contracture of the knee, elbow and/or wrist joints and often dislocation of the hips. They are classified as: myopathic; neuropathic; affecting connective tissue; restricting fetal movement.

The role of chemicals

Teratogenesis accords with the following principles.

1 Susceptibility may depend on the genotype of the zygote.
2 Maternal genotype affects drug metabolism, resistance to infection.
3 Susceptibility depends on developmental stage at time of exposure.
4 Severity of defect depends on dose and duration of exposure.
5 Individual teratogens have specific modes of action.
6 Abnormality is expressed as malformation, growth retardation, functional disorder or death.

Teratogenic medicines

These include:

- **Abortifacients**, e.g. the folic acid antagonist ***aminopterin***.
- **Anti-abortifacients**, e.g. ***diethylstibestrol*** causing malformations of reproductive systems.
- **Androgens** can cause masculinization of female external genitalia.
- **Anticonvulsants** used by epileptics; ***valproate*** (see above), ***trimethadone***, ***diphenylhydantoin***, ***phenytoin***, ***carbamazepine***.
- **Sedatives and tranquilizers: *thalidomide, lithium*.**
- **Anticancer drugs: *methotrexate, aminopterin*.**
- **Antibiotics**: ***streptomycin*** can cause inner ear deafness; ***tetracycline*** inhibits skeletal calcification.
- **Anticoagulants: *warfarin, dicumarol*.**
- **Antihypertensive agents*: ACE inhibitors*.**
- **Antithyroid drugs**.
- **Vitamin A analogues**, e.g. ***retinoids*** used to treat acne.

Thalidomide

Thalidomide, prescribed as a sedative, created severe abnormalities in 10 000 babies before medical recognition in 1961. The most common was **phocomelia**, with absence of long limb bones, ear defects, microphthalmia and CL ± P. Around 40% died of severe abnormalities of the heart, kidneys or GI tract. Thalidomide is currently used in the treatment of leprosy.

Non-prescription drugs

- **Fetal alcohol syndrome.** Children born to mothers who consumed excess alcohol during pregnancy can have mid-face hypoplasia, short palpebral fissures, a long smooth philtrum and mild developmental delay.
- **LSD** (lysergic acid diethylamide), **'angel dust'** or **PCP** (phenylcyclidine), **quinine** and birth control pills are all **teratogenic**.
- **Tobacco** smoking causes growth retardation and premature delivery.

Environmental chemicals

Lead, **methylmercury** and **hypoxia** are the most widely recognized hazards.

Physical agents

- **Prolonged hyperthermia** in early pregnancy can cause microcephaly, microphthalmia, and neuronal migration defects.
- **Ionizing radiation and X-rays** in large doses can cause microcephaly and ocular defects, the most sensitive period being 2–5 weeks. Radiation also has mutagenic and carcinogenic effects ('The 28 day rule', see Chapter 38).

30 Principles of multifactorial disease

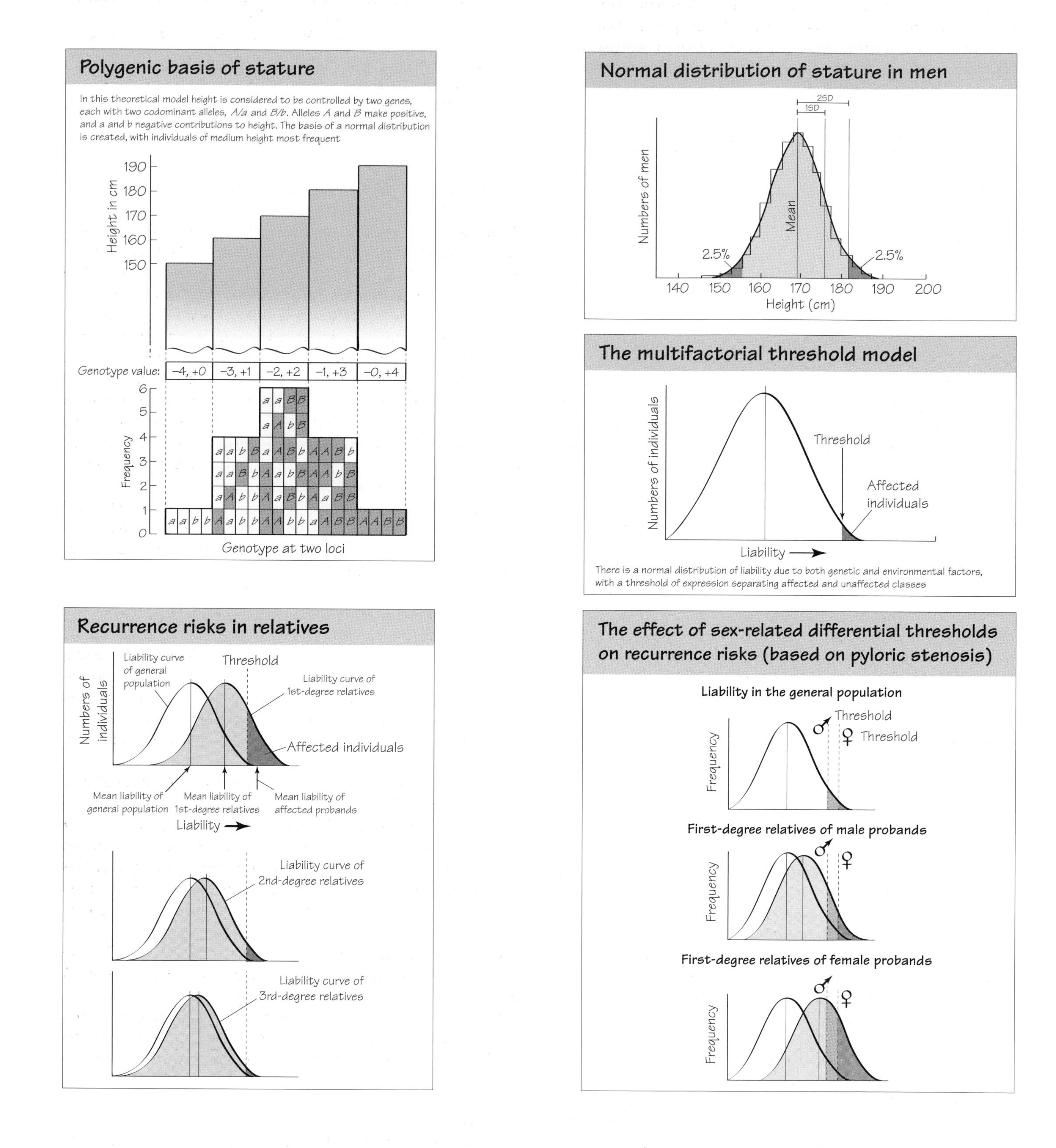

Overview

Mendelian traits show **discontinuous variation** in that alternative phenotypes are distinctly different. With some characters variation is **continuous**, with no natural boundaries. This chapter explains how discontinuous and continuous variation can be seen as two aspects of the same genetic system.

Table 30.1 Some continuously variable traits.

Height
Weight
Intelligence
Finger ridge count
Blood pressure
Skin colour
Head circumference

Continuous variation

Quantitative characters such as height, skin colour and intelligence quotient (IQ) typically show continuous variation, their frequency distributions approximating a **normal curve** definable by its mean and **standard deviation (SD)**. Such distributions are generated by the combined action of many genes, i.e. they are **polygenic** (see figure 'Polygenic basis of stature'), or together with environmental factors, **multifactorial**.

'**Variance**' is a measure of the variation in a character and equals the square of the SD.

In a normal distribution, 68% of the population is included within one SD of the mean, 95% within two and 99.7% within three SDs. The concept of a **normal range** is fundamental, especially in paediatrics, where height, weight, head circumference, etc. are measured routinely (see Chapter 49). Individuals that are outside two SDs from the mean (i.e. the 2.5% at either extreme) are regarded clinically as 'abnormal'.

Heritability (h^2)

Heritability refers to the proportion of variation in a character that can be ascribed to variation in genotype, as distinct from environment, and is expressed as a fraction of one (e.g. 0.8) or as a percentage (e.g. 80%).

The heritability of a continuous trait can be estimated from the **correlation coefficient** between the values in relatives. If the heritability is high, so is the correlation between first degree relatives. For discontinuous multifactorial traits, heritability can be derived from a variety of data, including concordance rates of twins (see Chapter 33).

Estimation of risk

If there is no discernible pattern of inheritance on which to base predictions, **empiric risks**, calculated from observed incidence in relatives, are used in counselling. Data on different kinds of relatives of many probands are combined and average incidence figures derived. In contrast to the situation with single gene disorders, recurrence risks are found to differ substantially between populations, because both allele frequencies and environmental factors vary between them.

The **relative risk** (λ) is the ratio of the risk for a class of family members to that for the general population. The relative risk for a sib is coded as **λs**. Despite the greater *empiric* risk for siblings of Type 2 diabetes patients, comparison of λs values reveals the greater responsibility of genotype in causation of Type 1 than Type 2 diabetes (Table 30.2).

Table 30.2 The greater responsibility of genotype in causation of Type 1 compared to that of Type 2 diabetes.

	Pop. incidence (%)	Freq. (empiric risk in sibs) (%)	λs (relative risk in sibs)
Type 1 diabetes (UK)	0.4	6.0	6.0/0.4 = 15.0
Type 2 diabetes (Europe)	10.0	35.0	35.0/10.0 = 3.5

Discontinuous variation, multifactorial threshold traits

Sometimes there are indications of genetic causation, but only a few family members are affected and the pattern of inheritance remains obscure. One explanation conceives an underlying normal distribution of **liability** to disease, due to an assemblage of harmful genetic and environmental factors, truncated by a threshold for disease manifestation. Disease liability for an individual depends on the combination of predisposing alleles and environmental conditions operating in that individual, and the proportion of the population beyond the threshold represents the population incidence. We all lie somewhere within the liability range for each condition, affected individuals beyond the threshold, and all those near the threshold having a greater than average probability of producing diseased offspring. Such conditions are known as **multifactorial threshold traits**.

Despite its intellectual appeal, the multifactorial threshold model should be viewed as an hypothesis rather than a fact and recent work suggests that very many fewer genes are often involved than was formerly imagined (see Chapter 31).

Rules for identification of a multifactorial threshold trait

1 ***Disorders can be common (> 1/5000 births; although they can also be rare!).*** Compare seriously disabling *monogenic* conditions, if dominant and fully penetrant, are usually eliminated by disease, reduced fertility, early death, or failure to mate, and are therefore very rare.
2 ***The disorder runs in families, but there is no distinctive pattern of inheritance.***
3 ***The concordance rate in MZ twins is significantly greater than in DZ*** (see Chapter 33).
4 ***The frequency of disease in second degree relatives is much lower than in first degree, but declines less rapidly for more distant relatives.***
5 ***Recurrence risk is proportional to the number of family members already affected.*** This is because the occurrence of several affected family members indicates a particularly high concentration of harmful alleles.
6 ***Recurrence risk is proportional to the severity of the condition in the proband.*** This is because severity of expression and recurrence risk both depend on the concentration of adverse alleles.
7 ***Recurrence risk is higher for relatives of the less susceptible sex.*** This is because disease expression in the less susceptible sex requires the higher concentration of harmful alleles (see Pyloric stenosis, below).

Examples

Cleft lip with or without cleft palate (CL ± P) (see also Chapter 31)
CL ± P is causally distinct from **cleft palate** alone (which occurs in 1/2000 malformed births). It is caused by failure of fusion of the

frontal and maxillary processes and includes chromosomal, teratogenic, monogenic and multifactorial forms.

A critical feature is the adhesive maturity of the cells on the surfaces of the lateral and medial processes in relation to their relative physical locations. Fusion of lateral and medial elements requires unimpeded movement of the palatal shelves past the tongue (see Chapter 31).

CL ± P affects about 1/1000 Europeans (0.1%), twice as many Japanese and half as many African-Americans. European recurrence risks in relatives are:

- first degree = 4%;
- second degree = 0.6%;
- third degree = 0.3% (Rule 4 above; also see figure 'Recurrence risks in relatives').

Severity of expression varies from unilateral cleft lip alone (UCL) to bilateral cleft lip with cleft palate (BCL + P). As Table 30.3 shows, the incidence of CL ± P (of all types) in first degree relatives is directly related to severity of expression in the proband (Rule 6 above).

Sixty to eighty per cent of CL ± P patients are male and the incidence in sibs of male probands is 5.5%; 20–40% of patients are female and the incidence in their sibs is 7% (Rule 7 above).

Table 30.3 The incidence of cleft lip with or without cleft palate (CL ± P) (of all types) in first degree relatives in relation to severity of expression in the proband.

Phenotype of proband	Percentage incidence in first degree relatives (= empiric risk for)
UCL	4
UCL + P	5
BCL	7
BCL + P	8

BCL, bilateral cleft lip alone; BCL + P, bilateral cleft lip with cleft palate; UCL, unilateral cleft lip alone; UCL + P, unilateral cleft lip with cleft palate.

Pyloric stenosis

Pyloric stenosis occurs in 5/1000 male but only 1/1000 female infants (see Chapter 29). Affected females are three times as likely as males to have affected offspring (Rule 7 above; see also Table 30.4). The sons of affected women have the highest risk, at about 20% (see figure 'The effect of sex-related differential thresholds on recurrence risks). The mean incidence in brothers of probands of both sexes combined is markedly higher than that in sisters. The mean incidence in the sibs (of both sexes) of female probands is markedly higher than when the proband is male. The highest risk category is male relatives of female probands.

Table 30.4 Recurrence risks (%) for pyloric stenosis in relation to gender of affected probands. (Adapted from Carter CO. (1976) Genetics of common single malformations. *Br Med Bull* **32**: 21–6.)

	Male probands		Female probands		Unweighted mean
	London	Belfast	London	Belfast	
Brothers	3.8	9.6	**9.2**	**12.5**	**8.8**
Sisters	2.7	3.0	3.8	3.8	3.3
Unweighted mean	4.8		**7.3**		

31 Multifactorial disease in children

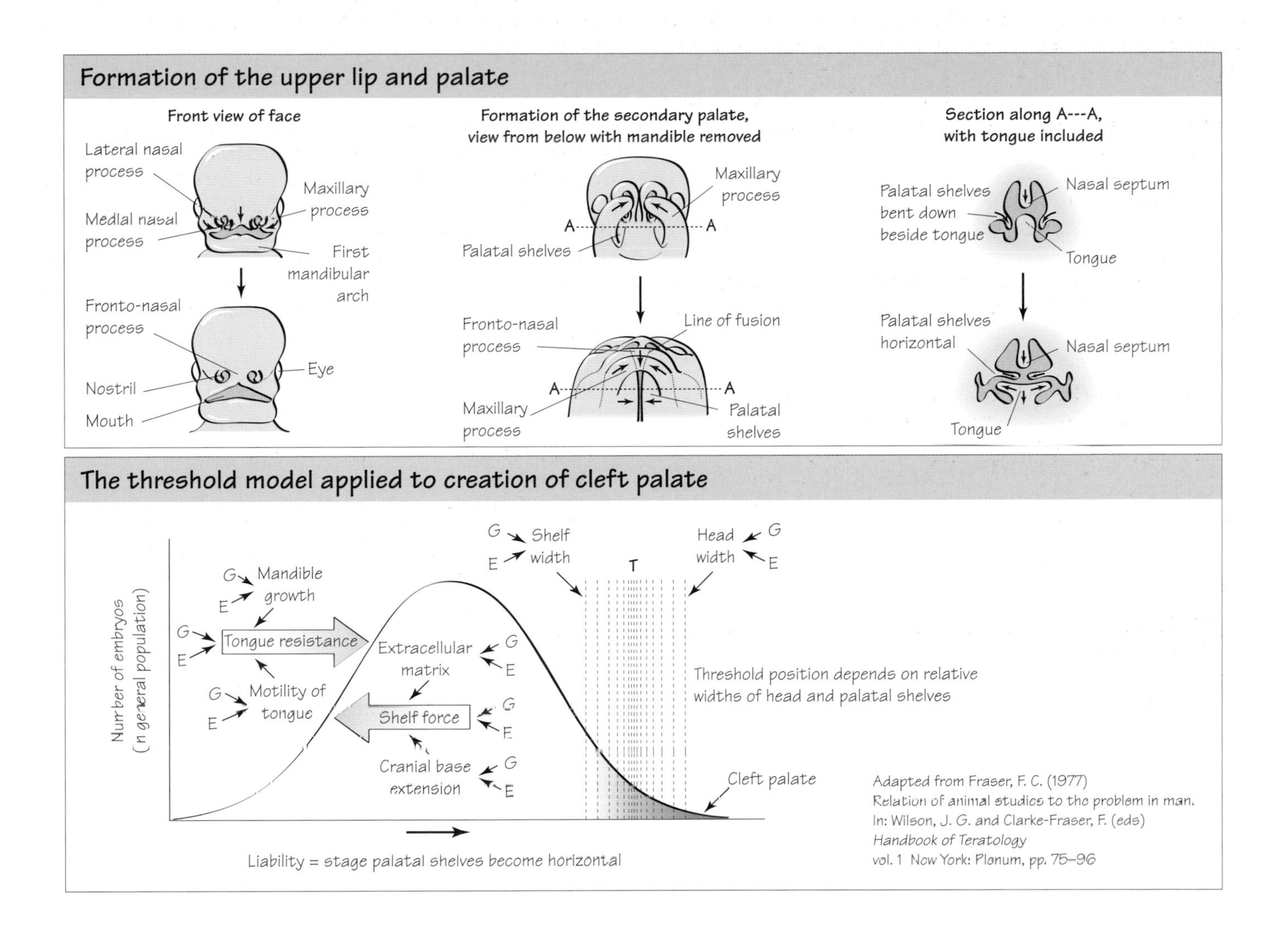

Overview

The diseases that collectively occupy the attention of most health care practitioners show clustering within families, but are not inherited by Mendelian rules. They are common because the causative alleles are also carried and transmitted by healthy individuals.

The traditional explanation was polygenic causation, with many genes of minor effect acting together (see Chapter 30), but with advancing knowledge this explanation seems less convincing.

In summary:

- In many diseases there is just ***one dominant allele, which is incompletely penetrant*** (see Chapter 20).
- In *most* common diseases there are ***probably no more than two AD disease alleles acting together*** (see Chapter 33).
- A few common diseases are **oligogenic**, i.e. there is ***more than one major disease allele acting with others of lesser effect***.
- Common inherited diseases are usually **genetically heterogeneous**, i.e. ***genes at different loci are responsible for similar disease symptoms in different families***.

Methodology

Recognizing the relative importance of genotype and environment in causation of the common diseases can make the difference between health and disease for many people and their analysis demands a variety of approaches.

Twin studies

If a disease has a major genetic component, identical or **monozygotic** (**MZ**) twin pairs tend to have a high degree of **concordance** for disease (i.e. if one is affected the other usually is also), whereas in non-identical **dizygotic** (**DZ**) twins concordance is much lower. If MZ and DZ concordances are similar, genotype is deemed unimportant (see Chapter 33).

Family studies

If there is genetic causation the relative risk for a patient's relatives is higher than in the general population and increases with degree of relationship (see Table 31.1 and Chapter 30).

Table 31.1 Empiric recurrence risks (%) for first, second and third degree relatives of patients with common childhood disorders. (Data from Jorde LB, Carey JC, Bamshad MJ & White RL. *Medical Genetics*, 3rd edition. Mosby, St Louis, Missouri 2003.)

Disorder	Population frequency (%)	First degree (%)	Second degree (%)	Third degree (%)
CL ± P	0.10	4.0	0.7	0.30
Talipes	0.10	2.5	0.5	0.20
Congenital dislocation of hip	0.20	5.0	0.6	0.40
Infantile autism	0.04	4.5	0.1	0.05

Table 31.2 Empiric recurrence risks (%) for some common multifactorial disorders of childhood, in relation to health status of parents.

Disorder	Unaffected parents having a second affected child (%)	Affected parent having an affected child (%)	Affected parent having a second affected child (%)
Asthma	10	26	–
Cleft palate	2	7	15
CL ± P	4	4	10
Congenital heart defects	1–4	1–4	10
Cryptorchidism	10	–	–
Dislocation of hip	6	12	36
Epilepsy (idiopathic)	5	5	10
Hypospadias	10	–	–
Pyloric stenosis:			
Male proband	2	4	13
Female proband	10	17	38
Renal agenesis	3	–	–
Spina bifida (see text also)	4–5	4	–
Talipes (club foot)	3	3	10

CL ± P, cleft lip with or without palate.

Adoption studies

Incidence of disease in children of affected parents adopted into unaffected families can show to what extent genetic predisposition is causative, as compared to a shared home environment.

Population studies

Study of migrant groups or different ethnic groups in the same environment can reveal genetic involvement.

Polymorphism association analysis

This approach seeks association of disease with specific alleles of a **candidate gene** (see Chapter 37).

Linkage studies

Linkage studies look for co-transmission of disease with polymorphisms of possible linked **genetic markers** (see Chapter 37).

Biochemical studies

Biochemical studies investigate abnormal activity of enzymes involved in implicated biochemical pathways.

Animal models

Animal models can provide insight into the biochemistry and help with gene mapping, but are notoriously misleading.

Examples

Neural tube defects (NTDs)

Frequency 6/1000 livebirths among Northern Chinese; 5/1000 in England and Wales, reduced now to 1/1000 by folic acid supplementation, ultrasound scanning and termination.

Features NTDs arise from failure of closure of the neural tube at the end of Week 3 (see Chapters 11, 28, 53, 60). An anterior defect can result in either **anencephaly** (partial or complete absence of the cranial vault, calvarium or cerebral hemispheres) or **encephalocele** (protrusion of the brain into an enclosed sack). Two-thirds of anencephalics are stillborn and term deliveries die within a few days; encephalocele is also rarely compatible with survival.

A posterior NTD can lead to lumbosacral **myelocele, meningomyelocele** (protruding spinal cord exposed, or covered by meninges) or **spina bifida** and about 75% of patients with posterior NTD have secondary hydrocephalus, which can lead to mental retardation.

Genetics NTD is associated with T13 and T18 and the AR **Meckel syndrome**. Isolated cases are mostly multifactorial. The empiric recurrence risk for siblings is 2–5%, reducible to 0.5% by medical intervention. For first degree relatives in general the risk is 1/30, for second degree 1/70, for third degree 1/150. In Hungary where the population incidence is 1/300, sibling risk was found to increase from 3%, to 12%, to 25% after one, two and three affected offspring (see also Table 31.2).

Management NTD can be diagnosed prenatally by ultrasound scanning and elevation of **α-fetoprotein (AFP)** in maternal serum, or amniotic fluid if the lesion is open (see Chapters 53, 60). It is claimed that 50–70% of NTDs could be avoided if women trying to conceive took 0.4 mg of folic acid daily, or 4–5 mg before and during early pregnancy if there is already an affected child.

Aetiology In Britain incidence is highest in Celtic people and correlates with multiparity, poor socioeconomic status, valproic acid exposure (see Chapter 28) and folic acid deficiency.

Crohn disease

Crohn disease is one of two main clinical subtypes of **inflammatory bowel disease** (the other being **ulcerative colitis**).

Frequency 1–2% in Western countries.

Genetics Maps to 16p12, 16q, 12q, 6p and 3p; λs: 25. Relative risk for heterozygous and homozygous genotypes: 2.5 and 40.0.

Aetiology The receptor product of the NOD2 (or CARD15) gene at 16p12 normally activates the cytoplasmic transcription factor, NF-κβ, making it responsive to the surface lipopolysaccharides of potentially harmful bacteria. This property is deficient in Crohn disease.

Management The most effective drugs target the NF-κβ complex.

Congenital heart defects (CHDs) (see also Chapter 28)

Frequency 7/1000 live births.

Features Abnormalities include ventricular septal defect (VSD: 1/400), atrial septal defect (ASD: 1/1000), patent ductus arteriosus (PDA: 1/800), pulmonary stenosis (1/2500), coarctation (constriction) of the aorta (1/1600) and aortic stenosis (constriction of the aortic valve; 1/2000).

Complex anomalies include **Tetralogy of Fallot** in about 1/1000 and **transposition of the great arteries**, in 1/16000. Tetralogy of Fallot involves: (i) *pulmonary stenosis*; (ii) *VSD*; (iii) *right ventricle hypertrophy*; and (iv) *right lateral displacement of the aorta*.

CHDs can result in inadequate oxygenation of blood and/or poor perfusion of tissues.

Genetics 90% are multifactorial, others chromosomal or monogenic.

Insulin dependent or Type 1 diabetes mellitus (IDDM; T1DM)

Features **Diabetes mellitus** is characterized by **hyperglycaemia,** causative of serious renal, retinal and vascular problems and ultimately coma and death (see Chapter 32 for Type 2 diabetes). Insulin dependent or **juvenile onset diabetes** affects 3–7% of Western adults, the peak age of onset being 12 years.

Genetics MZ concordance: 50%; DZ: 12% indicating a penetrance of 0.5 (see Chapter 33); λs: 15. Two loci are especially important: **IDDM-1** and **IDDM-2**, that together account for 40–50% of genetic predisposition, through autoimmune susceptibility (see Chapter 43) and insulin production. There is strong association (95%) with HLA-B 8 and B15, c.f. 50% of the general population (see also Table 43.1).

Aetiology Develops as a consequence of autoimmune destruction of β cells in the pancreatic islets, following viral infection. Predisposing environmental factors include diet, childhood viral exposure and some medications.

Disease susceptibility relates to mutant alleles involving substitution of aspartic acid by other amino acids at the 57th position in the DQ gene. Susceptibility is enhanced by > 20 other loci, including tandem repeats of a 14bp sequence upstream of the insulin gene at 11p15.

Obesity

Body Mass Index (BMI) is defined as (weight in kilograms) divided by (height in metres)^2. An 'obese' person has a BMI > 30, e.g. a person of height 5′8' (173 cm) who weighs over 90 kg, or 14 stone (156 lbs) has a BMI of $90/[1.73]^2 = 30$ at the borderline of obesity.

About 30% of American adults are classed as obese, providing an exacerbating factor for heart disease, stroke, hypertension and Type 2 diabetes (see Chapter 32).

Genetics Twin and adoption studies indicate heritability of 0.6–0.8, but the genetics is obscure.

Atopic diathesis

Atopic diathesis constitutes an exuberant IgE response to low levels of antigen (see Chapter 43). One in four of the population shares an AD allele that is possibly imprinted, as incidence is highest in offspring of affected mothers. Patients develop 'hay fever', eczema and asthma.

Infantile autism

Frequency 4–10%; 4 ♂ :1 ♀.

Features There is severe impairment in development of social responsiveness, very poor verbal and non-verbal communication and repetitive, stereotypic behaviour and interests, often associated with developmental delay. Onset is usually before the age of 4 years. It can be associated with chromosome imbalance, Fragile X syndrome and **tuberous sclerosis** (an AD tendency toward **hamartomas** caused by growth of blood vessels, especially in the brain).

Genetics MZ concordance: 80%; DZ concordance 20%. There are susceptibility loci on chromosomes 7q, 17q, 5p, 11, 4 and 9.

Combined recurrence risk for sibs of male probands is 3.5%, that for sibs of female probands, 7%.

32 The common disorders of adult life

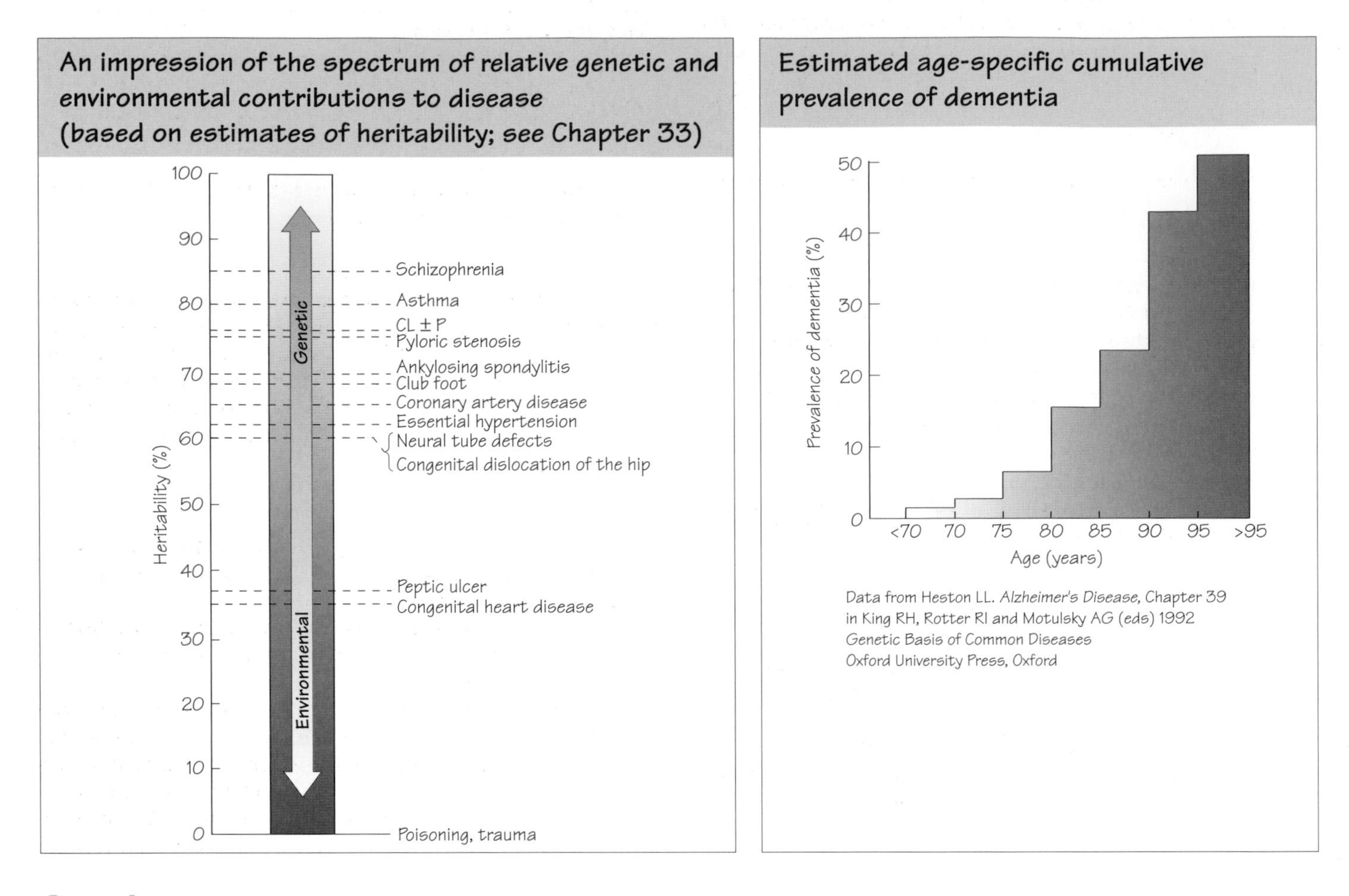

Overview

Among the leading causes of death in economically developed countries are **stroke**, **coronary artery disease** and **cardiomyopathy**, linked through obesity (see Chapter 31), **Type 2 diabetes**, **hypertension**, indolence, smoking, alcohol consumption, bad nutrition and other aspects of an economically privileged lifestyle. Schizophrenia, affective psychosis, mental retardation and Alzheimer dementia are also very common health problems of adult life with multifactorial origins (see Fig. 46.1).

Coronary artery disease (CAD)

Features CAD can account for up to half of deaths in developed countries.

Aetiology Lipid deposition in the coronary arteries causes fibrous conversion (**atherosclerosis**), failure of blood supply (**ischaemia**) and death of heart muscle (**myocardial infarction**). Predisposing conditions include **familial combined hyperlipidaemia (FCH)**, **familial hypercholesterolaemia (FH)** and point mutations in **apo B-100** (all AD), diabetes mellitus and hypertension.

Genetics Fifteen per cent of cases show AD inheritance at > 12 loci, including the gene for the **low density lipoprotein receptor (LDLR)** (see Chapter 17).

Risk increases several-fold if a first degree relative is affected, especially if female, if onset was before 55 years, or if additional relatives are affected.

Management Incidence is dramatically reduced by non-smoking, control of hypertension and fat intake, exercise and slimming.

Cardiomyopathy

About half of **cardiomyopathy** cases are familial involving hypertrophy of the left ventricle wall and caused by AD mutations in any of 10 genes that encode various components of the cardiac sarcomere. The most common are mutations in the genes for the **β-myosin heavy chain** (35%), **myosin-binding protein C** (20%) and **troponin T** (15%).

Dilated cardiomyopathy involves increase in size, with impaired contraction of the ventricles and circulation. There are AD, X-linked and mitochondrial defects and the proteins affected include **actin**, **cardiac troponin T**, **desmin** and components of the **destroglycan-sarcoglycan complex**.

In the **long QT (LQT) syndrome** there is elongation of the electrocardiogram QT interval, with potentially fatal cardiac arrhythmia. It shows familial patterns, but is also induced by drugs that block potassium channels. **Romano–Ward syndrome** is inherited as AD, **Jervell–Lange–Nielsen syndrome**, as AR.

Hypertension

High blood pressure affects 25% of adults of most developed countries and promotes heart disease, stroke and kidney disease. With no obvious cause it is called **essential hypertension**; induced by pregnancy, **pre-eclampsia**.

Frequency Up to 40% of 70 year olds are hypertensive.

Genetics Essential hypertension shows heritability of 20–40%. Monogenic AD inheritance is suggested in rare families.

Biochemical studies implicate the **sodium–potassium transmembrane pump**, the **angiotensin I converting enzyme** (**ACE**), the **angiotensin II type I receptor** and the gene coding for **angiotensinogen** involved in sodium reabsorption and vasoconstriction. At least eight rare mutations concerned are indicated.

Management Recommendations include avoidance of sodium intake, reduction of body weight and stress.

Stroke

Stroke or **apoplexy** refers to brain damage caused by sudden and sustained loss of blood flow to the brain. **Ischaemic stroke** arises from **embolism**, or arterial obstruction. **Haemorrhagic stroke** is due to rupture of a blood vessel in the brain. It may include loss of consciousness and **hemiplegia** and it is the third leading cause of death in Americans. It is associated with hypertension, obesity, atherosclerosis, diabetes and cigarette smoking.

MZ concordance is 10%, DZ 5%. It can be a consequence of sickle cell disease (see Chapter 34) and **c**erebral **a**utosomal **d**ominant **a**rteriopathy with **s**ubcortical **i**nfarcts and **l**eucoencephalopathy (**CADASIL**).

Type 2 diabetes mellitus and MODY

Type 2 (**T2DM**), **late-onset** or **non insulin dependent diabetes mellitus** (**NIDDM**), at a frequency of 4–10% of adults, is 10 times as common as T1DM (see Chapter 31). **Maturity onset diabetes of the young** (**MODY**) also affects 1–2% of diabetics in early adulthood.

Genetics Twin concordance indicates a strong genetic basis and high penetrance for T2DM (see Chapter 33). Linkage studies suggest possibly three susceptibility loci for T2DM; six or more for MODY, some families showing single gene AD inheritance.

Low intelligence (Table 32.1)

IQ (mental age/chronological age), is inherited as a polygenic trait (see Chapter 30). An IQ of 50–70 is shown by 3% of the population, at the lower end of the 'normal' range. **Severe non-specific mental retardation** (IQ < 50) usually has a single cause, with an overall risk of recurrence about 3%. This is increased to 15% if the parents are related, or to 25% after the birth of two affected children (see Table 32.1). Some male cases are XR, predicting an increased risk for subsequent male births.

Schizophrenia (Table 32.2)

Schizophrenia is a seriously disabling psychosis affecting 1% of the population. Twin concordance rates, family and adoption studies support a monogenic AD basis, with low penetrance, although this interpretation is by no means widely accepted. Gene mapping indicates genetic heterogeneity.

Table 32.1 Risk of recurrence of severe non-specific mental retardation in affected families.

Family category	Recurrence risk
One male offspring affected	1/25
One female offspring affected	1/50
Two offspring affected	1/4
Parents consanguineous	1/7

Suggested environmental triggers include prenatal viral infection, recreational drugs and social stress.

Affective disorder (Table 32.2)

Affective disorders include purely **depressive** or **unipolar**, and **manic depressive** or **bipolar illness**. The average lifetime risk for bipolar is about 1%, for unipolar 2–25% depending on cultural background. In women it is associated with adjustment of reproductive hormone regimes.

Twin, family and adoption studies point to a genetic basis. Mapping studies indicate genetic heterogeneity and there is evidence of anticipation (see Chapter 21).

Alzheimer disease

Alzheimer disease involves progressive **dementia** and memory loss and affects 40–50% of Americans in their 90s. It is less common in Hispanics and Africans than Europeans and Japanese.

There is defective cleavage of **amyloid-β precursor protein** (**APP**), causing **β-amyloid plaques** and neurofibrillary tangles in the brain, with progressive loss of neurones.

In the 3–5% of families with early onset AD inheritance is indicated, with at least seven susceptibility loci, including those for **presenilins-1** and **-2**. Another codes for a defect in the cleavage site within APP coded on Chromosome 21 (c.f. Down syndrome, Chapter 24). Late onset cases fit a multifactorial model best with the **epsilon 4** (**ε4**) allele of **apolipoprotein E**, involved in clearance of cleaved amyloid protein, the best characterized risk factor.

Alcoholism

Frequency 10% of (American) males, 4% of females.

Features Type 1 alcoholism is a feature of introverted, solitary behaviour. Age of onset is usually over 25 years and it is relatively easily cured. Type 2 is associated with extraversion and thrill-seeking; it usually begins before 25 and is less easily treated.

Genetics Risk of becoming an alcoholic is increased fourfold if there is an affected parent. The heritability of Type 1 is 0.2, that for Type 2, 0.9.

Unpleasant consequences of alcohol consumption due to hereditary metabolic deficiencies reduce heavy drinking and alcoholism in some ethnic groups (see Chapter 34).

Table 32.2 Empiric risks of recurrence of schizophrenia and affective psychosis in relatives. (Data from Kingston HM. *ABC of Clinical Genetics*, 3rd edn. BMJ Books, London 2002.)

	Population incidence (%)	Sibling (first degree relative) (%)	Offspring of one affected parent (first degree relative) (%)	Offspring of two affected parents (first degree relative) (%)	Second degree relative (%)	Third degree relative (%)
Schizophrenia	1	9	13	45	3	1–2
Affective psychosis (unipolar + bipolar)	2–3	13	15	50	5	2–3

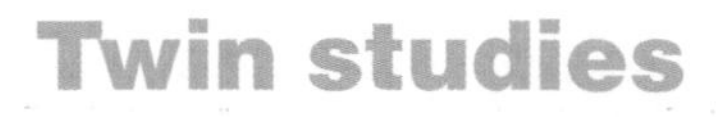

33 Twin studies

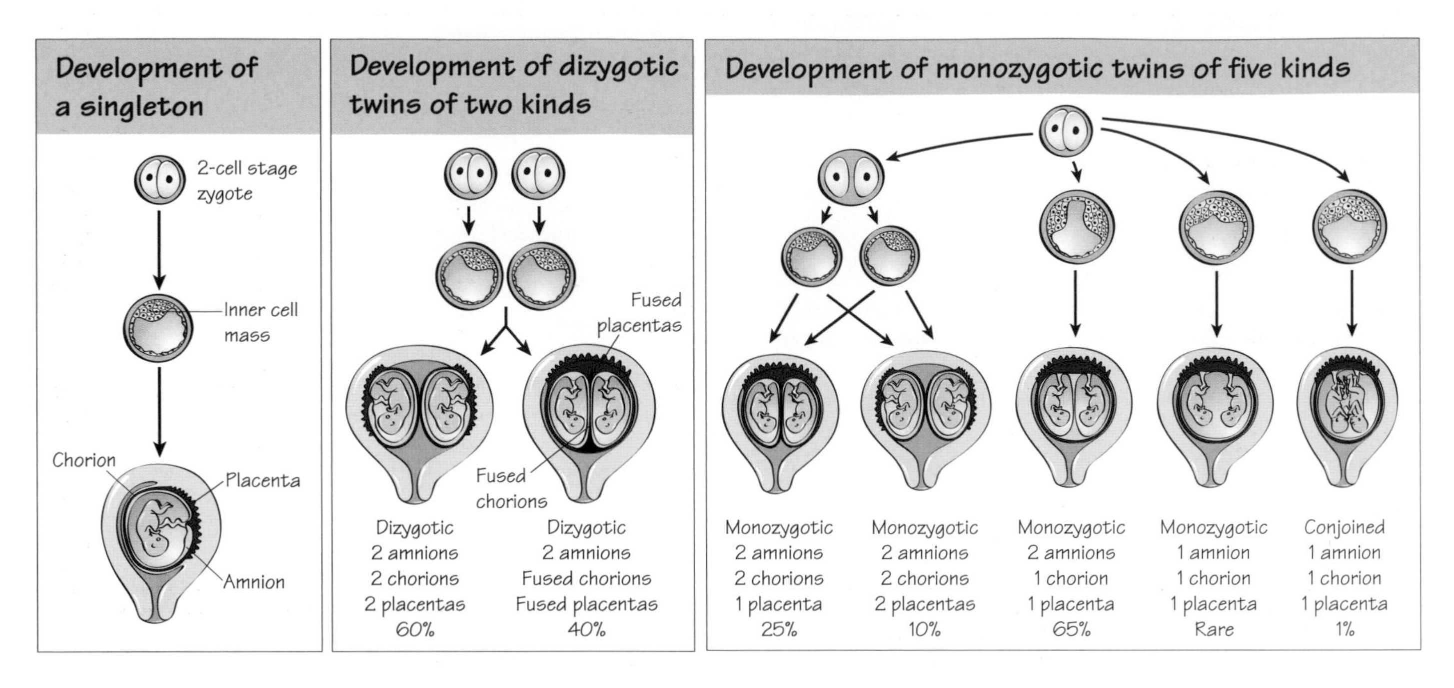

Overview

The main value of twins in genetic analysis is that they can reveal the relative importance of genotype ('nature') and environment ('nurture') in multifactorial disease.

There are two major categories of twins, **monozygotic** (**MZ**) or **identical**, and **dizygotic** (**DZ**) or **fraternal**. DZ twins originate from two eggs and two sperm; like ordinary sibs they share 50% of their alleles. MZ twins originate from a single zygote that divided into two embryos during the first 2 weeks of development. MZ twins are always of the same sex and their genomes are 100% identical.

Sixty-five per cent of MZ twins share a placenta and chorion, around 25% have separate chorions and almost all have separate amnions. They have non-identical, but very similar fingerprints. Their **'DNA fingerprints'** are identical (see Chapter 58).

Frequency of multiple births

Around 1/80 British pregnancies yield twins, about 1/260 births of MZ, 1/125 of DZ. Up to 1/20 births are of DZ in some African populations, but less than 1/500 in Chinese and Japanese. Multiple births involve various combinations of DZ- and MZ-like twinning events. Triplets occur in 1/7500 and quadruplets in 1/658 000 European births.

DZ twinning is increased at late births and greater maternal age, the peak being at age 35–40 years, possibly related to levels of **follicle stimulating hormone** (**FSH**). Women treated with ovulation-inducing agents like *clomiphene citrate* and *gonadotrophins* are at increased risk of multiple pregnancy. There is probably no familial tendency toward MZ twinning, but there is for DZ, with up to three times the normal rate in some families.

Analysis of discontinuous multifactorial traits

Concordance ratio

If both twins are affected by a condition they are said to be **concordant** for that condition. If only one is affected they are **discordant**. The **pair-wise concordance rate** is given by

$$\mathbf{C / (C + D)},$$

where C = the number of concordant pairs and D = the number of discordant pairs.

Since MZ twins are genetically identical, whereas DZ share only 50% of their genomes, the ratio of their concordances for a condition gives a rough indication of the relative importance of genotype in its causation.

If $\mathbf{C_{MZ} : C_{DZ} = 3\text{–}6 : 1}$, the genome is the major determinant, e.g. schizophrenia, CL ± P;

If $\mathbf{C_{MZ} : C_{DZ} = 2\text{–}3 : 1}$, both genetic and environmental factors are significant, e.g. blood pressure, mental deficiency;

If $\mathbf{C_{MZ} : C_{DZ} = 1\text{–}2 : 1}$, the main determinant is environmental, e.g. measles, tobacco smoking.

The Holzinger statistic

The Holzinger (H) statistic provides values from close to zero, for minimal genetic involvement, to close to unity for almost entirely genetic causation

$$\mathbf{H = \frac{C_{MZ} - C_{DZ}}{1 - C_{DZ}}}$$

Estimation of penetrance and gene counting

MZ concordance relates to penetrance (P) by the expression:

$$\mathbf{C_{MZ} = \frac{P}{2 - P}},$$

From which penetrance can be calculated.

When P is known the number of major causative alleles can be derived from DZ concordance:

Table 33.1 Twin concordances and derived values for some complex traits.*

Disorder	Population frequency /1000	MZ conc. (%)	DZ conc. (%)	n	P
Atopic diathesis	250	50	4	3	0.7
Autism	40–100	80	20	1 or 2	0.9
Bipolar affective disorder	4	79	24	1	0.9
CL ± P	1	30	5	2	0.5
Cleft palate	0.5	26	5	2	0.4
Congenital dislocation of hip	1	41	3	3 or 4	0.6
Coronary artery disease	Up to 500	46	12	1 or 2	0.6
Epilepsy	10	37	10	1 or 2	0.5
Essential hypertension	100	30	10	1	0.5
T1DM	2	30–40	6	2	0.5
Leprosy	Varies	60	20	1	0.75
Measles	Varies	97	94	0	–
Multiple sclerosis	1	20–30	6	2	0.4
T2DDM	30–70	100	10	2	1.0
Psoriasis	10	61	13	1 or 2	0.75
Pyloric stenosis	3	15	2	3	0.3
Rheumatoid arthritis	20	30	5	2	0.5
Schizophrenia	10	45	13	1	0.6
Spina bifida	5	6	3	1	0.1
Talipes equinovarus	5	32	3	3	0.5
Tuberculosis	Varies	87	26	1	0.9
Unipolar affective disorder	20–250	54	19	1	0.7

n, number of major genes acting in a monogenic or together in an oligogenic system, estimated from DZ concordance; P, approximate penetrance estimated from MZ concordance. (These data give no indication of genetic heterogeneity.)
* This table is meant to present only a general picture, actual frequencies and concordances vary in published reports.

$$C_{DZ} = \frac{P}{4-P},$$ for ONE major autosomal dominant;

$$C_{DZ} = \frac{P}{8-P},$$ for TWO dominants, or a pair of recessives;

$$C_{DZ} = \frac{P}{16-P},$$ for THREE dominants; or one dominant and a pair of recessives.

Analysis of continuously variable multifactorial traits

The most widely used estimate of genetic involvement is **heritability** (***h^2***), defined as ***the fraction of variation in a quantitative character that can be ascribed to genotypic variation***. It can furnish information on, for example, the effectiveness of a nutritional regime. It varies between populations and is derivable from (1) the standard deviations of the differences between co-twins, or (2) the coefficients of correlation (r) between them.

$$h^2 = \frac{V_{DZ} - V_{MZ}}{V_{DZ}}$$

stands for 'variance', the square of the standard deviation of the differences between members of twin pairs.

$$h^2 = \frac{r_{MZ} - r_{DZ}}{1 - r_{DZ}}$$

Health risks in twins

Twin pregnancies have a 5–10 fold increased incidence of perinatal mortality and a tendency toward premature birth. Deformations occur in both kinds of twins, but MZ also have twice the normal risk of malformation (see Chapter 28).

Monochorionic MZ twins often (~15%) share a blood supply. This can lead to **twin-to-twin transfusion syndrome** when one twin becomes severely undernourished while the other develops an enlarged heart and liver and **polyhydramnios**. There are marked differences in birth weights and both twins are at great risk of morbidity and mortality.

Conjoined twins

Conjoined, or **'Siamese' twins** develop from incompetely separated inner-cell masses and occur in about 1% of MZ pairs. They may be united at the same position of any part of the head or trunk.

Parasitic twins

A 'parasitic twin' is a portion of a body protruding from an otherwise normal host. Common attachment sites are the oral region, the pelvis and the **mediastinum** (the wall dividing the thoracic cavity).

Vanishing twins

Early loss and partial or complete resorption of one member of a twin pair is not unusual.

Reversed asymmetry

Asymmetric anatomical features sometimes show reversal in one twin. This is especially so in conjoined pairs and in those MZ twin pairs that result from late division (see Chapter 12).

Weaknesses of the twin study approach

1 Concordant pairs can be **ascertained** (i.e. recognized) through both individuals, discordant through only one, leading to **bias of ascertainment**.
2 The first two blastomeres may be fertilized by separate sperms.
3 Separate eggs may be fertilized by different fathers.
4 MZ discordance can arise from somatic mutation, or transfusion syndrome, rather than incomplete penetrance.

34 Normal polymorphism

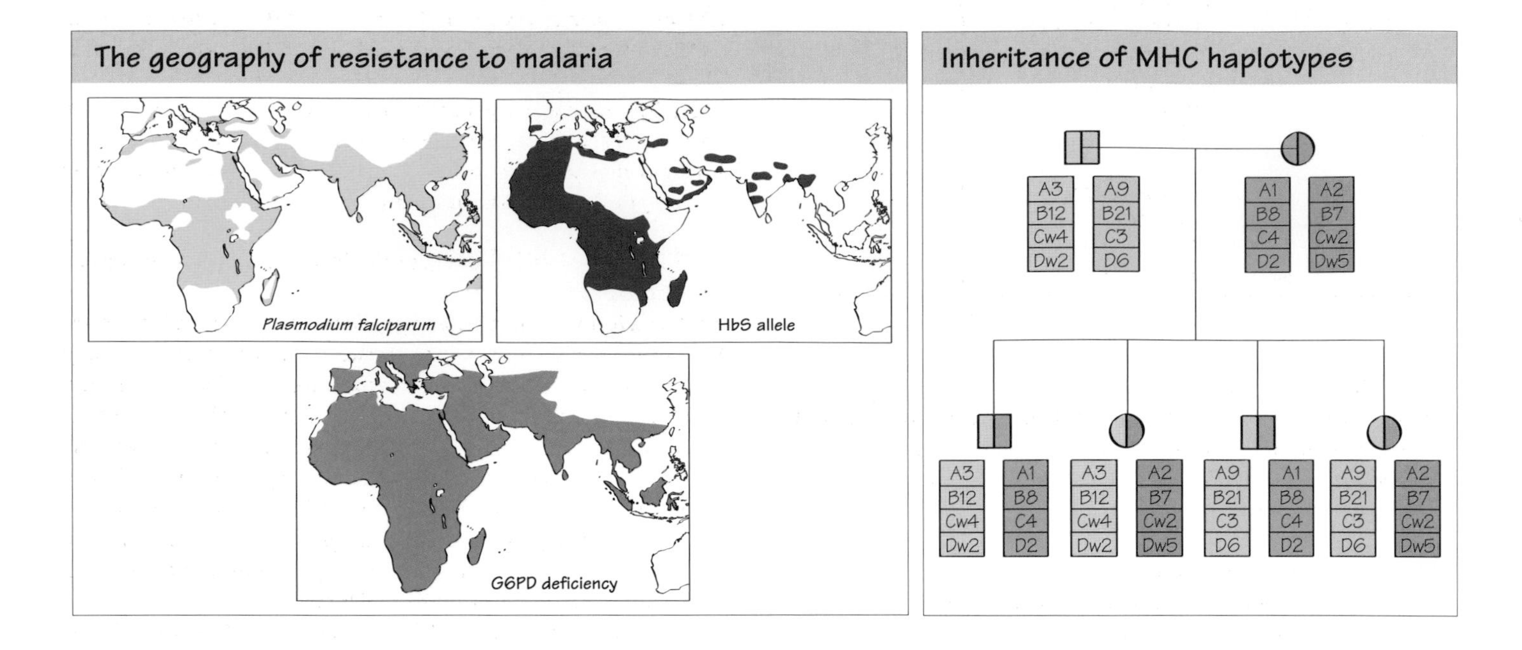

Overview

Genetic polymorphism is the occurrence of multiple alleles at a locus, where at least two are at frequencies greater than 1%. Over 30% of the genes that code for proteins are polymorphic. Part 3 deals with their analysis and application at the DNA level. Many polymorphisms owe their high frequency to selection of traits in specific populations.

Environment-related polymorphism

Sunlight

Skin colour relates to the prevailing intensity of sunlight in the region of origin of a population. Sunburn, skin cancer and toxic accumulation of vitamin D select for dark skin in sunny climates. Deficiency of vitamin D selects for pale skin in less sunny regions by causing **rickets**, formerly lethal at childbirth.

Food

Worldwide, most human adults cannot tolerate **lactose**, but traditional consumption of cows' milk has selected lactose tolerance in Europeans and some North Africans (see Chapter 44). Australian aborigines readily become hypertensive if they consume common salt. Other foods cause health problems for carriers of specific polymorphic variants (see Chapters 59, 60).

Alcohol

Ethyl alcohol is metabolized to acetaldehyde by **alcohol dehydrogenase (ADH)**, of which there are several types. Ninety per cent of Chinese and Japanese, and 5% of British people have a deficient form of ADH2, making them more prone to intoxication.

Acetaldehyde is further degraded by cytosolic **acetaldehyde dehydrogenase 1 (ALDH1)** and mitochondrial **ALDH2**. Up to 50% of Asians are deficient in ALDH2 and experience an unpleasant '**flushing**' reaction to alcohol caused by accumulation of acetaldehyde.

Malaria

Sickle cell anaemia (ID)

The ***HbS*** allele of β-globin causes reduced solubility of haemoglobin in homozygotes (*HbS*/*HbS*) and their red blood corpuscles collapse, characteristically into a sickle shape when oxygen concentrations are low. The 'sickled cells' clog capillaries causing problems that may result in death in childhood (see Chapters 20 and 39).

Heterozygotes (*HbS*/*HbA*) have '**the sickle cell trait**'. In low oxygen regimes they suffer capillary blockage, but they have the '**heterozygote advantage**' (see Chapter 19) of resistance to the malaria parasite, *Plasmodium falciparum*. By eliminating normal homozygotes (*HbA*/*HbA*) malaria creates high population frequencies of the HbS allele in malarial areas (see figure 'The geography of resistance to malaria').

Sickle cell disease is the classic example of a **balanced polymorphism**.

Thalassaemia (AR)

Thalassaemia is a quantitative or functional deficiency of α-, or **β-globin** (Tables 34.1, 34.2; also see Chapter 39). Homozygosity of some alleles is lethal, but heterozygosity of beta-thalassaemia and alpha-thalassaemia trait afford protection in malarial areas around the Mediterranean sea, the Middle East and South-East Asia.

Table 34.1 Genetic bases of alpha-thalassaemia.

Phenotype	Genotype	Quantity of α-globin produced (%)
Normal	αα/αα	100
'Silent carrier'	α–/αα	75
'Alpha-thalassaemia trait'	α–/α– or – –/αα	50
Haemoglobin H (β4)	α–/– –	25
Hydrops fetalis	– –/– –	0 (lethal)

Table 34.2 Genetic bases of beta-thalassaemia.

Affected population	Nature of defect	β-globin phenotype
Italian	δ/β fusion protein	β^0
Sardinian	Premature termination	β^0
African	RNA splicing	β^0
	RNA splicing	β^+
	Polyadenylation	β^+
Japanese	Promoter	β^+
Indian	Deletion	β^0
	Frameshift + premature termination	β^0
Asian	mRNA capping	β^+
South-East Asian	Substitution	β^+

G6PD deficiency (XR)

Deficiency of **glucose-6-phosphate dehydrogenase (G6PD)** is very common in malarial areas (see figure) as it prevents growth of *Plasmodium* parasites. Heterozygote advantage is confined to females, the trait being X-linked recessive.

The Duffy blood group (Co-D)

There are three alleles of the **Duffy blood group**, *FyA*, *FyB* and *FyO*, the latter reaching 100% frequency in some African populations. *FyA* and *FyB* provide an entry gate for malaria parasites into red cells, but *FyO* does not, so making homozygotes resistant.

Human immunodeficiency virus (HIV)

Some individuals that have slow disease progression from **HIV-1** infection to **acquired immunodeficiency syndrome (AIDS)** have a 32 bp deletion (Δ32), in the T-cell surface receptor called **CCR5** (see Chapters 42, 43). This causes a frameshift, inclusion of 31 novel amino acids and premature truncation of the protein (see Chapters 32, 39). The mutant protein lacks the regions involved in intra-cellular signal transduction and homozygotes fail to develop disease. The Δ32 allele is highest in Finns (16%) grading south through Europe to 4% in Sardinia and at 2–5% in the Middle East and India. It is virtually absent elsewhere.

Transfusion and transplantation

The ABO system

The ABO blood groups (see Chapter 20) are a vital consideration in blood transfusion and tissue transplantation because we naturally carry antibodies directed against those antigens that we do not ourselves possess (Table 34.3).

Group O are universal donors, Group AB are universal recipients.

Table 34.3 Transfusion relations between the ABO blood groups.

Blood group	UK frequency	Antigens on RBCs	Antibodies in serum	Can receive from	Can donate to
A	0.42	A	Anti-B	A or O	A or AB
B	0.09	B	Anti-A	B or O	B or AB
AB	0.03	A + B	None	**Everyone**	AB only
O	0.46	None	Anti-A + anti-B	O only	**Everyone**

RBCs, red blood cells.

The Rhesus system

The Rhesus system is genetically complex, but can be considered as involving two alleles, *D* and *d*. *DD* and *Dd* individuals display Rhesus antigens on their red cells and are said to be **Rhesus positive (Rh+)**. Rh+ individuals can be given Rh– blood, but **Rhesus negative (Rh–** *dd*) individuals develop an immune response if transfused with Rh+ blood.

If a Rh– woman is pregnant with a Rh+ (*Dd*) baby she can become immunized against red blood cells that leak across the placenta. Anti-Rh antibodies can then invade the body of the baby at birth, causing **haemolytic disease of the newborn**.

Cytochrome P450 (see also Pharmacogenetics section of Chapter 20)

The **Cytochrome P450** superfamily includes genes that encode more than 80 different membrane-bound haemoproteins involved in drug metabolism. An example is **debrisoquine hydroxylase**, encoded by the gene **CYP2D6**. Polymorphisms of this gene variably affect the hydroxylation of over 25% of all pharmaceuticals, including beta-blockers, neuroleptics and antidepressants. Deficient hydroxylation of drugs occurs in ~10% of UK residents and 30% of Hong Kong Chinese, conferring high susceptibility to some drugs such as the beta-blocking effect of **propanolol**. By contrast ultra-rapid hydroxylation occurs in 20% of Saudi Arabians and ~30% of Ethiopians.

The product of the related **CYP2C9** gene hydroxylates about 16% of medicinal drugs, including the anticoagulant **warfarin**, the anticonvulsant, **phenytoin** and the insulin-release stimulator **tolbutamide**. There are at least five polymorphic variants of CYP2C9 that cause drug toxicity or require specific therapeutic dose rates in members of some populations.

Enzymes encoded by the **CYP3A** gene family metabolize over 50% of clinically prescribed drugs and may be the most important contributor to population-specific variant drug response. **CYP3AB** is expressed at high levels in 30% of whites and Japanese, 40% of Chinese and 50% of African-Americans and South-East Asians.

Transplantation genetics

When tissues or organs are transplanted between individuals, the ultimate success of the operation depends on close similarity between the cell surface determinants of the recipient and those of the donor. As a general rule a recipient will reject a graft from a person who possesses a cell surface antigen that is not present in the recipient. The most important of these are the molecules of the human leukocyte antigen (HLA) (or major histocompatibility complex (MHC)) system (see Chapter 42).

The HLA system is very highly polymorphic, but the several genes involved are in tight linkage (on Chromosome 6) so tend to be inherited together as a '**haplotype**'. If a parental couple has a total of four different haplotypes, each offspring has a 25% chance of inheriting the same combination as any of his/her sibs (see figure 'Inheritance of MHC haplotypes'). MZ twins have a complete antigen match and DZ twins, although sharing only 50% of their genes, may accept reciprocal grafts if they previously shared a placental circulation (see Chapter 33).

The chance of a random HLA match between distantly related, or unrelated individuals is ~1/200 000; apart from corneal and bone grafts, which remain sequestered from the blood stream of the recipient. Successful transplantation generally requires pharmaceutical immunosuppression.

35 Allele frequency

Diallelic autosomal system with codominance, the MN blood groups

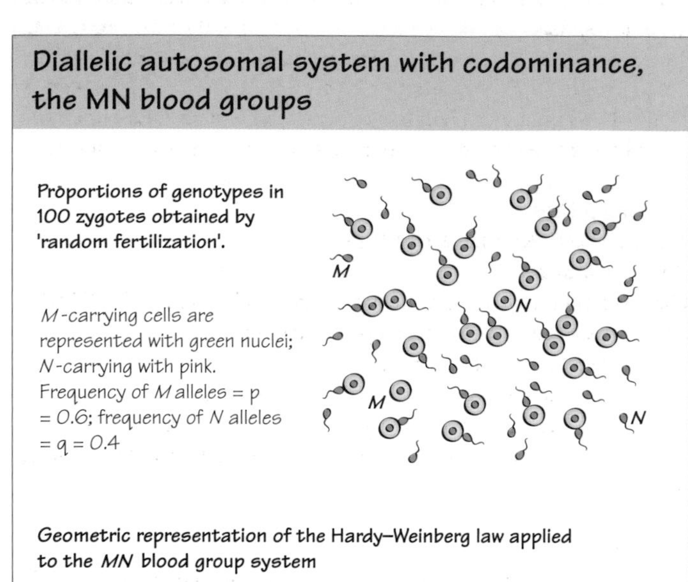

Geometric representation of the Hardy–Weinberg law applied to the *MN* blood group system

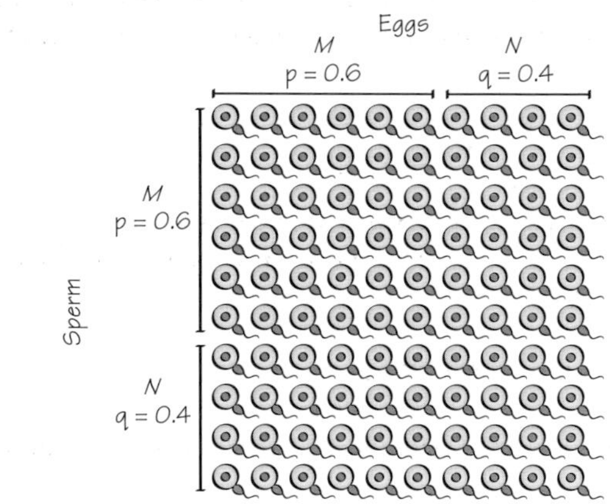

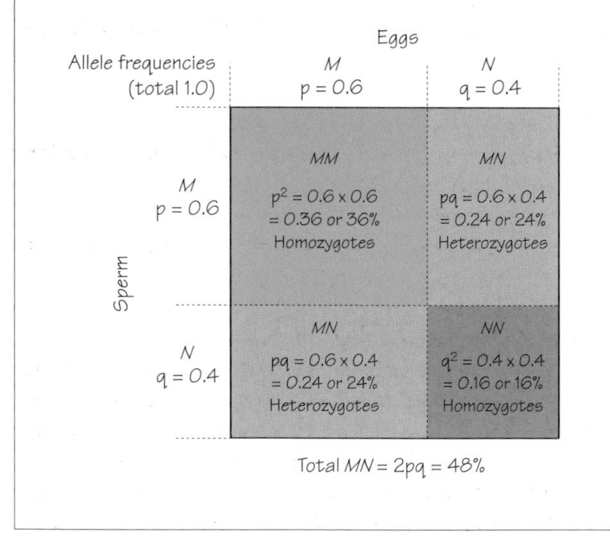

Diallelic autosomal system with dominance and recessivity, albinism

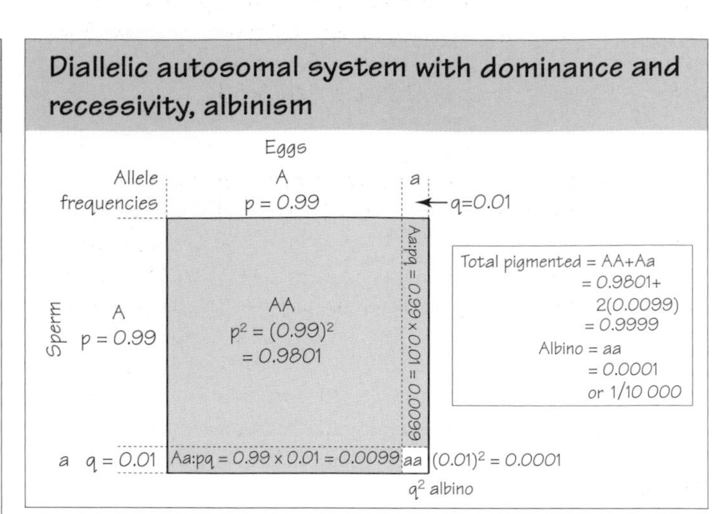

Triallelic autosomal system with codominance and dominance, the ABO blood groups

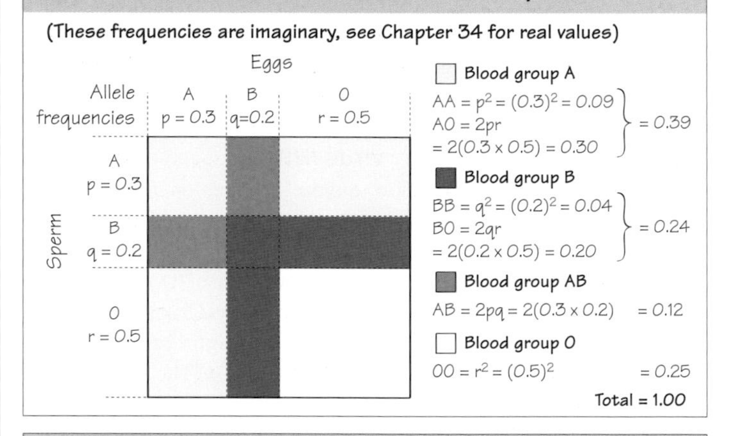

Relative frequency of recessive homozygotes and heterozygotes for some important recessive diseases

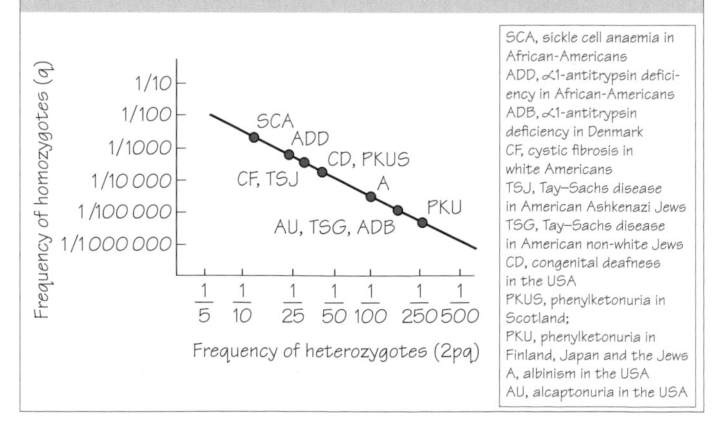

Overview

Within a *randomly mating* population the relative frequencies of heterozygotes and homozygotes are mathematically related to allele frequencies by what is known as the **Hardy–Weinberg law**. Extension of this theory reveals that ***allele frequencies will remain constant from generation to generation provided none is under positive or negative selection***. This is the '**Hardy–Weinberg equilibrium**'.

The Hardy–Weinberg law

Diallelic autosomal system with codominance

In the **MN blood group system** alleles ***M*** and ***N*** are codominant and there are three blood groups: **M**, **MN** and **N**, M and N individuals being homozygotes. We can calculate the frequency (p) of allele ***M*** in a population as the proportion of group M individuals plus half the proportion of group MN. Similarly, the frequency (q) of allele ***N*** equals the proportion of group N people plus half the proportion of group MN. Since there are no other alleles, $p + q = 1$. If Hardy–Weinberg conditions apply the frequencies of the genotypes are given by: $(p + q)^2 = p^2 + 2pq + q^2$, i.e. frequency of ***MM*** $= p^2$; frequency of ***MN*** $= 2pq$ and frequency of ***NN*** $= q^2$.

Diallelic autosomal system with dominance and recessivity (e.g. albinism)

If the frequency of a dominant allele ***A*** is p and that of a recessive allele ***a*** at the same locus is q and there are no other alleles, then the frequencies of the genotypes are ***AA***, p^2; ***Aa***, $2pq$; ***aa***, q^2. The frequencies of the phenotypes are **pigmented**: $p^2 + 2pq$, **albino**: q^2.

Triallelic autosomal system with codominance and dominance (e.g. the ABO blood groups)

If the population frequencies of alleles ***A***, ***B*** and ***O*** are p, q and r respectively, then $p + q + r = 1$ and the frequencies of the genotypes, from $(p + q + r)^2$, are ***AA***, p^2; ***BB***, q^2; ***OO***, r^2; ***AB***, $2pq$, ***AO***, $2pr$; ***BO***, $2qr$. The frequencies of the blood groups are **A**: $p^2 + 2pr$; **B**: $q^2 + 2qr$; **O**: r^2 and **AB**: $2pq$.

Diallelic X-linked system with dominance and recessivity (e.g. G6PD deficiency)

If the frequency of allele ***G*** is p and that of allele ***g*** is q, then the frequency of ***G*** phenotype males is p and that of ***g*** phenotype males is q. In females the frequencies of the genotypes are: ***GG***, p^2; ***Gg***, $2pq$; ***gg***, q^2, and the frequencies of the phenotypes are ***G***, $p^2 + 2pq$; ***g***, q^2.

Necessary conditions

1 Random mating. Two conditions can lead to over-representation of homozygotes: (i) assortative mating: usually selection of a mate on the basis of similarity with self, e.g. for deafness, stature, religion or ethnicity; and (ii) consanguinity, e.g. cousin marriage. Homozygosity exposes disadvantageous recessives to selection, which may alter their frequency in subsequent generations.

2 Absence of selection, i.e. no genotypic class may be less or more viable or fertile than the others. Allowance must therefore be made for disease alleles.

3 Lack of relevant mutation.

4 Large population size. In small populations random fluctuations in gene frequency (**genetic drift**) can result in **extinction** of some alleles, **fixation** of others.

5 Absence of gene flow. Migration of people slowly spreads variant alleles. An example is indicated by the cline in blood group B from 0.30 in East Asia to 0.06 in Western Europe.

Applications of the Hardy–Weinberg law

These include:

1 Recognition of reduced viability of certain genotypes.

2 Estimation of the probability of finding a tissue antigen match in the general population.

3 Estimation of the number of potential donors of a rare blood group.

4 Estimation of the frequency of carriers of autosomal recessive disease. The frequency of unaffected heterozygotes is invariably very much higher than that of affected recessive homozygotes (see figure).

Examples

Autosomal recessive conditions

Phenylketonuria

Phenylketonuria occurs in white Americans at a frequency of ~1/15 000; what is the frequency of heterozygous carriers?

- Homozygote frequency, $q^2 = 1/15\,000$;
- Disease allele frequency, $q = \sqrt{1/15\,000} = \sim 0.008$;
- Normal allele frequency, $p = 1 - q = 1 - 0.008 = 0.992$;
- **Heterozygote frequency, $2pq = 2 \times 0.992 \times 0.008 = 0.016$, = 1.6%, or ~1/60.**

Cystic fibrosis

Cystic fibrosis occurs in white Americans at a frequency of ~1/2500; what is the frequency of marriages (at random) between cystic fibrosis heterozygotes?

- $q^2 = 1/2500$;
- $q = \sqrt{1/2500} = 1/50 = 0.02$;
- $p = 1 - q = 1 - 0.02 = 0.98$;
- Carrier frequency $= 2pq = 2 \times 0.98 \times 0.02 = 0.04$.
- **Frequency of marriages between heterozygotes = $(2pq)^2 = (0.04)^2 = 0.0016$, or 0.16%.**

X-linked recessive conditions

Haemophilia

Haemophilia A occurs in 1/5000 male births; what is the frequency of female carriers?

- q = frequency of disease in males = $1/5000 = 0.0002$;
- $p = 1 - q = 1 - 0.0002 = 0.9998$;
- **Frequency of female carriers = $2pq = 2 \times 0.9998 \times 0.0002 = 0.0004$ = 0.04%, or 1/2500.**

Colour blindness

Colour blindness is present in 8% of British males; what is the frequency of affected females?

- Colour blindness allele frequency $= q = 0.08$.
- **Frequency of affected females = $q^2 = (0.08)^2 = 0.0064$ = 0.64%, or 1/156.**

Consequence of medical intervention

When medical intervention introduces major improvements in the biological fitness of carriers of lethal or seriously disabling alleles, this has serious effects on allele frequency. For example, one-third of all copies of X-linked disease alleles are in males. A major increase in the survival or fertility of male hemizygotes can therefore increase disease frequency by up to 33% *per generation*. Medical intervention can *double* the frequency of serious autosomal dominant disease *at each successive generation*. Recessive disease frequency could theoretically *quadruple* in $1/q$ generations; e.g. if $q = 1/25$, in 25 generations (see Chapter 61).

36 Genetic linkage

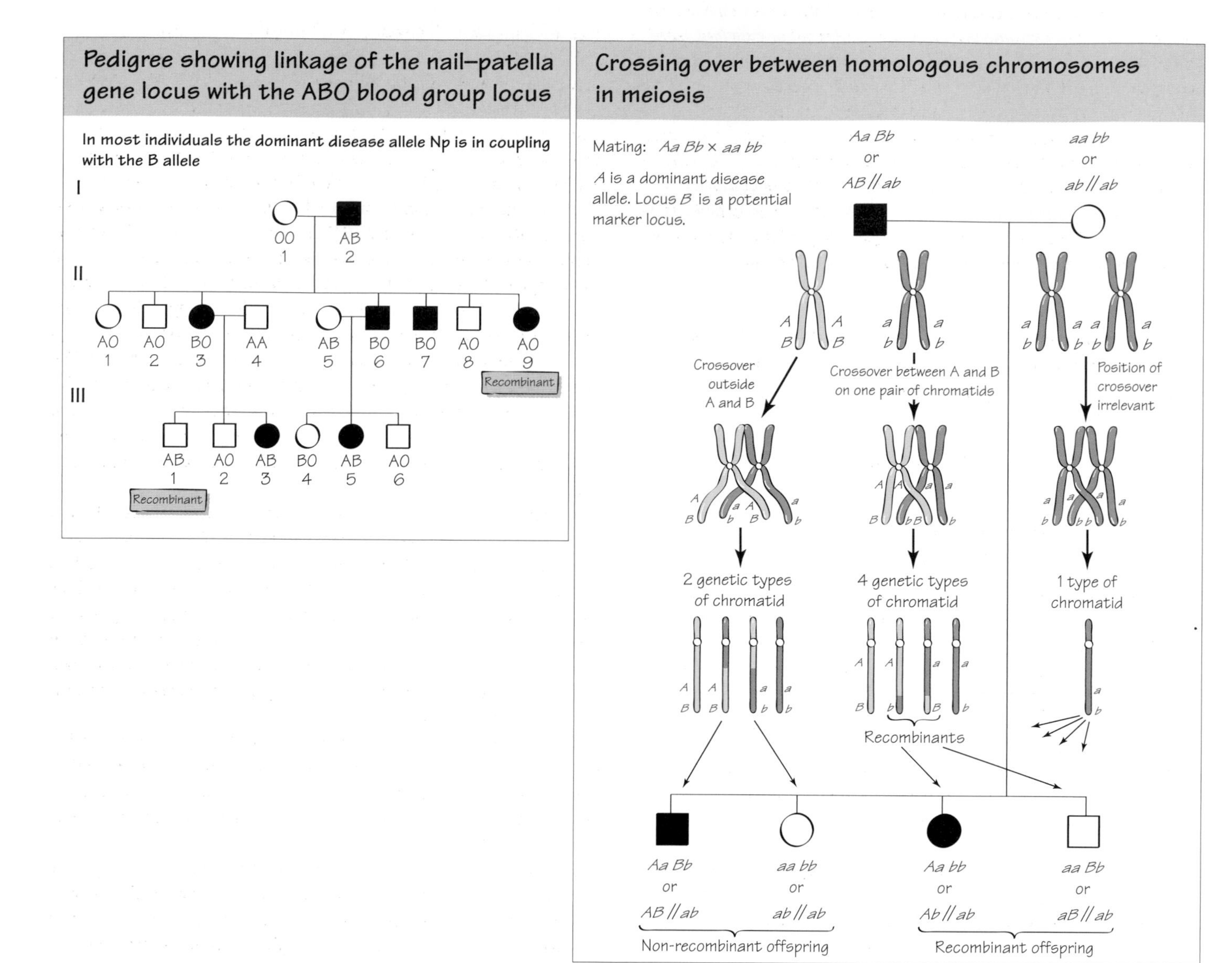

Overview

Genetic association refers to the appearance in many patients with disease of a second genetically determined character at a frequency higher than would be predicted on the basis of their independent frequencies. In a few cases this involves co-transmission of two causative genes, but in most it does not (see Chapters 43, 48). The term '**genetic linkage**' refers to the tendency for alleles close together on the same chromosome to be transmitted together to offspring, and this is the topic of this chapter. Genetic linkage is of very great value in genetic diagnosis.

Disease features can regularly occur together for several reasons, including pleiotropic expression of a single allele. The latter constitutes a syndrome. Distinction between a syndrome and the effects of linked genes depends largely on deducing logical causal relationships between the different features.

Genetic linkage

Assume two loci, ***A*** and ***B***, are close together on the same chromosome and we observe 'test matings' of type (i) ***AB//ab*** × ***ab//ab***, or type (ii) ***Ab//aB*** × ***ab//ab***, where '/' represents a chromosome. In type (i) matings, dominant alleles ***A*** and ***B*** are on the same chromosome and recessive alleles ***a*** and ***b*** on its homologue. The dominants and recessives are said to be '**in coupling**', or ***cis*** to one another. In matings of type (ii) the dominant and recessive alleles on opposite chromosomes are '**in repulsion**', or ***trans*** to one another.

Since loci A and B are close, chiasmata rarely occur between them and the parental combinations ***AB*** and ***ab***, or ***Ab*** and ***aB***, will be more frequently represented among offspring than the recombinant combinations ***Ab*** and ***aB***, or ***AB***, ***ab***, respectively.

Gregor Mendel was unaware of linkage and according to his principle of independent assortment (see Chapter 15), all four types of offspring: ***AaBb***, ***Aabb***, ***aaBb*** and ***aabb*** should be equally represented. When they are not, this is evidence of linkage.

If an allele of gene ***A*** causes disease, but is otherwise undetectable, whereas the alleles of gene ***B*** can be easily detected and distinguished, gene ***B*** can be used as a marker for the inherited disease. This is not completely reliable, as crossover occasionally occurs between them. For accurate prediction we need to know the **crossover frequency**, i.e. we need to '**map**' their relative positions. A marker locus five **map units** from a disease gene segregates from it in 5% of meioses, so predictions based on that marker are accurate in 95% of cases.

Historically important linkages are of ABO to **nail–patella syndrome** and of **secretor** to **myotonic dystrophy**. Currently the most useful markers are various types of DNA variant (see Part 3).

Genetic mapping

The genetic **map distance** between loci ***A*** and ***B*** can be deduced from the frequency of recombination between them, by the formula:

$$\frac{\text{Number of recombinant offspring} \times 100}{\text{Total number of offspring}}$$

i.e. in type (i) matings: $$\frac{(\boldsymbol{Aabb} + \boldsymbol{aaBb}) \times 100}{\boldsymbol{Aabb} + \boldsymbol{aaBb} + \boldsymbol{AaBb} + \boldsymbol{aabb}}$$

or, in type(ii): $$\frac{(\boldsymbol{AaBb} + \boldsymbol{aabb}) \times 100}{\boldsymbol{Aabb} + \boldsymbol{aaBb} + \boldsymbol{AaBb} + \boldsymbol{aabb}}$$

The unit of map distance is the **centiMorgan** (**cM**) and *map distances never exceed 50 cM*, as this corresponds to independent assortment, i.e. non-linkage.

Longer distances can be mapped by adding together the map distances between intermediate loci.

A gene map constructed from crossovers in males gives the same gene order as one constructed from the progeny of females, but the calculated 'distances' between them are often different. This is because chiasmata occur at different frequencies in the formation of ova and sperm. There are also 'hot spots' of high recombination frequency on some chromosomes.

The total map length of the genome, estimated from visible chiasmata in primary germ cells, is ~3000 cM in males and ~4200 cM in females. Since the haploid *physical* length of the genome is about 3000 million bp, 1 cM corresponds to about a million base pairs in males and 700 000 in females.

Other techniques of gene mapping and its diagnostic applications are discussed in Chapter 37 and Part 3.

LOD score analysis

The reliability of a suspected linkage can be confirmed by '**LOD score analysis**' of family pedigrees. The word LOD is derived from 'log of the odds'; the logarithm ($\log_{10}$) of the ratio of the probability that the observed ratio of offspring arose as a result of genetic linkage (of specified degree) to the probability that it arose merely by chance.

The **maximum LOD score** is the total value of the combined LODs, usually for a group of families, calculated at the most probable degree of linkage. *A value that exceeds +3 is accepted as evidence favouring autosomal linkage (or of +2 for linkage on the X); one of less than –2, of non-linkage.*

The Human Genome Mapping Project (HGMP)

Before the initiation of the HGMP in October 1990 a great deal was already known about the human gene map (see Chapter 37). The new project had three major goals: to create (i) a complete physical map of each chromosome; (ii) a fine scale map of molecular markers throughout the genome; and (iii) the complete 3000 million bp sequence.

The marker map is largely founded on the sites of **restriction fragment length polymorphisms** (**RFLPs**; see Chapter 56) and **variable number tandem repeats** (**VNTRs**; see Chapter 58) and they are spaced an average of 1 cM apart. This provides at least one molecular marker closely linked to every disease gene. In addition, many million **single nucleotide polymorphisms** (**SNPs**) were identified and located, which are especially useful in automated genome analysis (see Chapter 58). **Sequence tagged sites** (**STSs**) are DNA sequences flanked by PCR primers, that enable amplification of unique segments of DNA (see Chapter 57). These were invaluable for working on specific segments of the genome, such sites being found at intervals averaging around 100 kb.

Sequencing involved two simultaneous projects, one publicly and the other privately funded. The publicly funded effort used large fragments of cloned DNA, determined how they overlapped one another, and sequenced them. Identification of STSs within sequenced sections then enabled each detailed sequence to be positioned on the larger map. The private effort fragmented the DNA of one person, sequenced the fragments, and assembled them by identification of areas of overlap. The two were to some extent mutually dependent and resulted in similar sequences at around the same time.

Copies of expressed genes were also derived by reverse transcription of mRNA and mapped by correspondence of sequence. The complete map and sequence were revealed on April 14, 2003, exactly 50 years after Watson and Crick first proposed the accepted structure of DNA (see Chapter 4).

Possession of the human gene map and entire human DNA sequence has greatly increased accuracy and speed of diagnosis, and enhanced the prospect of gene therapy. It has accelerated the genetic engineering of protein pharmaceuticals and through **pharmacogenomics** promises to identify the most effective medications for individual patients (see Chapter 59).

This work offers the prospect of enormous advances in our understanding of how the various parts of the genome are expressed and integrated in their expression. It lays the foundations for the new discipline of **genomics**, which will place powerful new tools in the hands of physicians and permit new approaches to personalized prevention, diagnosis and treatment of disease.

Before the HGMP, the number of genes in our species was estimated at 100 000. We now believe it to be as low as 20 000 (considerably lower than that of many other species!), but we also now appreciate that many of those genes have multiple functions.

37 Gene mapping

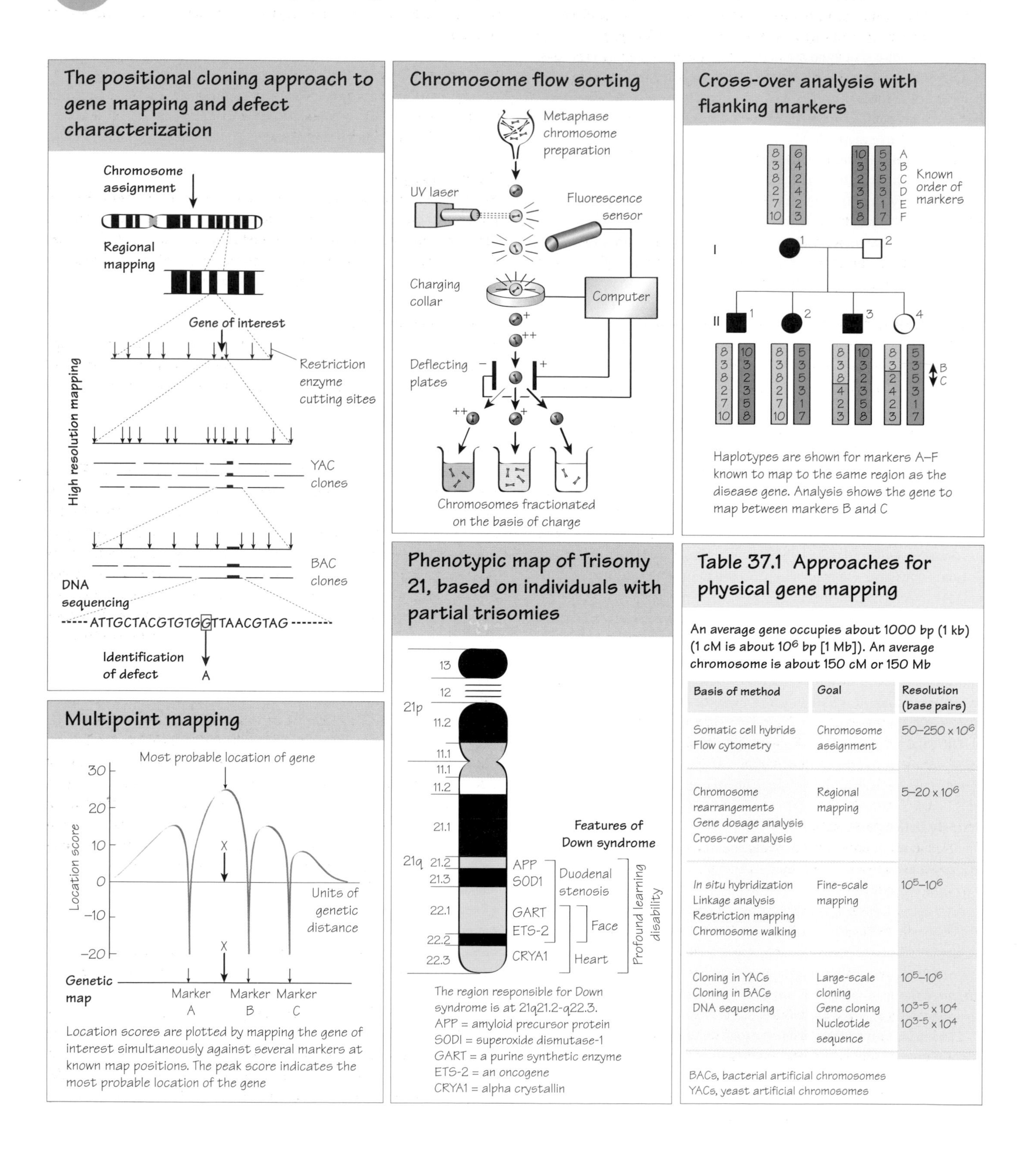

Haplotypes are shown for markers A–F known to map to the same region as the disease gene. Analysis shows the gene to map between markers B and C

Location scores are plotted by mapping the gene of interest simultaneously against several markers at known map positions. The peak score indicates the most probable location of the gene

The region responsible for Down syndrome is at 21q21.2-q22.3.
APP = amyloid precursor protein
SODl = superoxide dismutase-1
GART = a purine synthetic enzyme
ETS-2 = an oncogene
CRYA1 = alpha crystallin

Table 37.1 Approaches for physical gene mapping

An average gene occupies about 1000 bp (1 kb) (1 cM is about 10^6 bp [1 Mb]). An average chromosome is about 150 cM or 150 Mb

Basis of method	Goal	Resolution (base pairs)
Somatic cell hybrids Flow cytometry	Chromosome assignment	$50–250 \times 10^6$
Chromosome rearrangements Gene dosage analysis Cross-over analysis	Regional mapping	$5–20 \times 10^6$
In situ hybridization Linkage analysis Restriction mapping Chromosome walking	Fine-scale mapping	$10^5–10^6$
Cloning in YACs Cloning in BACs DNA sequencing	Large-scale cloning Gene cloning Nucleotide sequence	$10^5–10^6$ $10^{3-5} \times 10^4$ $10^{3-5} \times 10^4$

BACs, bacterial artificial chromosomes
YACs, yeast artificial chromosomes

Overview

There are two fundamentally different approaches to mapping human genes: **genetic mapping** involves measurement of the tendency of genes to co-segregate through meiosis (see Chapter 36); **physical mapping** deals with the assignment of genes to specific physical locations.

Gene mapping exercises generally progress through four stages:

1 chromosome assignment;
2 regional mapping;
3 high resolution mapping;
4 DNA sequencing (see Chapter 55).

Chromosome assignment

Patterns of transmission

Four locations are indicated by unique patterns of transmission. These are the X and Y chromosomes, the pseudo-autosomal region and the mitochondria (see Chapters16–23).

Chromosome flow-sorting, flow cytometry

A culture of dividing cells is arrested at metaphase (see Chapter 9) and the chromosomes released and stained with a fluorescent DNA stain. The preparation is then squirted through a fine jet, vertically downwards through an ultraviolet (UV) laser beam. As each chromosome fluoresces it acquires an electrical charge and is deflected by an electrical potential across its path. Deflection is proportional to intensity of fluorescence and this allows preparations of individual chomosomes to be amassed.

Such chromosome preparations can be used for making chromosome paints (see Chapter 50 and book cover) or chromosome-specific 'dot-blots' on nitrocellulose membranes. Sequences can then be assigned to chromosomes merely by testing their capacity to hybridize with the dot-blots (see Chapter 56).

Somatic cell hybrids

A **somatic cell hybrid** is produced by fusing together two somatic cells or by incorporating a foreign genome into a cell. By careful selection, cloning and long-term maintenance it is possible to create cultures of mouse–human cells containing a single human chromosome along with most of the mouse genome. Chromosome assignment of the genes for human proteins synthesized in such cultures is then a matter of recognizing the human chromosome present.

Regional mapping

Family linkage studies

The frequency of cross-over between loci relates inversely to the physical distance between them, by a mathematical expression called **the mapping function**.

Autosomal traits have been assigned on the basis of co-transmission with cytogenetic features such as translocation breakpoints, or linkage to already assigned markers, an early objective being the identification of DNA markers at 10 cM intervals throughout the genome (see Chapter 36).

When many loci are involved, advanced computer programs integrate linkage data in '**multipoint maps**' to produce '**location scores**' (c.f. LOD scores for single genes; see Chapter 36).

Restriction mapping

DNA is digested with a restriction enzyme and subjected to electrophoresis, etc., as described for Southern blotting (see Chapter 56). By use of several enzymes that cleave DNA at different sites, it is possible to order the fragments by recognizing regions of overlap.

Cross-over analysis

This approach aims to map a gene by defining its haplotype with respect to adjacent markers before and after cross-over (see figure 'Cross-over analysis with flanking markers').

Gene dosage

Normally every individual has two copies of every autosomal gene. Exceptions include heterozygotes for a deletion, and trisomics. Among these, the amount of primary gene product varies threefold. The location of a gene can sometimes be determined by relating quantity of enzyme to the chromosomal breakpoints (see figure).

In situ hybridization

The technique of FISH provides a spectacular approach to gene mapping (see Chapter 50). If a probe recognizes a specific gene sequence, both chromosomal and regional assignment is straightforward.

High resolution mapping

Cloning

A range of advanced techniques, such as **chromosome microdissection**, **jumping** and **walking**, involve mass production of DNA fragments of a variety of lengths. Before PCR was developed (see Chapter 57) the only way to amplify a chosen gene sequence was by cloning in a microorganism. The basic idea is to insert the gene into a bacterial **plasmid**, or **bacteriophage** and allow this to proliferate in a bacterial culture (see Chapter 56). Larger DNA fragments are cloned in artificial bacterial vectors called **cosmids** and **bacterial artificial chromosomes** (**BACs**), very large ones (50–1000 kb) in **yeast artificial chromosomes** (**YACs**).

Fibre-FISH

Chromosomes are extended at interphase and this can be exploited to map genes by an adaptation of FISH called **fibre-FISH** or **DIRVISH** (**dir**ect **vis**ualization **h**ybridization). A liquid preparation of interphase DNA is applied to a microscope slide, which is tilted, causing the liquid to run down the slide and the chromosomes to become stretched along its length. Fluorescent probes directed against genes known to map to the same region are added to the slide and allowed to hybridize, when the order of the fluorescent spots indicates that of the genes along the chromosome.

Two basic strategies for mapping genes

The **positional cloning approach** involves mapping the disease gene by conventional linkage analysis with respect to the nearest reliable marker.

An alternative is the **candidate gene approach**. In this, one identifies genes known to map to the indicated region, or to have a role in relevant physiology. Patients are then screened for variants of these candidate genes. In both cases the gene is eventually isolated and the molecular defect(s) associated with disease deduced by sequencing (see Chapter 55).

38 Mutagenesis and DNA repair

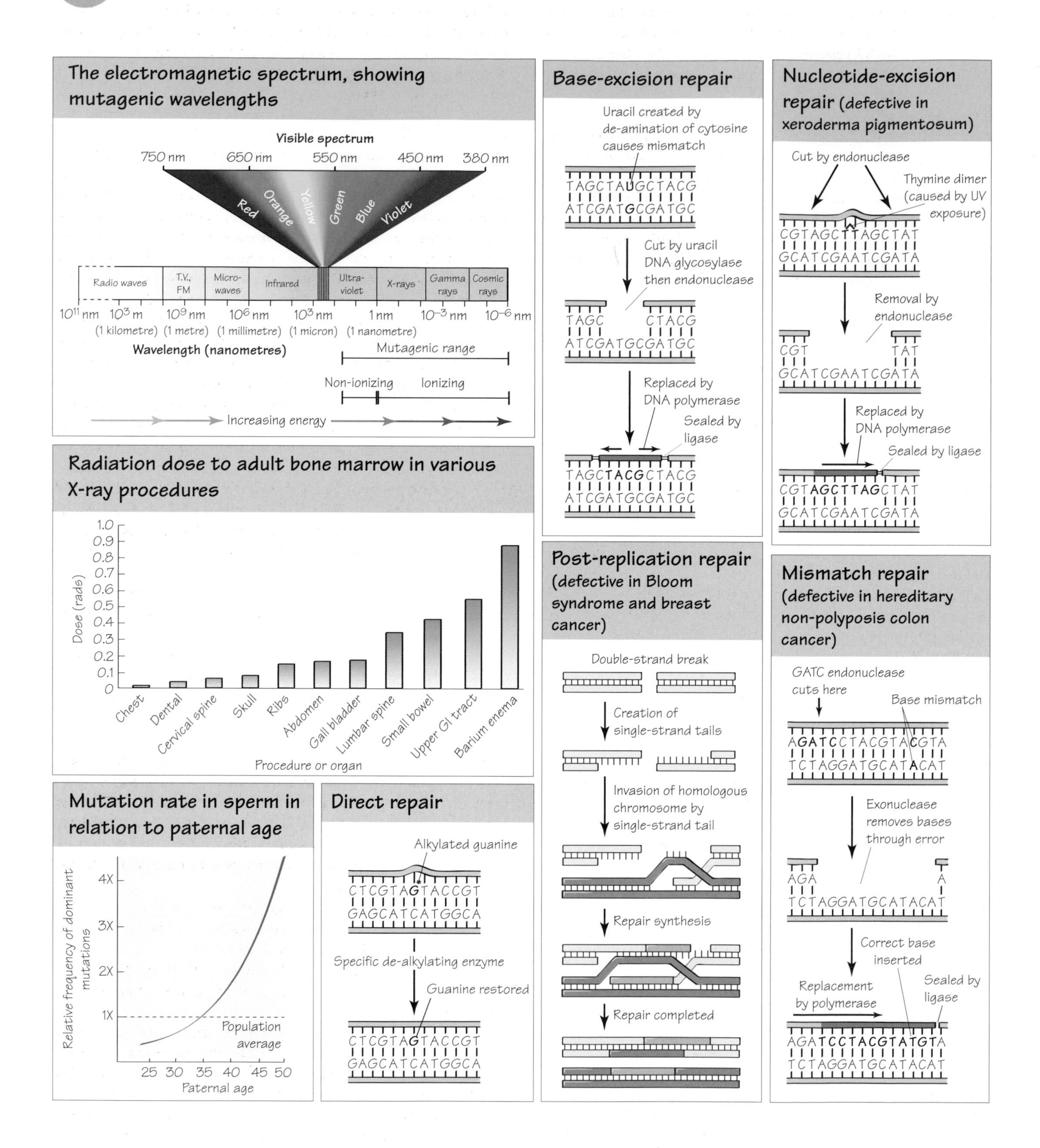

Overview

Apart from the effects of ultraviolet (UV) light, mutagenesis of the DNA in somatic cells is no different from that in the germline. Some is **spontaneous**, caused by a base adopting a variant molecular form or **tautomer** during DNA replication; most is initiated by chemicals and 10–15% by radiation. For the natural mutation rate, see Chapter 16.

Chemical mutagenesis

Environmental **mutagens** include constituents of smoke, paints, petrochemicals, pesticides, dyes, foodstuffs, drugs, etc. **Promutagens**, such as *nitrates* and *nitrites* are converted into mutagens by body chemistry. Examples of the major categories of mutagen are given below.

1 **Base analogues.** *2-amino-purine* is incorporated into DNA in place of adenine, but pairs as cytosine, causing a **substitution** of thymine by guanine in the partner strand. *5-bromouracil* (5-BU) is incorporated as thymine, but can undergo a tautomeric shift to resemble cytosine, resulting in a **transition** from T-A to C-G.

2 **Chemical modifiers.** *Nitrous acid* converts cytosine to uracil, and adenine to hypoxanthine, a precursor of guanine. *Alkylating agents* modify bases by donating alkyl-groups.

3 **Intercalating agents.** The antiseptic *proflavine* and the *acridine dyes* become inserted between adjacent base pairs, producing distortions in the DNA that lead to **deletions** and **additions**.

4 **Other.** A wide range of other chemicals cause DNA **strand breakage** and **cross-linking**.

The principal means of exposure are inhalation, skin absorption and ingestion.

Electromagnetic radiation

Particulate discharge from radioactive decay includes alpha-particles (helium nuclei), beta-particles (electrons) and gamma-rays. The mutagenicity of subatomic particles depends on their speed, mass and electric charge.

The mutagenicity of electromagnetic radiation increases with decreasing wavelength. All radiation beyond UV causes ionization by knocking electrons out of their orbits.

Ultraviolet light

UV light is the non-visible, short wavelength fraction of sunlight responsible for tanning. It exerts a mutagenic effect by causing **dimerization** (linking) of adjacent pyrimidine residues, mainly T-T (but also T-C and C-C). It does not cause germline mutations, but is a major cause of skin cancer, especially in homozygotes for the red hair allele (see Chapter 15), who have white, freckled skin. Their phaeomelanin pigment provides a poor sun screen and also releases free radicals on UV exposure.

Most UV radiation from the sun is blocked by a thin layer of ozone in the upper atmosphere, but this is currently under destruction by industrial *fluorocarbons*.

Atomic radiation

1 **Natural background radiation.** This varies with local geology. The most abundant radioisotopes are Potassium-40 and Radon-222 gas. Radon contributes 55% of all natural background radiation and may be responsible for 2500 deaths per annum in the UK.

2 **Cosmic rays.** These present a major theoretical hazard for aircrews, as their intensity increases with altitude. Exposure during a return flight between England and Spain may equal five chest X-rays.

3 **Man-made radiation.** This includes fallout from nuclear testing and power stations. Radiation workers are at particular risk and bone-surface-seeking isotopes present a major risk of leukaemia.

4 **X-rays.** X-rays account for 60% of man-made and 11% of total radiation exposure. They mutagenize DNA either directly by ionizing impact, or indirectly by creating highly reactive **free radicals** that impinge on the DNA. These can be carried in the bloodstream and harm cells not directly exposed.

Biological effects of radiation

Electromagnetic radiation damages proteins and above 100 rads kills cells. (One **rad** is the amount of radiation that causes one gram of tissue to absorb 100 ergs of energy.) At the chromosomal level it causes **major deletions**, **translocations** and **aneuploidy** (see Table 60.1). It causes **single-** and **double-strand breaks** in DNA and **base pair destruction**. X-rays damage chromosomes most readily when they are condensed, which is why they are most harmful to dividing cells, including the progenitors of sperm. The offspring of older men have a many-fold risk of genetic disease, as the DNA in their sperm has been copied many times (see figure). The high testicular temperature caused by clothing (6°C above unclothed) has been estimated to be responsible for half the present mutation rate in human sperm.

For the first 7 days of life the embryo is ultra-sensitive to the mutagenic and lethal effects of X-rays; over weeks 2–7 teratogenic effects come to the fore. Childhood leukaemia can be induced by exposure at gestational weeks 8 to 40.

At 100 rads X-rays cause a 50% reduction in white blood cell count, while whole-body irradiation of 450 rads kills 50% of people. Therapeutic doses of up to 1000 rads are used against cancer cells. Radiation damage is cumulative and there is no lower baseline of effect.

Safety measures when using X-rays

1 Patients' previous X-ray exposure should be reviewed before requesting further X-rays.

2 The '28-day rule': a woman of child-bearing age should be X-rayed only if she has had a period within the last 28 days.

3 Patients with DNA repair deficiencies should NEVER be X-rayed.

DNA repair

Apart from direct repair, all the DNA repair systems in human cells require **exonucleases**, **endonucleases** (defective in **Cocayne syndrome**), **polymerases** and **ligases**. **Ataxia telangiectasia** and **Fanconi anaemia** patients have defects in DNA damage detection and are extremely sensitive to X-rays (see also Chapter 41).

1 **Direct repair.** A specific enzyme reverses the damage, e.g. by de-alkylation of alkylated guanine.

2 **Base-excision repair.** The damaged base, plus a few others on either side, are removed by cutting the sugar-phosphate backbone and the gap filled by re-synthesis directed by the intact strand.

3 **Nucleotide excision repair.** This removes **thymine dimers** and chemically modified bases over a longer stretch of DNA. Defects cause **xeroderma pigmentosum**.

4 **Mismatch repair.** This corrects base mismatches due to errors at DNA replication and involves nicking the faulty strand at the nearest GATC base sequence. Defects occur in **hereditary non-polyposis colon cancer**. The genes involved are sometimes called '**mutator genes**'.

5 **Postreplication repair.** This corrects double-strand breaks either unguided, or by using the homologous chromosome as a template. Defects include **Bloom syndrome** (a **'chromosome breakage syndrome'**), **breast cancer** and possibly **prostate cancer**.

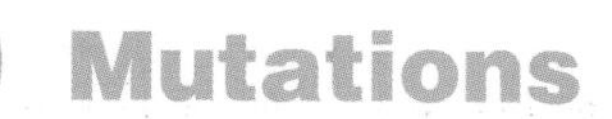
39 Mutations

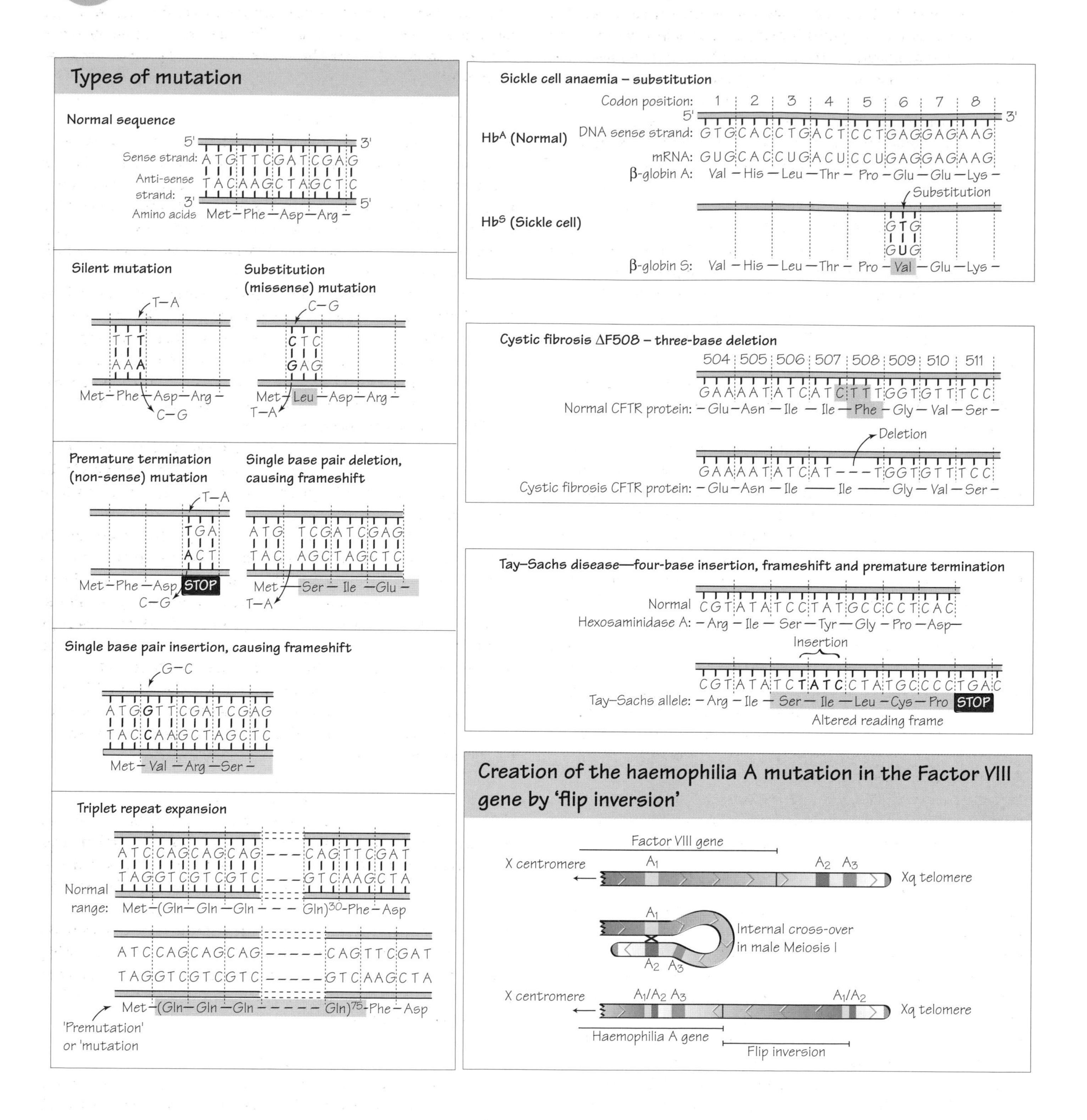
Types of mutation
Normal sequence
5' 3'
Sense strand: ATG TTC GAT CGA G
Anti-sense strand: TAC AAG CTA GCT C
3' 5'
Amino acids Met – Phe – Asp – Arg –
Silent mutation
T–A
TTT
AAA
Met – Phe – Asp – Arg –
C–G
Substitution (missense) mutation
C–G
CTC
GAG
Met – Leu – Asp – Arg –
T–A
Premature termination (non-sense) mutation
T–A
TGA
ACT
Met – Phe – Asp STOP
C–G
Single base pair deletion, causing frameshift
ATG TCG ATC GAG
TAC AGC TAG CTC
Met – Ser – Ile – Glu –
T–A
Single base pair insertion, causing frameshift
G–C
ATG GTT CGA TCG AG
TAC CAA GCT AGC TC
Met – Val – Arg – Ser –
Triplet repeat expansion
ATC CAG CAG CAG – – – CAG TTC GAT
TAG GTC GTC GTC – – – GTC AAG CTA
Normal range: Met – (Gln – Gln – Gln – – – Gln)30 – Phe – Asp
ATC CAG CAG CAG – – – – – CAG TTC GAT
TAG GTC GTC GTC – – – – – GTC AAG CTA
Met – (Gln – Gln – Gln – – – – – Gln)75 – Phe – Asp
'Premutation' or 'mutation
Sickle cell anaemia – substitution
Codon position: 1 2 3 4 5 6 7 8
5' 3'
HbA (Normal)
DNA sense strand: GTG CAC CTG ACT CCT GAG GAG AAG
mRNA: GUG CAC CUG ACU CCU GAG GAG AAG
β-globin A: Val – His – Leu – Thr – Pro – Glu – Glu – Lys –
Substitution
HbS (Sickle cell)
GTG
GUG
β-globin S: Val – His – Leu – Thr – Pro – Val – Glu – Lys –
Cystic fibrosis ΔF508 – three-base deletion
504 505 506 507 508 509 510 511
GAA AAT ATC ATC TTT GGT GTT TCC
Normal CFTR protein: – Glu – Asn – Ile – Ile – Phe – Gly – Val – Ser –
Deletion
GAA AAT ATC AT – – – TGG TGT TTC C
Cystic fibrosis CFTR protein: – Glu – Asn – Ile — Ile — Gly – Val – Ser –
Tay–Sachs disease—four-base insertion, frameshift and premature termination
Normal CGT ATA TCC TAT GCC CCT CAC
Hexosaminidase A: – Arg – Ile – Ser – Tyr – Gly – Pro – Asp –
Insertion
CGT ATA TCT ATC CTA TGC CCC TGA C
Tay–Sachs allele: – Arg – Ile – Ser – Ile – Leu – Cys – Pro STOP
Altered reading frame
Creation of the haemophilia A mutation in the Factor VIII gene by 'flip inversion'
Factor VIII gene
X centromere
A1
A2 A3
Xq telomere
Internal cross-over in male Meiosis I
A1
A2 A3
X centromere
A1/A2 A3
A1/A2
Xq telomere
Haemophilia A gene
Flip inversion

Overview

Mutations are permanent modifications of DNA. They include aneuploidies (see Chapters 24, 25), chromosome rearrangements (see Chapter 26), **point mutations**, involving **substitution**, **deletion** or **insertion** of a base pair, DNA **duplications** and **inversions** and RNA processing mutations.

Large deletions and insertions can be created by **unequal crossing over** between misaligned segments of repetitious DNA causing, for example, anomalous colour vision (see figure in Chapter 22).

Dynamic mutations are progressive and involve expansion of **triplet repeat sequences** (see Chapter 21).

Substitutions, deletions, insertions, frameshifts and duplications

Substitution involves replacement of a base pair. If the amino acid coded by the new codon is the same, it is a **silent mutation**, or if different, a **missense mutation**. Most missense mutations are harmful, but a notable exception is the substitution of the sixth codon in the β-globin chain responsible for sickle cell anaemia (see Chapter 34), which in heterozygotes confers resistance to *falciparum* malaria.

Substitution can create a STOP codon, causing translation to come to a premature halt. This is called a **premature termination** or **non-sense mutation**.

If a deleted or inserted segment is of other than a multiple of three bases, apart from loss or gain of coding information, the translation reading frame is also disrupted in a **frameshift mutation**. This causes the protein produced to be entirely erroneous 'downstream' (3′) of the deletion. The most common mutation causing **Tay–Sachs disease** (see Chapter 18) is a four-base insertion causing a frameshift and leading to premature termination, so that no functional **hexosaminidase A** is synthesized.

Duplications of whole genes can lead to disease, e.g. Charcot–Marie–Tooth disease. This is a peripheral nervous system disease involving progressive atrophy of distal limb muscles. It can be caused by a variety of types of mutation, but about 70% have a large duplication of chromosome 17 that includes the gene PMP22 encoding a peripheral myelin protein. This contributes to demyelination, whereas deletion of the same region causes a paralytic response to pressure.

Transcriptional control

Mutations in the flanking regions of genes can have quantitative effects by inhibiting binding of RNA polymerase or transcription factors, as in the **Factor IX** gene 5′ region, causing **haemophilia B**.

RNA processing

Splicing mutants either directly affect hnRNA donor or acceptor sites (see Chapter 7), or activate cryptic competitive splice sites in introns or exons. The acceptor sequence at the end of the first intron of β-globin is UUAGGCU, while within that intron is a sequence that differs by two bases: UUGGUCU. In some beta-thalassaemia patients the latter is modified to UUAGUCU. Since this differs by only one base from the normal acceptor, it gets misidentified as the acceptor, the hnRNA is cut in the wrong place and the mRNA erroneously retains some intron bases. This in turn introduces a frameshift, causing 'CUU AGG' to be read as '-CU **UAG** G-'. Translation ceases prematurely because UAG is a STOP signal, resulting in **β⁺-thalassaemia** (see below).

In one RNA processing mutation an A-to-C transition of the first nucleotide of the β-globin messenger inhibits capping, while in another, substitution of U by C in the trailer sequence AAUAAA inhibits polyadenylation (see Chapter 7). Both fail to suppress rapid degradation of the messenger.

Mobile elements

SINE and Alu DNA repeats (see Chapter 4) can propagate independently and insert at other locations, causing frameshift mutations. This has caused isolated cases of neurofibromatosis, Duchenne muscular dystrophy, beta-thalassemia, breast cancer, familial polyposis coli and haemophilia.

Haemoglobinopathies

The thalassaemias are collectively the most common single gene disorder, in all of which there is reduced level of synthesis of either the α- or β-globin chain (see Chapter 34). In the absence of a complementary chain with which to form the haemoglobin tetramer (α2β2), the chain produced at the normal rate is in relative excess and precipitates out, damaging the red cell membranes and leading to their premature destruction.

There are at least 80 different **beta-thalassaemia** alleles, in addition to the RNA splicing error above (see Table 34.2). Most of these are point mutations and most patients are '**compound homozygotes**', with two *different* deficient alleles. Carriers of one beta-thalassaemia allele have slight anaemia and are said to have **β⁺-thalassaemia**, or **thalassaemia minor**. If no β-globin is present, the condition is **β°-thalassaemia**, or **thalassaemia major**.

In **hereditary persistence of fetal haemoglobin**, the β-globin gene has been deleted and the neighbouring γ-globin gene responsible for **fetal haemoglobin** (α2γ2) remains transcriptionally active at a high level after birth.

Alpha-globin is coded by *two pairs* of genes per diploid genome. In the 'heterozygous' state, called **alpha-thalassaemia trait**, there are two mutant and two normal genes; either –α/–α, or – –/αα (see Table 34.1). The latter is relatively common in South-East Asia and gives rise to completely α-globin deficient homozygotes (– –/– –) with **hydrops fetalis**. The (–α) haplotype is more common than normal (αα) among Melanesians, having been selected by malaria (see Chapter 34).

In **Haemoglobin Constant Spring** the UAA α-globin STOP codon is mutated to CAA, coding for glutamine, and translation continues for a further 31 frames to another STOP. The mutant mRNA is unstable, causing mild alpha-thalassaemia.

Haemophilia A (see also Chapter 22)

Fifty per cent of severe cases of haemophilia A (i.e. with $< 1\%$ Factor VIII activity) involve a novel mutation called a **flip inversion**. This occurs as a consequence of two unusual conditions: (i) the existence of several copies of a small gene called A located near the Xq telomere, plus another within intron 22 of the Factor VIII gene; and (ii) the fact that the long arm of the X has no pairing homologue in male meiosis. As a consequence, internal recombination sometimes occurs following looping back of the end of the X. Breakage and rejoining within the A genes causes inversion of the intervening segment of the Factor VIII gene, with loss of function.

Nomenclature of mutations

Mutations are named by conventional abbreviations. For example, the most common mutation responsible for cystic fibrosis (see Chapter 18) is **ΔF508**. The symbol 'Δ' denotes a deletion, F stands for phenylalanine, and 508 indicates the location of the mutation in the coding sequence of the gene for the '**cystic fibrosis trans-membrane regulator**' (**CFTR**). The **G380R** achondroplasia mutation is a substitution of glycine (G) by arginine (R) at amino acid 380 within the FGFR3 gene (see the single letter amino acid code, Chapter 8 and Chapter 17).

40 The molecular biology of cancer

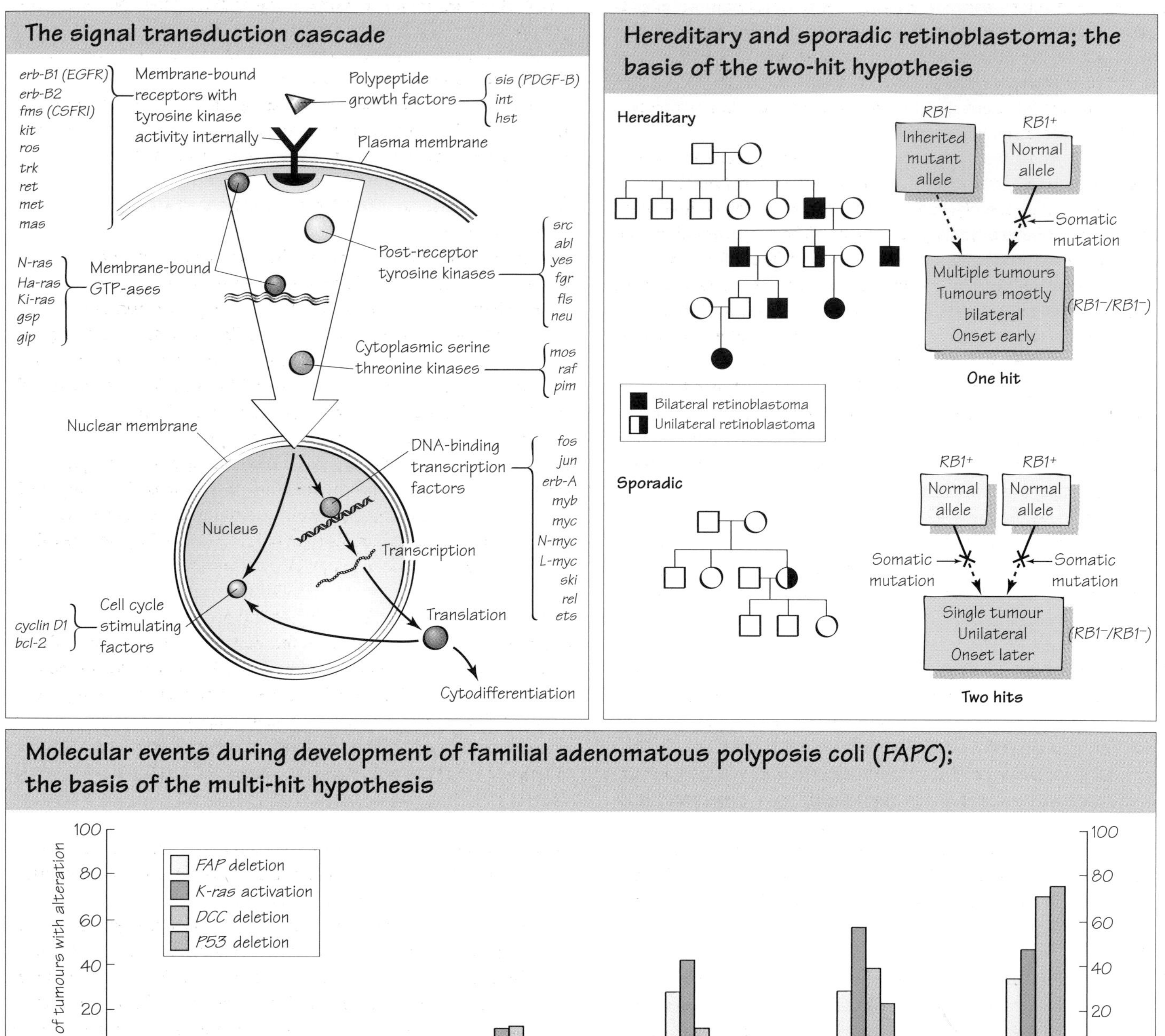

Molecular events during development of familial adenomatous polyposis coli (FAPC); the basis of the multi-hit hypothesis

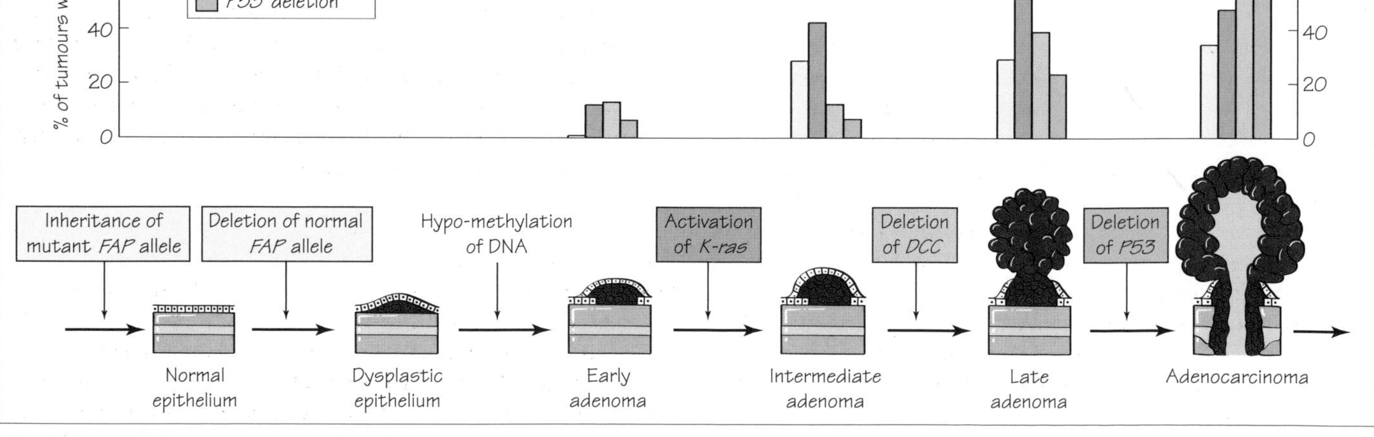

Overview

Normal progress through the cell cycle is promoted by polypeptide **growth factors** that bind to specific receptors on the cell surface. Their presence is conveyed to the nucleus by a series of phosphorylations of **kinases** (phosphate-attaching enzymes) that constitute the **signal transduction cascade** (**STC**). Phosphorylated **DNA binding proteins** then bind to specific sites in the DNA and promote transition to the next phase of the cycle. The genes that code for the (normal) proteins involved in the STC are **proto-oncogenes**. Cancer-causing derivatives are called **oncogenes**.

Progress through the cycle is moderated by the protein products of the **mitosis suppressor** (or '**tumour suppressor**') **genes** (see Chapter 9) and cancers are frequently initiated by their failure, sometimes indicated by **loss of heterozygosity** at that locus. The properties of tumour suppressor genes and oncogenes are compared in Table 41.1.

Cancer cells can invade neighbouring tissues or undergo **metastasis**, i.e. break up and move in the blood to establish **secondary tumours**.

If a tumour shows sustained proliferation and spread it is said to be '**malignant**', being capable of causing death, most often by pressure or occlusion. Malignant cells typically lack **contact inhibition of movement**, **density dependent inhibition of growth** and the normal requirement of a rigid substratum for mitosis, allowing them to invade and proliferate to abnormal extent. '**Benign**' tumours usually do not spread, either by local invasion or metastasis.

Environmental triggers

Most mutagens (see Chapter 38) can trigger **carcinogenesis**; non-mutagenic cancer-promoting chemicals generally operate by activation of kinases.

Viruses

Viruses can '**transform**' normal cells into cancer cells by insertion of a viral promoter beside a host proto-oncogene (as with **Epstein–Barr virus** in some cases of Burkitt lymphoma), or by introduction of a viral genome that already carries an oncogene. Some of the latter are replication-competent **transforming viruses**, but in most cases an additional '**helper virus**' is needed for replication.

DNA viruses implicated in human cancer include **papilloma**, Epstein–Barr and **hepatitis B**. Oncogenic RNA retroviruses include **T-cell leukaemia virus** and **Kaposi sarcoma associated herpes virus**.

The signal transduction cascade

1 Growth factors. Growth factors promote transition from G0 to G1 (see Chapter 9). The best-known is *c-sis*, identical to the B subunit of **platelet derived growth factor**. Two others, *hst* and *int-2*, have been found amplified in stomach cancers and malignant melanomas respectively.

2 Growth factor receptors. Growth factor receptors span the cell membrane and have tyrosine kinase properties at their cytoplasmic ends. An example is *c-erb-B*, which encodes **epidermal growth factor receptor**. Activation of *erb-B2* independently of growth factor stimulation is associated with cancer of the stomach, pancreas and ovary.

3 Post-receptor tyrosine kinases. The target of kinase activity of the growth factor receptor is characteristically a **post-receptor tyrosine kinase**, which in turn phosphorylates another cytoplasmic kinase that phosphorylates a third, and so on.

4 Serine threonine kinases. Some steps in the STC involve phosphorylation of serine or threonine residues by, for example, the *raf* protein. Mutant versions of *raf* maintain continuous transmission of the growth-promoting signal.

5 GTPases. Phosphate for kinase activity is largely supplied by ATP, but the intracellular membranes carry GTPases also, including multiple *ras* proteins. Mutations resulting in increased or sustained GTPase activity lead to continuous growth.

6 DNA binding proteins and cell cycle factors. DNA-binding oncoproteins control expression of genes concerned with the cell cycle. Over-production of *myc* and *myb*, which stimulate transition from G1 to S-phase, prevents cells from entering G0.

Loss of factors that normally cause **apoptosis** (cell death) results in tumour build up and activation of *bcl-2*, through chromosome rearrangement, inhibiting apoptosis in some lymphomas.

Conversion of proto-oncogenes to oncogenes

1 Point mutation. Thirty per cent of tumours contain mutated versions of a *ras* protein that is unable to adopt the inactive form.

2 Translocation. Examples are the Philadelphia chromosome (see Chapter 27) and translocations of *myc* on Chromosome 8, to alongside the promoters of the Ig heavy chain on Chromosome 14, the κ light chain on 2 or the λ light chain on 22 (see Chapter 42). These are found in at least 90% of cases of Burkitt lymphoma (see Chapter 41).

3 Insertional mutagenesis. See 'Viruses' above.

4 Amplification. In 10% of tumours are tiny, supernumerary pieces of DNA called **double-minute chromosomes** composed of amplified copies of a proto-oncogene, e.g. of *N-myc* in some neuroblastomas and *erb-B2* in breast cancers. If inserted into chromosomes they are detectable as **homogeneously staining regions**, or **HSRs**.

'The guardian of the genome', p53

Point mutations and deletions of the tumour suppressor gene **TP53** occur in 70% of all tumours. Its protein, p53, contributes to the G1 block and so allows time for DNA defects to be detected and repaired. Protein p53 also mediates commitment to apoptosis.

Li–Fraumeni syndrome, due to a germline defect in TP53, is notable for its assortment of tumours (see Chapter 41).

The two-hit hypothesis

Retinoblastoma, can be: (a) sporadic, unilateral, with average age of onset 30 months; or (b) familial, bilateral, with average age of onset 14 months and accompanied by other cancers.

The normal allele for retinoblastoma is a tumour suppressor that blocks mitosis of retinal cells at the G1/S transition. Knudson's **two-hit hypothesis** proposed that cancer develops only if *both* RB alleles are inactive. In familial cases one lesion is inherited. Only one further mutation *in any retinal cell* is necessary, so it occurs much earlier than in normal homozygotes (see figure 'Hereditary and sporadic retinoblastoma: the basis of the two-hit hypothesis').

The multi-hit hypothesis

Cancer of the colon

In **familial adenomatous polyposis** (**coli**) or (**FAP**(**C**)), inheritance of a single mutant tumour suppressor allele is associated with multiple benign polyps (**adenomas**) of the colon lining. Progression toward an **adenocarcinoma** begins with deletion of the normal allele. Subsequent steps involve activation of the *K-ras* oncogene and deletion of P53 (see Chapter 41). Deletion of the **Deleted in Colorectal Carcinoma** (**DCC**) gene initiates cell surface changes and further mutation promotes metastasis and early death. The specific mutations described are characteristic, but can occur in any order (see figure).

41 Familial cancers

A pedigree for Li–Fraumeni syndrome showing breast cancer, sarcomas and other malignancies, with general susceptibility to cancer inherited in a dominant fashion (From Li, F. P. (1998) *Cancer Research* 48; 5381–6)

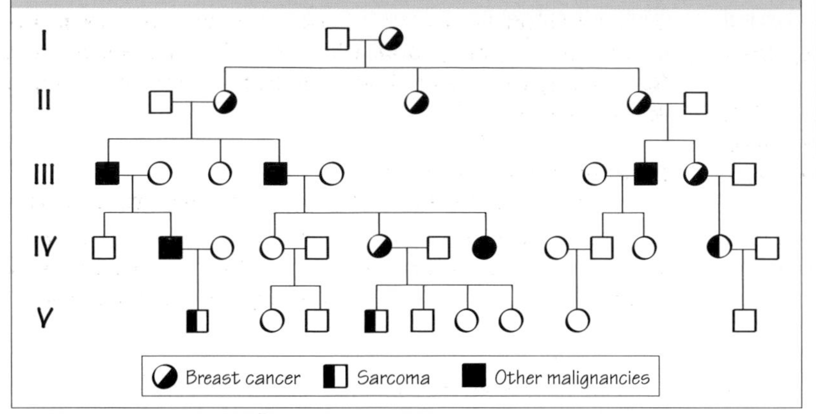

Table 41.1 Comparison of the properties of oncogenes and tumour suppressor genes

Oncogenes	Tumour suppressor genes
(Over-) active in tumour	Normal allele inactive in tumour
(Over-) activity associated with translocation or substitution	Abnormality due to deletion or specific mutation of normal allele
Abnormality rarely inherited	Abnormality can be inherited
Dominant at cellular level	Recessive at cellular level
Broad tissue specificity	Considerable tumour specificity
Frequently causative of leukaemia and lymphoma	Causative of solid tumours

Typical 8:14 translocation causing Burkitt lymphoma

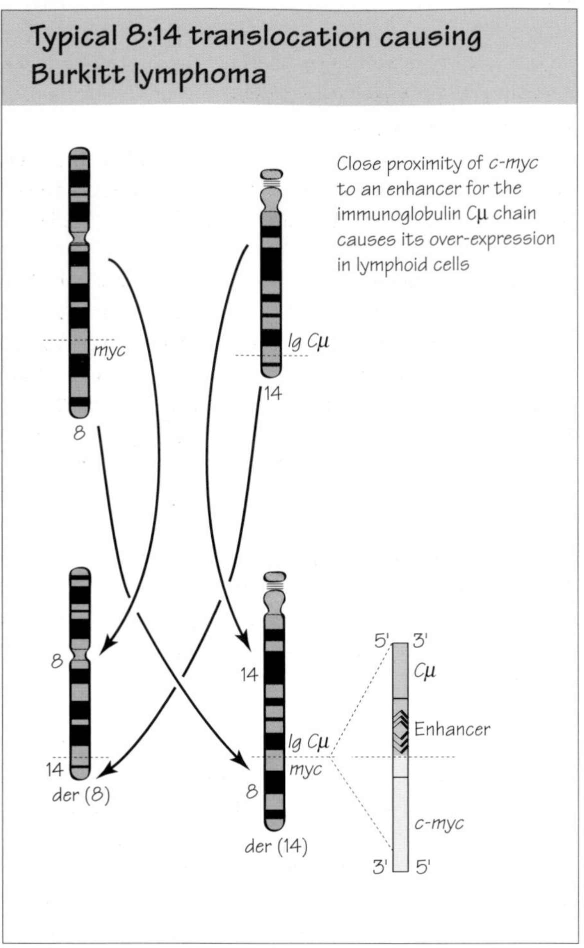

Overview

All cancer is genetic at the level of the cell. **Oncogenesis**, i.e. cancer development, is a multi-stage process during which a cell accumulates damage in several critical genes related to mitosis and/or cell differentiation, such as the proto-oncogenes (see Chapter 40). A small proportion develop as a consequence of genetic predisposition that includes pale (e.g. northern European) skin pigmentation, red hair with associated freckling (see Chapter 15) and defective DNA repair genes (see Chapter 38). Dominant inheritance patterns are generally due to a defective tumour suppressor gene (coding for a mitosis suppressor protein, see Table 41.1; see also 'comparative genome hybridization', Chapter 50).

Indicators of inherited cancer

Familial clusters can be caused by shared environments; the following are pointers to *genetic* causation of cancer.

1 Several close relatives with the same, or genetically associated cancers.
2 Two family members with the same rare cancer.
3 Unusually early age of onset.
4 Bilateral tumours in paired organs.
5 Non-clonal multifocal or successive tumours in the same tissue, or in different organ systems of the same individual.

DNA repair genes

Recessive DNA repair defects

See Chapter 38.

Damage detection errors

Ataxia telangiectasia AR; frequency: 1/50 000. There is hypersensitivity to X-rays, rearrangement of Chromosomes 7 and 14, cerebellar degeneration and enlargement of capillaries (**telangiectasis**) in the conjunctivae and facial skin. A 35% risk of lymphoreticular malignancy leads to early death in 30% of cases.

Fanconi anaemia AR; 1/350 000. There is undue sensitivity to DNA cross-linking agents, with chromosome breakage, and a 5–10% risk of leukaemia and carcinomas.

Nucleotide excision repair defects

Xeroderma pigmentosum (XP) AR, at least seven types; 1/250 000. Errors in pyrimidine dimer excision lead to multiple skin cancers, with corneal scarring and early death.

Post-replication repair errors

Bloom syndrome AR There is a 10-fold increased rate of sister chromatid exchange typically associated with short stature and increased risk of leukaemia, lymphoma and carcinoma. The defective gene is a **DNA helicase**.

Tumour suppressor genes

Dominant DNA repair defects

DNA mismatch repair

Hereditary non-polyposis colon cancer (HNPCC) AD. **HNPCC** accounts for 2–5% of cases of inherited colorectal cancer, germline mutations being associated with an 85% risk, compared to a population risk of 6%.

At least five genes are involved in mismatch repair. Protein MSH2 binds with MSH6 (or MSH3) and slides along the DNA to detect single-base mismatches (or mismatch loops). MLH1 and PMS2 (or PMS1) then bind to the complex and coordinate subsequent repair activity. Defects in any of these result in HNPCC, those in MSLH and MSH2 being the most common; malignancies also occur in other organs and affected women have a 40–60% risk of endometrial cancer.

Post-replication repair

Familial breast cancer, BRCA1, BRCA2 AD; ~1/200. One in eight British women develop breast and/or ovarian cancer, about 5% of these having inherited susceptibility. BRCA1 and 2 account for well over half of these. The age-related penetrance for ovarian cancer is 40–60% for BRCA1, 10–20% for BRCA2.

Prostate cancer Possibly AD. This is the second most common cancer in white males (after skin cancer), with a lifetime risk of 10% and a median onset age of 72 years. Five to ten per cent of cases and possibly 40% of early onset cases (< 55 years) are probably inherited. Men carrying **BRCA1** or **BRCA2** have a 16% risk by age 70 years (c.f. 4% of the general population). There are several additional susceptibility loci, including that for **ribonuclease L**, thought to be a tumour suppressor.

Cell cycle block defects

Familial retinoblastoma AD with 90% penetrance; frequency: 1/18 000 (see Chapter 40).

Li–Fraumeni syndrome AD. This is due to an inherited defect in the gene for protein p53 (see figure and Chapter 40).

Intracellular signal defects

Neurofibromatosis Type 1 (NF1; von Recklinghausen disease) AD; 1/3000; 50% are new mutations. Loss of the NF1 normal protein allows accumulation of **ras-GTP**, with increased cell turnover (see Chapter 40). There are numerous prominent benign neurofibromas and malignant tumours of the CNS. Expression is highly variable within families.

Neurofibromatosis Type 2 (NF2) AD; 1/35 000. There are bilateral Schwann cell tumours (**schwannomas**) of vestibular, cranial and spinal nerves and intracranial and spinal meningiomas.

Familial adenomatous polyposis (FAP) AD; frequency 1/10 000. There are multiple benign polyps of the colon, with 90% risk of malignancy and **retinal hypertrophy** in 80% of families (see Chapter 40).

Transcriptional control defects

Von-Hippel–Lindau syndrome AD; 1/36 000. There are **haemangioblastomas** of the retina and cerebellum, early onset renal carcinomas and **phaeochromocytomas** (tumours of sympathetic nervous tissue).

Wilms tumour (nephroblastoma) AD; 1/10 000. This is a highly malignant kidney tumour; 1% of cases are familial. It forms part of the **contiguous gene syndrome WAGR** (**W**ilms tumour, **A**niridia, **G**enitourinary anomalies and mental **R**etardation) caused by a major deletion (see Chapter 27).

Cytodifferentiative errors

Basal cell naevus (Gorlin) syndrome AD; 1/57 000. There are skin naevi from puberty and a predisposition to basal cell carcinoma, medulloblastoma and ovarian fibromas. There are also dental malformations, cleft palate and bifid ribs. Patients are unduly sensitive to radiation.

Oncogenes

Growth factor reception

Multiple endocrine neoplasia, Type 2 (MEN 2) There are three subtypes: **MEN2A** (representing 90%), **MEN2B** and **familial medullary thyroid carcinoma** (**MTC**) a tumour of the calcitonin-producing cells of the thyroid. All three carry a high risk of thyroid cancer and are associated with gain-of-function mutations, most involving replacement of a cysteine responsible for a disulphide bond, causing constitutive activation of the RET receptor and an increase in intestinal innervation. The *c-ret* proto-oncogene (*ret* = ***re****arranged during* ***t****ransfection*) encodes a cell-surface receptor tyrosine kinase that transduces glia-cell-derived neurotropic signals for growth and differentiation (see Chapter 40).

Individuals with the MEN2A mutation have an extremely high risk of MTC in early life, which should be treated by surgical thyroidectomy before the age of 5 years. Those in families with MEN2 are also at risk of phaeochromocytoma, and hypoparathyroidism. MEN2B is broadly similar, but with onset in childhood.

Signal transduction

Chronic myeloid (or myelogenous) leukaemia (CML) Translocation of *c-abl*, normally on 9q, to a position beside the '**breakpoint cluster region**' (***BCR***) on 22q initiates synthesis of a chimaeric '**fusion protein**' with increased tyrosine kinase activity. Reciprocal exchange of the 22q telomere leaves a characteristic modified version of 22, the '**Philadelphia chromosome**', in the affected cell line (see Chapter 27).

DNA binding

Burkitt lymphoma This is a B-lymphocyte tumour of the jaw, the most common childhood cancer of equatorial Africa. The DNA-binding proto-oncogene *c-myc* at 8q24 becomes activated by translocation adjacent to an immunoglobulin enhancer at 14q32, 2p11 or 22q11 (see figure and Chapter 40).

42 Immunogenetics

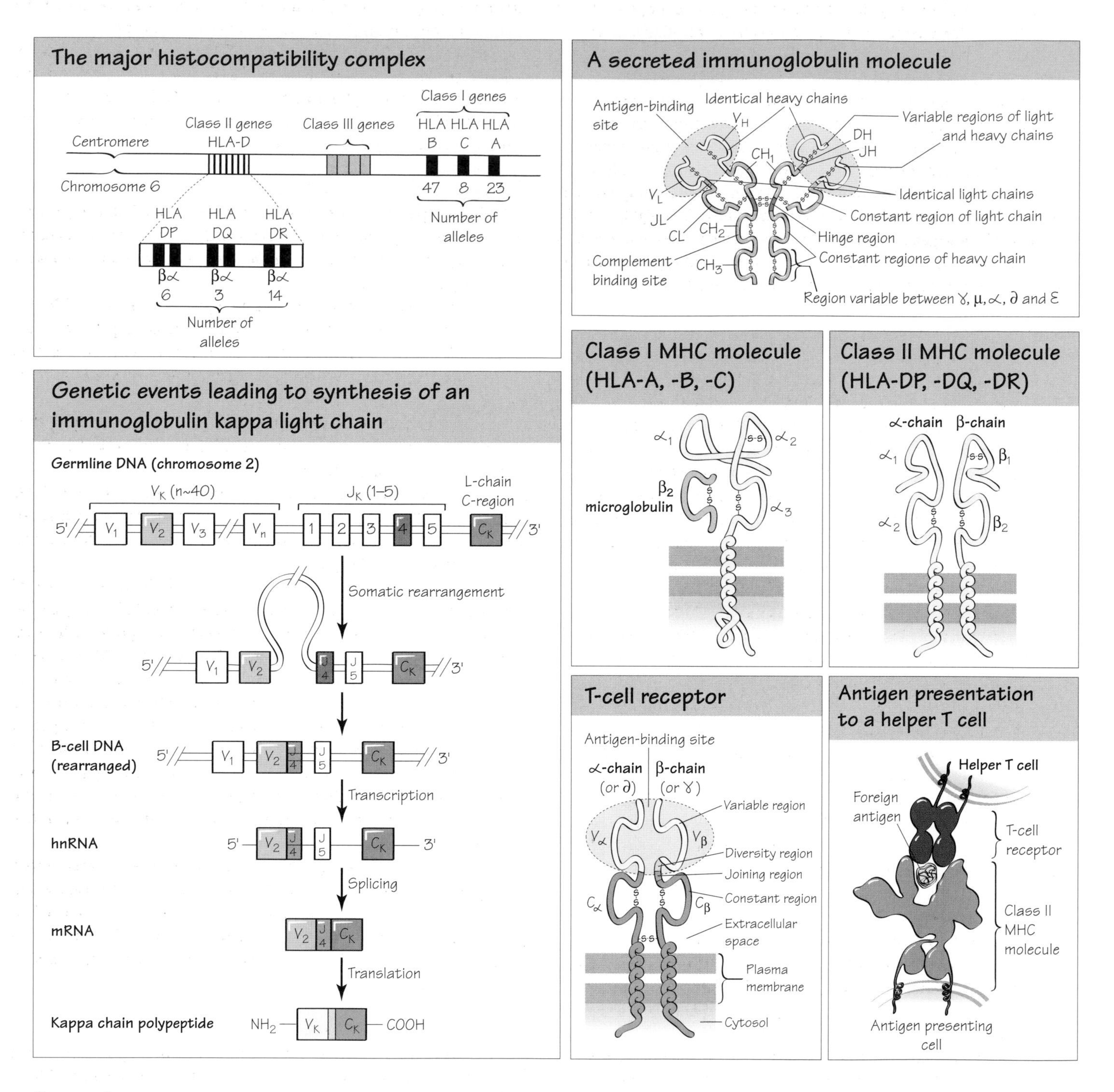

Overview

Immunogenetics concerns the genetics of the **immune system**, which defends the body against invading pathogens and rejects malignant cells and incompatible tissue grafts (see also Chapter 34).

Immune defence mechanisms include **innate** and **specific acquired immunity**. Both involve **humoral** and **cell-mediated** components, which combat extracellular and intracellular infections respectively.

Three classes of bone-marrow stem cells are involved. One migrates to the spleen and lymph nodes and becomes **B lymphocytes**, or **B cells**. The second migrates to the thymus and develops into **T lymphocytes**: **T4 cells** (**helpers** and **inducers**), **T8 cells** (**cytotoxic** and **suppressor cells**) and **natural killer cells**. T cells competent to attack the body's own components are selected and eliminated, generating **immune tolerance** to 'self antigens'. **Macrophages** move directly into the circulation.

The innate immune system

The innate immune system attacks non-specifically, on exposure to alien macromolecules in general. It depends on the joint action of:

phagocytes, that consume and destroy microorganisms, **natural killer cells** that recognize and destroy virally infected cells, and **complement**. Complement is a complex of some 20 proteins that coats the surfaces of microbes, so attracting the attention of phagocytes, or generating a **membrane attack complex** that induces lysis of the microorganism.

The adaptive immune system

The adaptive immune system is highly specific to the minor molecular characteristics of pathogens and depends on interaction between **B** and **T lymphocytes**. Three kinds of molecule are especially important: **MHC proteins**, **immunoglobulins** and **T-cell receptors (TCRs)**.

Mature B cells secrete soluble **antibodies**, or **immunoglobulins**, into the blood and lymph circulations. These react in a highly specific fashion with **antigens** such as peptide or polysaccharide components of invading pathogens. **Helper T cells** help other lymphocytes to respond more effectively. **Cytotoxic T cells** destroy infected cells.

The humoral component

The humoral response begins when phagocytes that contribute to the innate system engulf invading microbes and display their component molecules on their own surfaces. These are **antigen presenting cells** or **APCs**. These normally display **Class II MHC molecules**, but after ingesting a foreign protein they incorporate its components into a groove in the MHC molecule. Circulating helper T cells display receptors which interlock neatly with MHC molecules, but disruption by a foreign antigen causes the T cell to respond. That the APC contains foreign molecules is advertised also by surface **co-stimulatory molecules**, which interact with other receptors on the helper T cell.

This stimulates the helper T cell to secrete **cytokine** molecules, which impact on B lymphocytes. The helper T cell detaches from the APC, but takes the MHC-peptide complex with it. Each B lymphocyte displays immunoglobulin molecules and if these are capable of binding the antigen it is stimulated to proliferate.

The very few B cells carrying antibodies with a loose, but appropriate specificity, then proliferate and minor variations in the immunoglobulin coding sequences are rapidly and sequentially introduced. The process is driven by the affinity of antibody binding to antigen, so that within 5–7 days B cells are produced that bind that specific antigen with high affinity. This subset of B cells then secretes their immunoglobulin receptors into the bloodstream, as **plasma cells**. Each mature plasma cell can secrete 10 million antibody molecules per hour.

The cellular component

Foreign peptides in infected body cells move to the surface complexed with **MHC Class I molecules** (c.f. Class II in the humoral response). Receptors on the surface of the **cytotoxic T cell** then bind to these and release chemicals capable of destroying around 50 infected body cells per hour.

One class of APCs migrates to secondary lymphoid sites in the tonsils, lymph nodes, etc., and alerts the appropriate subset of T cells. Their secretion of cytokines stimulates proliferation of T-cell subsets that bind specifically to infected cells, which then undergo selective evolutionary progression essentially similar to that of B lymphocytes.

In virally infected cells **interferon** destabilizes viral mRNA.

Memory cells

Specification for a specific response is retained by both **memory B** and **memory T cells**. **Vaccination** involves creating a bank of appropriate memory cells without exposure to harmful live pathogen.

The major histocompatibility complex (MHC)

MHC proteins are present on the surfaces of all nucleated cells. ***They show wide polymorphism, but are uniform within an individual.*** In the context of transplantation they act as antigens (see Chapter 34).

A Class I MHC protein consists of a heavy chain encoded by genes HLA-A (23 alleles), -B (47 alleles), or -C (8 alleles), which links with a molecule of **β_2-microglobulin**. Class II (HLA-D: 23 alleles) proteins are heterodimers of α and β subunits. The Class III genes encode components of the **complement** system.

The immunoglobulins

Within each person a different species of immunoglobulin (Ig) is produced for every potential foreign antigen. ***This enormous diversity is created by unique kinds of genetic rearrangement within individual B lymphocytes*** (see figure).

At initial exposure to a foreign peptide possibly one in a million B lymphocytes happens by chance to produce antibody capable of binding specifically to that peptide. Binding stimulates B-cell proliferation and hypermutation in the Ig genes, in which minor DNA sequence variations are introduced at each cell division.

An Ig molecule has two **heavy** (H) chains and a pair of **kappa** (κ) or **lambda** (λ) **light** (L) chains. The latter consist of **constant** (C), **variable** (V) and **joining** (J) **regions**.

There are five classes of heavy chain defined by their C-regions: **IgG**, **IgM**, **IgA**, **IgD** and **IgE**, with heavy chains **gamma** (γ); **mu** (μ); **alpha** (α); **delta** (δ) and **epsilon** (ε) respectively. There is also a '**hinge**' and V, J and **diversity** (D) **regions**.

There are around 40 alternative sequences within the κ L-chain V region, five in the J, and one C gene, on Chromosome 2. The λ genes on Chromosome 22 show similar complexity. For the heavy chains, there are nine C genes (γ, μ, etc., on Chromosome 14), plus about 20 D between the arrays of V and J genes. As the V, D and J regions are assembled, slight variation occurs at the junctions. **Somatic hypermutation** also occurs, involving an increase in the mutation rate of the V, D and J genes.

The different B cells of one individual synthesize billions of different specificities of antibody by differential splicing of these alternative sequences, their transcripts being edited further at the RNA stage. Different pairs of H and L chains then link as symmetrical tetramers.

Within one B cell, antigen-binding specificity can be transferred between different heavy chains. This is called **class switching**. When a B cell produces both IgG and IgM of the same specificity it acquires competence to respond to antigen. Possibly as many as 10 million million distinct immunoglobulin molecular subspecies can be produced in one individual.

The T-cell receptor (TCR)

The TCRs play key roles in antigen recognition and helper activity, but a T cell responds to a foreign antigen only if it is complexed with an MHC molecule.

The TCRs are dimers composed usually of a TCR α- and β-chain (or else a TCR γ- and δ-chain). Their genes also have C, V, J and D segments that are spliced alternatively to create extensive diversity, but they do not undergo hypermutation and are not secreted into the circulation.

The immune system in pregnancy

Immune rejection of a fetus by maternal cytotoxic and natural killer cells is avoided by down-regulation of their MHC antigens.

43 Genetic disorders of the immune system

Characteristic posture of a patient with ankylosing spondylitis (very strongly associated with HLA-B27)

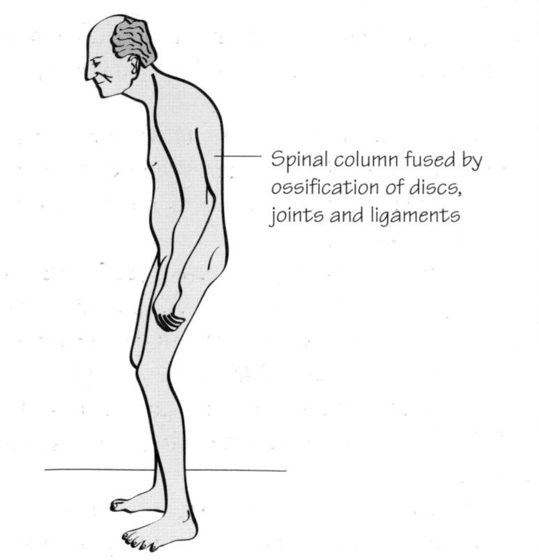

Phagocytosis and intracellular destruction of micro-organisms by macrophages

In normal cells hydrogen peroxide (H_2O_2) is released at phagocytosis, but not in patients with chronic granulomatous disease

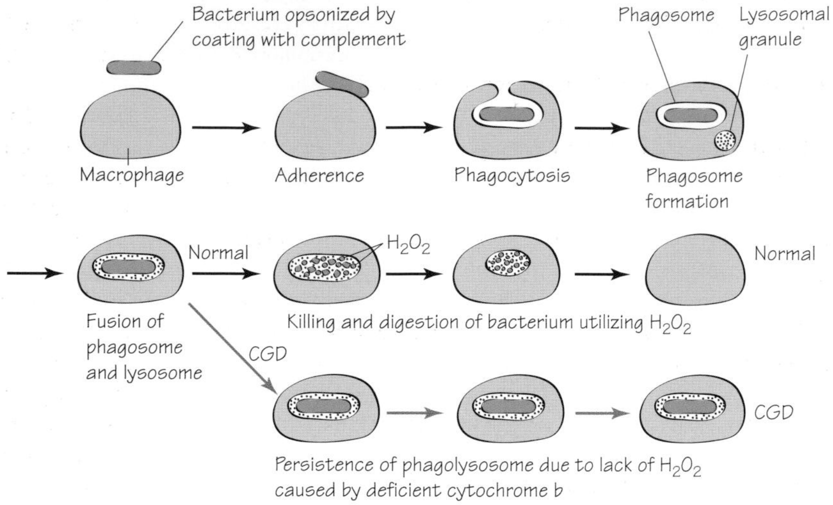

Overview

Immunological **hypersensitivity** can cause **anaphylactic shock**, a rare and terrifying, sometimes fatal response to foreign substances, this being an exaggerated version of the more common allergic response to foreign antigens. Both involve attachment of antigen-specific IgE to **mast cells**. Physiological shock occurs when there is massive release by the mast cells of mediators such as histamine that impinge on smooth muscle, mucus glands and blood vessels. Death can occur from respiratory failure or vascular collapse. Antigens that trigger such '**atopic**' responses are called **allergens**. A dominant autosomal allele that promotes **atopia** is carried by one in four northern Europeans (see Chapter 31).

Immunodeficiency results when one or more components of the immune system is missing or defective. More than 100 **primary immunodeficiency** syndromes have been described caused mainly by genetic defects affecting cells of the immune system. **Secondary immunodeficiency** can occur when the immune system is harmed by external factors such as **human immunodeficiency virus** (**HIV**). Immunodeficiency should be considered when babies have an unexplained failure to thrive, diarrhoea, recurrent or chronic infections, or unexplained **hepatosplenomegaly** (enlarged liver and spleen). Recurrent *bacterial* infection suggests humoral (B-cell) deficiency, whereas unusual susceptibility to *viral* infection is indicative of deficiency in cell-mediated immunity.

The immune system presents a serious challenge to blood transfusion and tissue/organ transplantation (see Chapter 34). **Autoimmune disease** occurs when the immune system turns against the tissues of the same individual.

Disorders of humoral innate immunity

Complement system defects

Genetics Mostly AR; HAO is AD.

Features Defects in complement C3 can cause failure of **opsonization** (coating) of bacteria, or upset the membrane attack complex (see Chapter 42), causing susceptibility to bacteria, especially *Neissaria*.

Hereditary angioneurotic oedema (**HAO**) involves fluid accumulation in soft tissues and airways due to uncontrolled production of C2a, caused by deficiency of C1 inhibitor.

Management Infusion of plasma, or for HAO, C1 inhibitor, and daily therapy with attenuated androgens such as **danazol**.

Disorders of cell-mediated innate immunity

Chronic granulomatous disease (CGD)

Genetics 1 XR, > 3 AR

Features Phagocytes ingest foreign pathogens, but fail to destroy them, causing a persistent cellular immune response. **Granulomas** (nodular lesions) form containing macrophages (see figure). Patients develop pneumonia, lymph node infections and abscesses in the skin, liver, etc.

Aetiology The XR form involves defective cytochrome b that confers failure to generate hydrogen peroxide.

Management Antibiotics.

Leucocyte adhesion deficiency

Genetics AR

Features A life-threatening, acute infection of skin and mucus membranes, with impaired pus formation.

Aetiology Absence of the β2 component of the leucocyte **integrin** molecule involved in cell adhesion produces phagocytes unable to recognize and ingest microorganisms.

Management Antibiotics, bone marrow transplantation.

Chediak–Higashi syndrome

Genetics AR

Features Partial albinism, recurrent bacterial infections, malignant lymphoma.

Aetiology A defect in lysosome assembly causes deficiency specifically of natural killer cells.

Disorders of humoral specific acquired immunity

X-linked agammaglobulinaemia (XLA)

Genetics XR

Features At 5–6 months boys develop multiple bacterial infections. Death can occur from chronic lung infection.

Aetiology Defective B-cell tyrosine kinase prevents maturation of B cells. Since IgG can cross the placenta, infants may be unaffected for several months.

Management Prophylactic intravenous immunoglobulin.

Hyper-IgM syndrome

Genetics XR

Features Raised levels of IgM and IgD; other immunoglobulins decreased. Patients are susceptible to recurrent **pyogenic** (pus-generating) infections.

Aetiology There is a defect in a T-cell surface ligand (TNFSF 5), causing failure of Ig class switching.

Common variable immunodeficiency

The aetiology of the most common B-cell deficiency is heterogeneous and generally unexplained. **AR B-cell immunodeficiency** can be caused by mutation of the Ig heavy and light chains.

Disorders of cell-mediated specific acquired immunity

DiGeorge syndrome

Genetics AR, AD and sporadic

Features See Chapter 27.

Aetiology DiGeorge syndrome is part of a spectrum of phenotypes caused by abnormalities of the third and fourth gill pouches consequent upon contiguous gene deletion in Chromosome 22q11.2. Complete or partial absence of the thymus reduces production of T cells allowing recurrent viral infections, which however usually decrease with age. (see also Chapters 12, 50).

Severe combined immune deficiency (SCID)

Genetics 50–60% XR, AR

Features Lethal susceptibility to both viral and bacterial infections due to profound deficiency of both humoral and cell mediated immunity.

Aetiology The XR forms have mutations in the γ-chain common to several cytokine receptors, so that T cells and natural killer cells fail to receive signals for normal maturation. This in turn upsets B-cell development, which requires T-cell interaction.

Mutation of the intracellular signalling molecule **Jak3** (**Janus kinase 3**), with which the cytokine receptors interact, also causes failure of T-cell maturation, as does deficiency of **protein-tyrosine phosphatase receptor type C** (**CD45**), since CD45 normally suppresses Jak. Deficiencies in **adenosine deaminase** (**ADA**) and **purine nucleoside phosphorylase** (**PNP**) both cause accumulation of purine breakdown products that kill T cells.

SCID can also be caused by mutations in genes involving VDJ recombination and formation of T-cell and B-cell receptors (see Chapter 42).

Management The ADA-deficient and XR forms can be treated by bone marrow transplantation and attempts are being made at gene therapy (see Chapter 60).

Bare lymphocyte syndrome (BLS)

Genetics AR

Features Lymphocytes lack surface MHC display.

Aetiology Type I: mutations in the TAP2 gene prevent export of Class I MHC molecules to the surface. Type II has defects in MHC Class II specific transcription factors, causing deficiency of functional helper T cells.

Wiskott–Aldrich syndrome

Genetics XR

Features Boys have eczema, diarrhoea and recurrent infections, **thrombocytopenia** (low platelet count), low IgM levels and failure of cytotoxic T cell and helper T-cell function. Death can occur from haemorrhage or B-cell malignancy.

Aetiology The basic defect is in the lymphocyte cytoskeleton.

Management Bone marrow transplantation.

Ataxia telangiectasia

Genetics AR

Features Problems with balance and coordination, with **oculocutaneous telangiectasia** (dilated blood vessels in the conjunctivae, ears and face). There are low serum IgA and IgG levels and susceptibility to sinus and pulmonary infection. Lymphocyte chromosomes show rearrangements of Chromosomes 7 and 14, at the T cell receptor loci (see Chapter 42).

Aetiology There is a failure of repair of DNA damage, which can lead to thymus hypoplasia and an increased risk of leukaemia and lymphoma (see Chapter 38).

Autoimmunity and HLA-disease association

In autoimmune disease, tolerance to 'self antigens' (see Chapter 42) breaks down, cytotoxic T cells proliferate and destroy the patient's own tissues. It can be organ-specific, e.g. **Hashimoto thyroiditis**; or **systemic**, e.g. **lupus erythematosus (SLE)**. Autoimmune diseases are most common in females and typically show association with specific MHC/HLA alleles. Table 43.1 lists some important HLA-disease associations with the relative risk of disease associated with HLA carrier status (see also Chapter 48).

Ankylosing spondylitis (AS, poker spine)

AS is a chronic inflammatory condition that leads to fusion of the spine and sacro-iliac junctions. Over 90% of AS patients carry HLA-B27. Five per cent of Europeans overall carry HLA-B27 and, although only 1% of these have AS, their theoretical risk is 90 times that of those who are B27-negative. This genetic association is thought to involve interference with the normal immune response to the bacterium *Klebsiella*.

Table 43.1 Important HLA associations of some common diseases.

HLA	Disease	Frequency in patients (%)	Frequency in general popn	Relative risk
A3	Haemochromatosis	75	13	20
B17	Psoriasis	38	8	7
B27	Ankylosing spondylitis	> 90	8	> 100
	Reiter syndrome	75	8	35
B47	CAH	17	0.4	51
Cw6	Psoriasis	> 50	9	> 10
DR2	Narcolepsy	~100	16	> 100
	Goodpasture syndrome	88	32	16
	Multiple sclerosis	57	21	5
	SLE	> 70	16	> 12
DR3	SLE	50	25	3
	Coeliac disease	60	12	11
	T1DM	50	12	7
DR4	T1DM	38	13	4
DR3//DR4	T1DM			33
DR5	Juvenile RA	50	16	5
	Pernicious anaemia	25	6	5

CAH, congenital adrenal hyperplasia; HLA, human leucocyte antigen; T1DM, insulin dependent diabetes mellitus; popn, population; RA, rheumatoid arthritis; SLE, systemic lupus erythematosus. Relative risk = ad/bc, where a = number of patients with the antigen, b = number of controls with the antigen, c = number of patients without the antigen, d = number of controls without the antigen.

Explanations for HLA-disease association

1 Close genetic linkage of disease susceptibility genes to the MHC complex. For example, **primary haemochromatosis** and congenital adrenal hyperplasia (see Chapter 23) are caused by disease alleles that arose relatively recently and have not yet had time to segregate by chromosomal crossover from their original close neighbour in the MHC. These disease alleles therefore show **linkage disequilibrium** with specific **HLA haplotypes**.

2 Close similarity of structure of HLA antigens and environmental antigens (cross-reactivity).

3 Incomplete development of tolerance.

4 Exposure of 'privileged sites' sequestered during acquisition of tolerance.

Immune system subversion

Cytomegalovirus (CMV)

Some CMV strains evade T-cell detection by down-regulating expression by the host of Class I MHC protein and substituting their own non-functional versions.

Human immune deficiency virus (HIV)

Some HIV strains gain entry to macrophages and helper T cells via a cytokine receptor. A deleted version of the receptor, common in some north-eastern Europeans, confers resistance to HIV (see Chapter 34).

Transplantation genetics

See Chapter 34.

44 Biochemical genetics: part 1

Table 44.1 Important inherited metabolic defects.

Name	Frequency	Inheritance	Defective biomolecule
Carbohydrate metabolism disorders			
Classical galactosaemia	1/35 000–1/60 000	AR	Galactose-1-phosphate uridyl transferase
Hereditary fructose intolerance	1/20 000	AR	Fructose-1,6-biphosphate aldolase/ fructose-1-phosphate aldolase
Diabetes mellitus, Type 1	1/400 (Caucasians)	Polygenic	Unknown
Diabetes mellitus, Type 2	1/20	Polygenic	Unknown
MODY	1/400		Various
Gluconeogenesis			Pyruvate carboxylase/fructose-1,6-biphosphatase/glucose-6-phosphatase
Lactose intolerance	1/10 (Caucasians); 90+% in others	AD	Lactase-phlorizin hydrolase
Glycogen storage disorders			
Hepatic			
Von Gierke disease, GSD1	Rare	AR	Glucose-6-phosphate
Cori disease, GSD3	Rare	AR	Amylo-1,6-glucosidase
Anderson disease, GSD4	Rare	AR	Glycogen 'brancher enzyme'
Hepatic phosphorylase deficiency, GSD6	Rare	AR/XR	Hepatic phosphorylase
Muscular			
Pompe disease, GSD2	Rare	AR	Lysosomal α-1,4-glucosidase
McArdle disease, GSD5	Rare	AR	Muscle phosphorylase
Lipid metabolism disorders			
Familial hypercholesterolaemia	1/500	AD	Low-density lipoprotein receptor
MCAD deficiency	1/20 000	AR	Medium-chain acyl-CoA dehydrogenase
LC4AD deficiency	Rare	AR	Long-chain acyl-CoA dehydrogenase
Smith–Lemli–Opitz syndrome	1/10 000	AR	δ 7 sterol reductase
Porphyria			
Hepatic			
Acute intermittent porphyria	Rare	AD	Uroporphyrinogen synthetase
Hereditary coproporphyria	Rare	AD	Coproporphyrinogen oxidase
Porphyria variegata	Common in South Africa	AD	Protoporphyrinogen oxidase
Erythropoietic			
Congenital erythropoietic porphyria	Rare	AD	Uroporphyrinogen-3 synthase
Erythropoietic porphyria	Rare	AR	Ferrochelatase
Purine and pyrimidine metabolism disorders			
Lesch–Nyhan syndrome	Rare	XR	Hypoxanthine-guanine phosphoribosyl transferase
Severe combined immunodeficiency	1/70 000	AR	Adenosine deaminase
Sphingolipidosis			
Tay–Sachs disease	1/62 500 (UK); 1/625 (Ashkenazim)	AR	Hexosaminidase-A
Gaucher disease Type1	~1/22 000; 1/3200 (Ashkenazim)	AR	β-glucosidase
Gaucher disease Type2	Rare	AR	β-glucosidase
Niemann–Pick disease	Rare	AR	Sphingomyelinase
Mucopolysaccharidosis			
Hurler syndrome, MPS 1	1/10 000	AR	α-L-iduronidase
Hunter syndrome, MPS 2	1/100 000 males	XR	Iduronate sulphate suphatase
Sanfilippo syndrome MPS 3A	1/25 000 (all types)	AR	Heparan-S-sulphaminidase

Table 44.1 (*Continued*)

Name	Frequency	Inheritance	Defective biomolecule
MPS 3B		AR	*N*-acetyl-α-D-glucosaminidase
MPS 3C		AR	Acetyl-CoA: α-glucosaminidase-*N*-acetyltransferase
MPS 3D		AR	*N*-acetyl-glucosamine sulphatase
Morquio syndrome, MPS 4A	1/100 000 (all types)	AR	Galactosamine-6-sulphatase
MPS 4B		AR	β-galactosidase
Maroteaux–Lamy syndrome, MPS 6	Rare	AR	Aryl sulphatase B
Sly syndrome, MPS 7	Rare	AR	β-glucuronidase
Amino acid metabolism disorders			
Phenylketonuria	1/10 000	AR	Phenylalanine hydroxylase
Tyrosinemia Type 1	1/100 000	AR	Fumaryl-acetoacetate hydrolase
Tyrosinemia Type 2		AR	Tyrosine aminotransferase
Tyrosinemia Type 3		AR	4-hydroxyphenyl-pyruvate dioxygenase
Oculocutaneous albinism	1/35 000	AR	Tyrosinase; P protein
Maple syrup urine disease	1/180 000	AR	Branched-chain α-ketoacid decarboxylase
Cystinuria	1/7000	AR	SLC3A1 / SLC7A9
Cystinosis	1/100 000	AR	CTNS
Homocystinuria	1/340 000	AR	Cystathione β-synthetase
Alkaptonuria	1/250 000	AR	Homogentisic acid oxidase
Urea cycle disorders			
Ornithine transcarbamylase deficiency	1/70 000–1/100 000	XR	Ornithine transcarbamyl transferase
Carbamyl phosphate synthetase deficiency	1/70 000–1/100 000	AR	Carbamyl phosphate synthetase
Arginosuccinic acid synthetase deficiency	1/70 000–1/100 000	AR	Arginosuccinic acid synthetase
Heavy metal transport defects			
Menkes disease	1/250 000	XR	ATP7A
Wilson disease	1/50 000	AR	ATP7B
Acrodermatitis enteropathica	Rare	AR	SLC39A4
Haemochromatosis	1/200–1/400 (Caucasians)	AR	HFE
Steroid metabolism defects			
Congenital adrenal hyperplasia	1/10 000; 1/400 (Yupic Alaskans)	AR	21-hydroxylase / 11β-hydroxylase / 3β-dehydrogenase
Androgen insensitivity (testicular feminization)		XR	Androgen receptor
Organic acid disorders			
Methylmalonic acidemia	1/20 000	AR	Methylmalonyl-CoA mutase

Overview

Biochemical genetics is such an extensive discipline that we are devoting two chapters to it (Chapters 44 and 45), in addition to one on biochemical diagnosis (Chapter 51).

Metabolic disorders result from defects in the genetic coding of enzymes, in the production of cofactors, or the uptake, transport or storage of metabolites.

Most of the 200 or so known 'inborn errors of metabolism' are inherited as recessives, because the gene product is usually diffusible and there is generally sufficient residual activity in the heterozygous state for normal function. However, if that reaction is rate-limiting, or the product of the gene is part of a multimeric complex, the disorder can manifest in the heterozygous state and be classed as dominant.

Energy generation

Some 20 mitochondrial and several AR nuclear disorders of oxidative phosphorylation are known. All are rare and their management is generally aimed at promoting alternative pathways of energy generation.

Carbohydrates

Carbohydrates account for the major part of the human diet. All are eventually broken down by glycolysis, following conversion to the monosaccharides, glucose, galactose and fructose, or stored as glycogen. The failure to utilize these three sugars effectively accounts for most defects of carbohydrate metabolism.

Galactose

Galactosaemia is one of the most common monogenic disorders of carbohydrate metabolism, caused by deficiency in **galactose-1-phosphate uridyl transferase**, **galactokinase** or **UDP-galactose-4-epimerase**. Newborn infants present with vomiting, lethargy, failure to thrive, sepsis and jaundice; hepatic insufficiency, developmental delay, poor growth, mental retardation, lens cataract and ovarian failure later become apparent. Newborn screening is by direct enzyme assay on a drop of dried blood, diagnosis is established by enzyme assay and treatment by elimination of dietary galactose.

Fructose

Symptoms of **fructose intolerance** begin when fructose is introduced into the diet and include failure to thrive, jaundice, vomiting, lethal hepatic and renal insufficiency and convulsions. Diagnosis is confirmed by demonstration of fructosuria and enzyme assay on intestinal mucosa or liver biopsy. Management requires exclusion of dietary fructose.

Glucose

There are many errors of glucose metabolism, notably several forms of diabetes mellitus (see Chapters 29, 30, 31, 32, 43 and 46). Disorders of gluconeogenesis present with episodes of hypoglycemia and lactic acidosis due to inability to synthesize glucose during fasting. Treatment includes supportive care during crises and avoidance of low blood sugar.

Lactose

The lactose molecule consists of one molecule of glucose linked to one of galactose. It is a major component of milk and in babies is largely metabolized by the intestinal brush-border enzyme **lactase-phlorizin hydrolase**. In populations with traditional consumption of animal milk, enzyme activity persists in most adults, due to homozygosity of an AR allele. Lactose intolerance, characterized by nausea, bloating and diarrhoea, is however common in most tropical and subtropical populations for whom milk should be processed (e.g. by *Lactobacillus* fermentation) before consumption.

Glycogen

Errors in the synthesis or breakdown of the glucose polymer, **glycogen**, cause **glycogen storage disorders (GSDs)** primarily affecting either the liver or skeletal muscle.

Primarily hepatic

Von Gierke disease, GSD 1

Features Hepatomegaly, sweating and rapid pulse.

Management Maintenance of blood sugar.

Cori disease, GSD 3

Features Hepatomegaly and/or muscle weakness.

Aetiology Deficiency of amylo-1,6-glucosidase (the 'glycogen debrancher enzyme').

Management Maintenance of blood sugar.

Anderson disease, GSD 4

Features Hypotonia and progressive liver failure.

Aetiology Deficiency of '**glycogen brancher enzyme**' leads to unmetabolizable, long glycogen chains.

Management Liver transplant.

Hepatic phosphorylase deficiency, GSD 6

Genetics Hepatic phosphorylase is a multimeric complex coded by both X-linked and AR genes.

Features Hepatomegaly, hypoglycaemia and failure to thrive in the first 2 years.

Aetiology There is failure of glycogen degradation.

Management Carbohydrate supplements that improve growth.

Primarily muscular

Pompe disease, GSD 2

Features Hypotonia in the first few months, muscle weakness with heart enlargement and heart failure in the 2nd year.

Aetiology Alpha-1,4-glucosidase deficiency in the lysosome leads to glycogen accumulation in voluntary and cardiac muscle.

Management Diagnosis by cellular enzyme assay; enzyme replacement therapy by intravenous infusion.

McArdle disease, GSD 5

Features Teenagers present with muscle cramps on exercise.

Management Muscle cramps tend to decline if exercise is continued.

Lipid

Familial hypercholesterolaemia

This is one of the commonest monogenic AD disorders in Western society, responsible for **coronary artery disease** (see Chapters 5, 17, 32).

Medium-chain acyl co-enzyme A dehydrogenase (MCAD) deficiency

MCAD deficiency is characterized by episodic hypoglycaemia, often provoked by fasting that causes accumulation of fatty acid intermediates. There is failure to produce ketones and exhaustion of glucose supplies, causing potentially lethal cerebral oedema and encephalopathy. Most patients are of north-west European origin.

Long-chain L-3 hydroxyacyl co-enzyme A dehydrogenase (LC4AD) deficiency

LCHAD deficiency is one of the most severe, although rare, disorders of fatty acid oxidation, causing severe liver disease, cardiomyopathy, peripheral neuropathy, etc., culminating in sudden death. Mothers can develop 'fatty liver of pregnancy' and related disorders.

Smith–Lemli–Opitz (SLO) syndrome

An AR defect in the enzyme catalysing the final step in cholesterol biosynthesis causes SLO syndrome, characterized by congenital abnormalities of the brain and heart, hypospadias or ambiguous genitalia and digital anomalies (polydactyly and syndactyly; see Chapters 12, 17 and 23). Treatment involves cholesterol supplementation of the diet.

Porphyrin

Porphyrin metabolism mainly concerns the synthesis of haem. All defects are AD as they are rate-limiting in their pathways, except **congenital erythropoietic porphyria** which is AR. All have neurological or visceral involvement and cutaneous photosensitivity.

Hepatic porphyrias

Acute intermittent porphyria (AIP)

Features Abdominal pain, weakness, vomiting, confusion, emotional upset and hallucinations; frequently affects women in relation to the menstrual cycle. Can be precipitated by steroids, anticonvulsants, barbiturates, etc., and is fatal in 5%.

Aetiology Partial deficiency of uroporphyrinogen synthetase leads to urinary excretion of precursors of porphobilinogen and δ-aminolaevulinic acid.

Hereditary coproporphyria
Features Similar to a AIP, but a third of patients also have photosensitive skin.

Porphyria variegata
Features Prevalent in South Africa especially in Afrikaaners; neurological and visceral illness triggered by drugs, variable skin photosensitivity, faecal excretion of protoporphyrin and coproporphyrin.

Erythropoietic porphyrias

Congenital erythropoietic porphyria
Features Extreme photosensitivity with blistering of the skin and extensive scarring; haemolytic anaemia; red coloration of teeth which fluoresce red under ultraviolet light.

Management Protection from sunlight, blood transfusion, splenectomy.

Erythropoietic porphyria
Features Photosensitivity, chronic liver disease.

Management Treatment of photosensitivity with β-carotene.

Purines

Lesch–Nyhan syndrome

Genetics XR

Features Uncontrolled movements, spasticity, mental retardation and compulsive self-mutilation.

Aetiology Deficiency of **HGPRT** results in high levels of phosphoribosyl pyrophosphate and accumulation of uric acid, etc.

Diagnosis Uric acid in urine; HGPRT in skin fibroblasts.

Management Allopurinol alleviates symptoms.

SCID

See Chapter 43.

45 Biochemical genetics: part 2

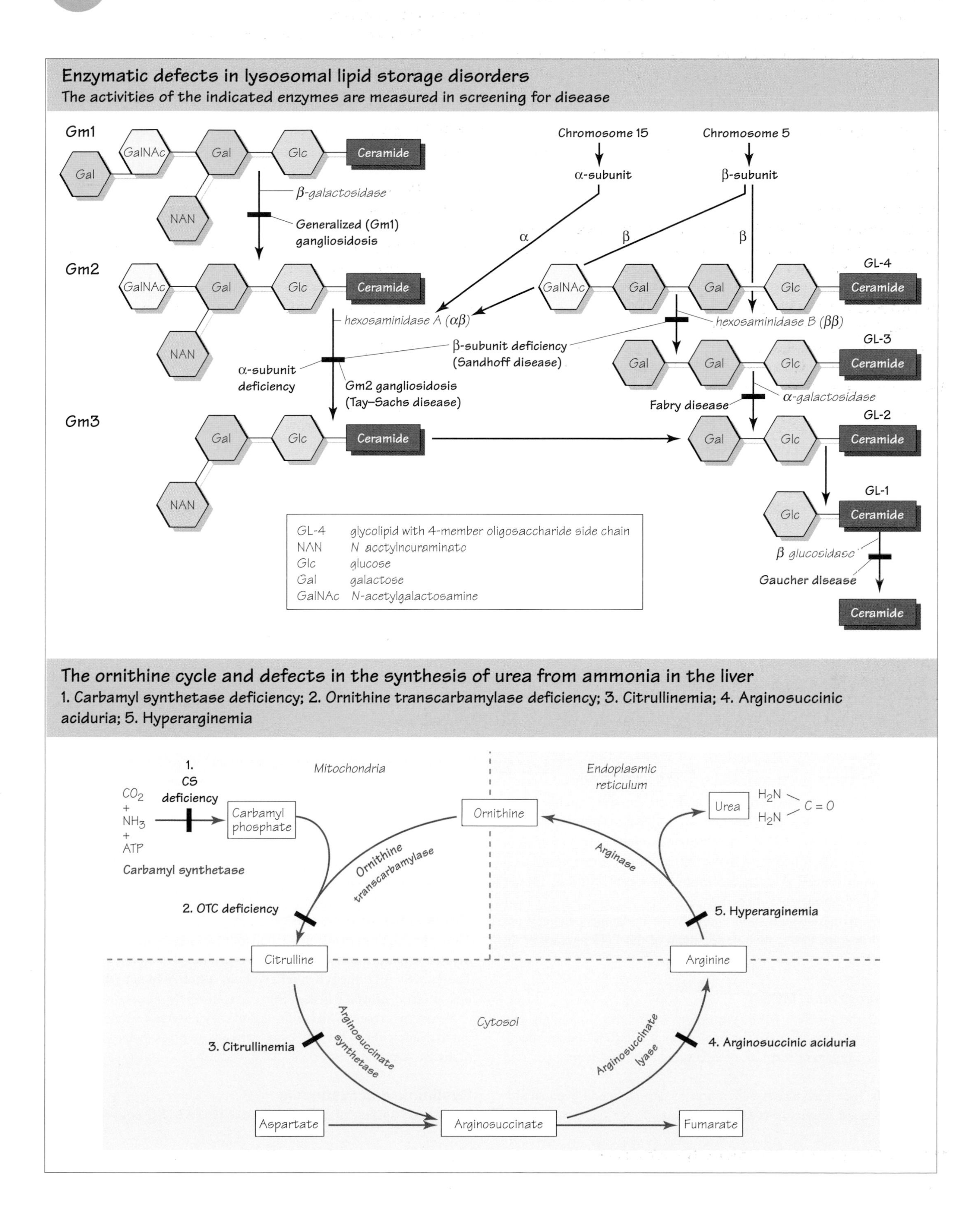

Sphingolipidoses, lipid storage disorders (LSDs)

The sphingolipidoses involve inability to degrade glycosylated membrane phospholipid in the lysosomes, with its accumulation primarily in the brain, liver and spleen. There are at least 10 specific enzyme deficiencies, all AR.

Tay–Sachs disease

Frequency 1/625 in Ashkenazi Jews, ~1/6250 in others.

Features Presents in the first 6 months with poor feeding, lethargy and poor muscle tone. Progressive neurological dysfunction leads to loss of sight and hearing and to spasticity, rigidity and death from respiratory infection in the second year.

Aetiology Defective α-subunit of **hexosaminidase-A** allows accumulation of GM2 ganglioside.

Diagnosis Cherry-red spot in macula; low hexosaminidase activity in serum.

Gaucher disease

Frequency 1/3600 in Askenazi Jews, 1/25 000 in others (90% are Type 1).

Features **Type 1**: adult onset, febrile episodes, hepatosplenomegaly, bone lesions, skin pigmentation (NB. CNS is unaffected).

Type 2: infantile onset, hepatosplenomegaly, failure to thrive, neurological deterioration, with spasticity and fits; death from pulmonary infection in the second year.

Diagnosis Deficient glucosylceramide β-glucosidase.

Management Pain relief, splenectomy, enzyme replacement by intravenous infusion, enzyme augmentation, bone marrow transplantation.

Niemann–Pick disease

Features Infants fail to thrive, hepatomegaly, lethal by the age of 4 years.

Diagnosis Cherry-red spot in macula, 'foam cells' in bone marrow, **sphingomyelinase** deficiency.

Mucopolysaccharidoses (MPSs)

All the MPSs involve chronic and progressive multi-system deterioration, due to accumulation of sulphated polysaccharides (glycosaminoglycans). This causes problems with hearing, vision, joint and cardiovascular function. Affected children develop coarse facial features, short stature, skeletal deformities and joint stiffness. Hunter syndrome is X-linked, the others AR.

Bone marrow transplantation and enzyme replacment therapy are successful in some cases, though treatment of the CNS remains problematic.

Hurler syndrome, MPS 1

This is the most severe MPS, presenting with corneal clouding and spinal curvature in the first year, with mental deterioration and death from cardiac failure or respiratory infection by the mid-teens.

Diagnosis Increased urinary excretion of dermatan and heparan sulphates, reduced activity of **α-L-iduronidase**.

Hunter syndrome, MPS 2

This usually presents at 2–5 years with a variety of problems, including hearing loss and abnormal vertebrae, progressive physical and mental deterioration and death usually in the teens.

Diagnosis Excess dermatan and heparan sulphates in the urine, decreased activity of **iduronate sulphate sulphatase** in serum or white blood cells.

Sanfilippo syndrome, MPS 3, types A, B, C and D

This is the most common MPS. Symptoms appear in the second year: intellectual loss, convulsions and death in early adulthood.

Diagnosis Increased urinary heparan chondroitin sulphate and deficiency of either one of four specific degradative enzymes (see Table 44.1).

Morquio syndrome, MPS 4, types A and B

Children present in the second or third year with skeletal abnormalities that can later cause spinal cord compression. Intelligence is normal and survival long-term.

Diagnosis Keratan sulphate in the urine; deficiency of **galactosamine-6-sulphatase** (type A) or **β-galactosidase** (type B).

Maroteaux–Lamy syndrome, MPS 6

Hurler-like symptoms in early childhood, but retention of normal intelligence. Survival into adulthood or until only the third decade.

Diagnosis Increased urinary dermatan sulphate excretion, cellular **aryl sulphatase B** deficiency.

Sly syndrome, MPS 7

Diagnosis Increased urinary excretion of glycosaminoglycans; **β-glucuronidase** deficiency in serum and cells.

Amino acid metabolism

Phenylketonuria

See Chapters 19, 51.

Tyrosinemia

Hereditary **tyrosinemia Type 1**, relatively common in French-Canadians, is caused by deficiency of **fumarylacetoacetate hydrolase**. Accumulation of substrates causes neurological, kidney and liver dysfunction. **Type 2** is characterized by corneal erosion, thickening of the palms and soles and mental retardation, **Type 3** with neurological dysfunction.

Albinism

See Chapters 18 and 35.

Maple syrup urine disease

The urine smells of maple syrup due to increased excretion of the three **branched chain amino acids** (**BCAAs**) valine, leucine and isoleucine. The defective enzyme is **branched chain α-ketoacid dehydrogenase**, measurement of which in the urine can confirm the diagnosis.

Newborns present with vomiting and irregular muscle tone, proceeding to death within a few weeks. Treatment involves dietary restriction of the BCAAs.

Cystinuria and cystinosis

Abnormal transport of cystine produces two AR diseases, **cystinurea** and **cystinosis**. Cystinurea is very common (1/7000) and involves failure of excretion of cystine, causing renal **calculi** (kidney stones) sometimes with infection, hypertension and renal failure.

Management of cystinuria Consumption of large volumes of water, alkalinization of the urine and use of cystine chelating agents such as penicillamine.

Cystinosis is rare (1/100 000) and involves accumulation of crystalline cystine in the lysosomes of most tissues.

Homocystinuria

Homocystinuria (frequency: 1/340 000) is caused by deficiency of the enzyme **cystathione β-synthetase**, with elevation of serum homocystine. It is associated with mental retardation, seizures, thromboembolic episodes and osteoporosis. The combination of scoliosis, pectus excavatum, arachnodactyly and lens dislocation may cause confusion with Marfan syndrome (see Chapter 17), though mental retardation in homocystinuria provides a distinction.

Diagnosis Cyanide nitroprusside test for homocysteine in urine and plasma.

Management Low methionine diet with cystine supplementation.

Alkaptonuria

Alkaptonuria (frequency: 1/250 000) is caused by a deficiency in **homogentisic acid oxidase**. The acid is excreted in the urine, to which it gives a dark colour on exposure to air. Dark pigment is deposited in the ear wax, cartilage and joints (**ochronosis**), a condition that can lead to arthritis.

Urea/ornithine cycle disorders

The urea/ornithine cycle consists of five major chemical reactions, deficiency of any of which can lead to progressive neurological impairment, lethargy, coma and death from build-up of ammonium ions and glutamine (see figure 'The ornithine cycle and defects in the synthesis of urea from ammonia in the liver'). These operate in the mitochondria, endoplasmic reticulum and cytosol. The most common is **ornithine transcarbamylase** deficiency (X-LR) in the mitochondria.

Management Largely dietary.

Metals

Copper, Cu

Copper is absorbed by intestinal epithelial cells and transported to the liver for incorporation as a cofactor of several enzymes. Excess Cu is excreted in the bile. Cu transport protein **ATP7A** is present in many tissues except liver, usually in the Golgi body, where it provides Cu for various enzymes. However, when Cu levels exceed a certain threshold, it moves to the plasma membrane and pumps Cu into the bloodstream, to return to the Golgi body when levels normalize. **ATP7B** plays a similar role in the liver, controlling excretion of Cu into the biliary tree.

Menkes disease

Menkes disease (MND) is caused by an XR error of ATP7A and characterized by mental retardation, seizures, hypothermia, twisted and hypopigmented hair, loose skin, arterial rupture and death in early childhood. Cu export by the gastrointestinal epithelium into the bloodstream fails, so there is an overall Cu deficiency.

Treatment Subcutaneous administration of copper.

Wilson disease

Wilson disease results from abnormality of ATP7B (AR) causing excessive Cu excretion into the biliary tract. It causes liver **cirrhosis** (fibrous discoloration, with destruction of parenchyma cells) and neurological abnormalities, such as **dysarthria** (inability to articulate words correctly), **dysphagia** (difficulty in swallowing) and diminished coordination. Adults also develop arthritis, cardiomyopathy, kidney damage and hypoparathyroidism.

A diagnostic sign is the **Kayser–Fleischer ring** caused by deposition of copper in Descemet's membrane at the margin of the cornea. There is increased copper in the urine, but the most sensitive indicator involves incorporation of isotopes of copper into cultured cells.

Treatment Copper chelating agents such as **D-penicillamine** and **trientine**.

Zinc, Zn

Acrodermatitis enteropathica is caused by a defect in the uptake of zinc by the intestinal epithelial cells. Patients show growth retardation, diarrhoea, immune dysfunction, scaly dermatitis of the genitals and buttocks, limbs and around the mouth. It can be fatal soon after weaning. Management requires supplemental zinc.

Iron, Fe

Hereditary haemochromatosis is one of the commonest recessive genetic disorders in Caucasians, 1/200–1/400 being affected homozygotes and one in eight carriers (the condition is incompletely penetrant). Excess iron is absorbed by the small intestine and accumulates in the liver, kidney, heart, joints and pancreas, causing fatigue, joint pain, diminished libido, diabetes, increased skin pigmentation, cardiomyopathy, liver enlargement and cirrhosis.

Diagnosis By abnormal serum **ferritin** and **transferrin** saturation levels. Liver biopsy samples can be stained for iron stores; confirmation by DNA test.

Treatment Serial **phlebotomy** (bleeding) to reduce iron stores.

Steroid metabolism defects

See Chapter 23.

Organic-acid disorders

Methylmalonic acidemia

Deficiency of **methylmalonyl-CoA mutase** or the **cobalamin** coenzyme causes accumulation of toxic methylmalonic acid, leading to poor feeding, vomiting and lethargy, low white blood cell (**neutropenia**) and platelet (**thrompocytopenia**) counts, hypoglycemia and hyper-ammonemia. Cobalamin-deficient patients respond to vitamin B_{12} (see Chapter 51).

Treatment Fluid replacement, correction of metabolic acidosis and cessation of protein intake; vitamin B_{12} for selected patients.

46 Clinical applications of genetics: an overview

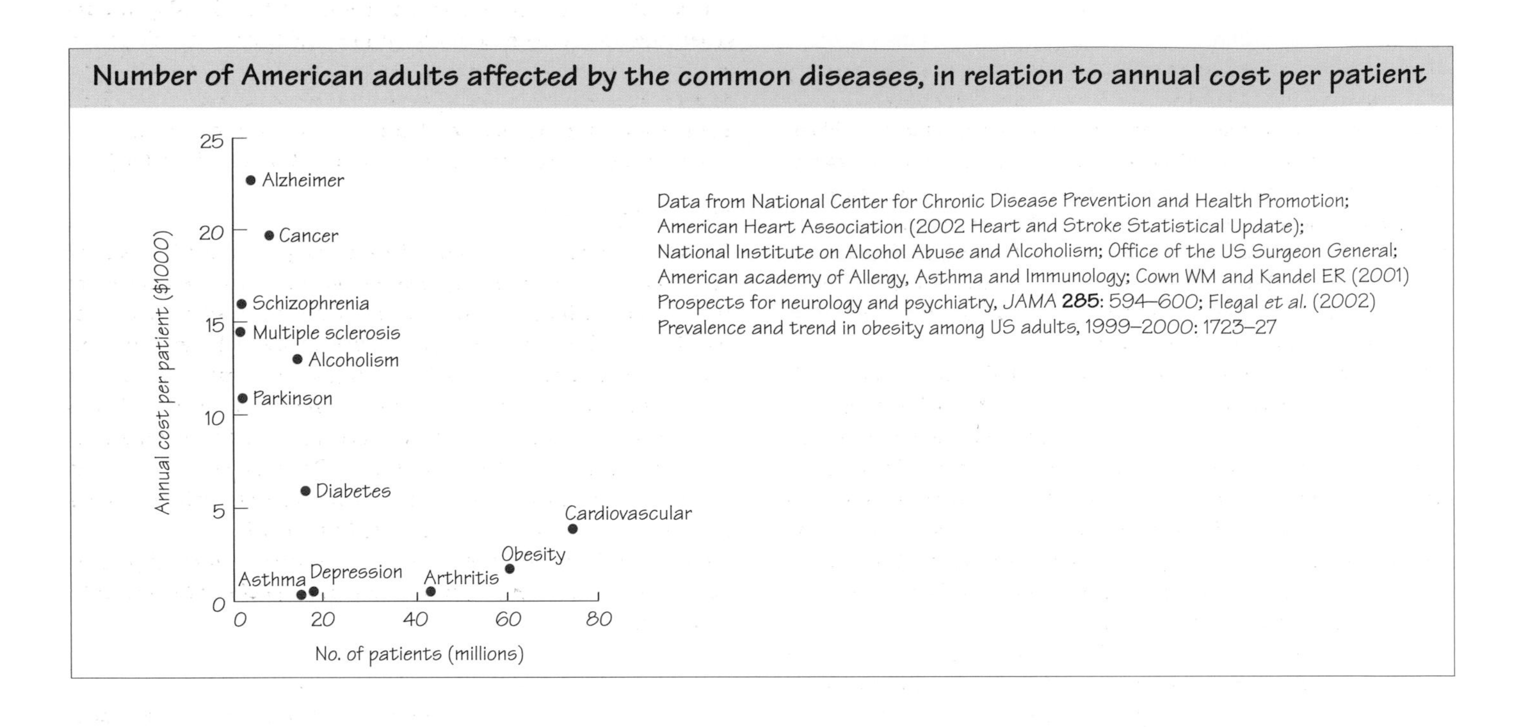

Overview

Genetics underpins and potentially overlaps all other clinical topics, but is especially relevant to reproduction, paediatrics, epidemiology, therapeutics, internal medicine and nursing. It offers unprecedented opportunities for prevention and avoidance of disease because genetic disorders can often be predicted long before the onset of symptoms. This is known as **predictive** or **presymptomatic genetics**. Healthy families can be screened for persons with a particular genotype that might cause later trouble for them or their children.

Genetic advice to patients and their families should however be **non-directive**, **non-judgemental** and **supportive**, and can be summarized by four words: **communication**, **comprehension**, **care** and **confidentiality**.

Communication

For the genetic counsellor and the health visitor good communication skills are vital, as what they convey to a family can have profound implications not only for their present happiness, but for the health of that family for ever more. When assembling information they should preserve a warm and non-judgemental attitude, take adequate time and remember to consider their own body language. It is common for people to experience fear, denial, anger or guilt, but reassurance from an authoritative figure outside the family can help them come to terms with such feelings.

Family myths often grow up around genetic disorders and these must be explored and disentangled before concepts such as X-linked, dominant or recessive inheritance will be accepted. Family secrets such as incestuous or extra-marital relationships may be revealed during the investigation and may be critical to the assessment of genetic risk. Such problem areas must be treated with extreme discretion.

Comprehension

An important principle is that ***where possible, diagnosis should precede counselling***, but in some cases supportive counselling is needed before a definitive diagnosis has been achieved. Examples include unknown dysmorphic syndromes, children with dysmorphic features who are too young to have 'grown into' a recognizable syndrome and conditions in which there is marked genetic heterogeneity.

Initial contact with the consultand usually involves construction of a 'family tree' or **pedigree diagram** (see Chapter 47). Physical examination for dysmorphic features can play a significant part in genetic diagnosis and guidance on this is given in Chapter 49.

Looking at chromosomes provides a broad overview of the genome (see Chapter 50), in contrast to the molecular genetics approach where tests are for one or a few specific mutations (see Chapters 55–58). The assessment of risks can be exceedingly complex, but instructive examples are given in Chapter 48. DNA fingerprinting, as described in Chapter 58, is of enormous value in paternity testing and other forensic aspects of medicine.

Prenatal diagnostic tests require informed consent, and consultands should be made fully aware of the limitations of such tests. 'Valid consent' requires that anything that represents a significant risk that would affect the judgement of a reasonable person has been explained.

The genetic counsellor will generally have been trained in psychology as well as general medicine, clinical genetics and possibly other medical specialities, but his or her comprehension is further informed by a team of experts. This generally includes additional medically trained clinical geneticists, laboratory scientists including cytogeneticists and molecular biologists, and genetic nurses.

Care

After taking family details and constructing a family tree it is necessary to assess what the consultand actually wants to know: there may be specific concerns that are not obvious to the counsellor. Individuals should, when possible, be offered the choice of more than one alternative; for example, between presymptomatic testing and medical surveillance alone. The concept of 'high risk' is subjective, but comparison of genetic risks with statistics on other aspects of health can help put things in perspective (see Table 52.1). A risk of > 1/10 would generally be considered high, but by comparison with other hazards, one of < 1/20 is considered by some authorities as low.

Genetically based disease varies between ethnic groups (Table 46.1) and some knowledge of a family's educational, social and religious backgrounds is important also as these affect their reactions and decision making. Consultation can create new uncertainties and individuals may adopt a coping style known as 'functional pessimism' to protect themselves from future disappointments. Guilt and depression can arise in those who receive favourable test results when their relatives are less fortunate. Long-term emotional support should therefore be offered at the same time as any offer of predictive testing.

Population screening for disease alleles, combined with appropriate courses of action have yielded dramatic reductions in disease incidence (see Chapter 60). However, 'eugenic' concepts that conceive genetic improvement at the *population* level and issues such as cost-saving (see figure) or contribution to research should not be used to influence decisions made by consultands regarding their own lives or those of their offspring. Potential ethical problems are minimized if the *rights of individuals* are given priority.

It should be remembered that diagnosis of high liability toward genetic disease is not necessarily an irrevocable condemnation to ill health. As stressed in Chapter 1, phenotypic characters are the product of interaction between genotype and environment, acting over time; and in some cases optimal health can be maintained by avoidance of genotype-specific environmental hazards (see Chapters 59 and 60).

Table 46.1 Genetic isolates with high frequency of certain autosomal disorders.

Population	Disease
Old order Amish (Pennsylvania)	Chondroectodermal dysplasia Ellis–van Creveld syndrome Cartilage-hair hypoplasia
Kuna (San Blas) Indians (Panama)	Albinism
Hopi Indians (Arizona)	Albinism
Pima Indians (US Southwest)	Type 2 diabetes
Finns	Congenital chloride diarrhoea Aspartylglycosaminuria Congenital nephrotic syndrome Mulibrey nanism
Yupik Eskimo	Congenital adrenal hyperplasia
Afrikaaners (South Africa)	Porphyria variegata Familial hypercholesterolaemia Lipoid proteinosis Huntington disease Sclereosteosis
Ashkenzi Jews	Tay–Sachs disease Gaucher disease Dysautonomia Canavan disease
Karaite Jews	Werdnig–Hoffmann disease
Ryukyan Islands (Japan)	Spinal muscular atrophy
Cypriots, Sardinians	Beta-thalassaemia

Confidentiality

Genetic information about one individual may have implications for other family members and agreement should always be sought for disclosure of such information. If a patient refuses to allow this, his or her wish would normally be respected. Exceptionally the genetic counsellor may decide to breach confidentiality, when the potential harm to another family member outweighs that to those first considered. Breach of confidence is however never undertaken lightly and not without considerable negotiation. The World Health Organization considers the counsellee to have a moral obligation to inform relatives if this allows them in turn to choose whether or not to be screened.

Genetic information should never be disclosed to third parties, such as insurance companies and employers, without the subject's written consent.

Communicating bad news

Families receive bad news in many ways, but they generally remember in detail the way that news was delivered.

1 Prepare yourself.
2 Choose a private area with adequate seating.
3 Talk to both parents together.
4 Communicate the diagnosis as early as possible.
5 Remember the baby's sex, refer to him or her by name and avoid pejorative terms (remembering that connotations can vary between cultures).
6 Be as encouraging as realistically possible.
7 Answer questions fully, but avoid technical overload.
8 Listen.
9 Accept every emotional response as natural.
10 Recognize the right of individuals not to have their anxiety increased.
11 Refer the family to sources of support.
12 Spend time with the family.

Summary

Genetic counselling can be summarized as helping the consultand to:

• comprehend the diagnosis, possible course and available management of the disorder;
• appreciate the contribution of heredity and the risk of recurrence;
• understand the reproductive options available;
• choose a course of action appropriate to the family goals, ethical and religious standards and to act on that decision;
• help the family make the best possible adjustment to the disorder.

Following face-to-face consultation it is usual for the clinician to write to the family to reiterate the main points and re-address difficult aspects. This letter can become a valuable resource for the family, as it documents advice on risk. Pamphlets and booklets relating to the condition and about lay advocacy groups may also be provided and follow-up visits are appreciated.

47 Pedigree drawing

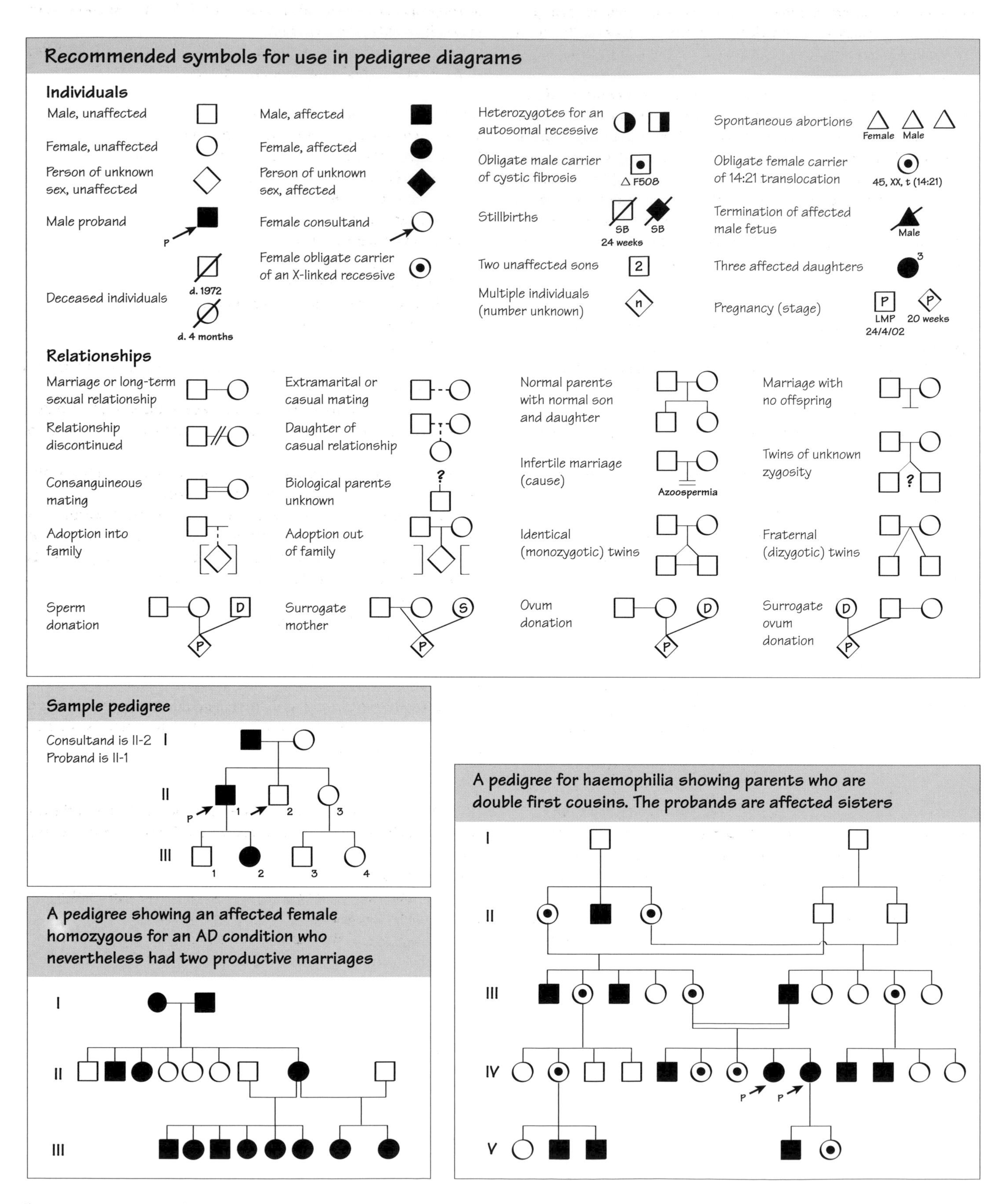

Overview

The collection of information about a family is the first and most important step taken by doctors, nurses or genetic counsellors when providing genetic counselling. A clear and unambiguous **pedigree diagram**, or '**family tree**', provides a permanent record of the most pertinent information and is the best aid to clear thinking about family relationships.

Information is usually collected initially from the **consultand**, i.e. the person requesting genetic advice. If other family members need to be approached it is wise to advise them in advance of the information required. Information should be collected from both sides of the family.

The affected individual who caused the consultand(s) to seek advice is called the **propositus** (male), **proposita** (female), **proband**, or **index case**. This is frequently a child or more distant relative, or the consultand may also be the proband. A standard medical history is required for the proband and all other affected family members.

The medical history

In compiling a medical history it is normal practice to carry out a **systems review** broadly along the following lines:

- **cardiovascular system**: enquire about congenital heart disease, hypertension, hyperlipidaemia, blood vessel disease, arrhythmia, heart attacks and strokes;
- **respiratory system**: asthma, bronchitis, emphysema, recurrent lung infection;
- **gastrointestial tract**: diarrhoea, chronic constipation, polyps, atresia, fistulas and cancer;
- **genito-urinary system**: ambiguous genitalia and kidney function;
- **musculoskeletal system**: muscle wasting, physical weakness;
- **neurological conditions**: developmental milestones, hearing, vision, motor coordination, fits.

Rules for pedigree diagrams

Some sample pedigrees are shown (see also Chapters 16–23). Females are symbolized by circles, males by squares, persons of unknown sex by diamonds. Affected individuals are represented by solid symbols, those unaffected, by open symbols. Marriages or matings are indicated by horizontal lines linking male and female symbols, with the male partner preferably to the left. Offspring are shown beneath the parental symbols, in birth order from left to right, linked to the mating line by a vertical, and numbered (1, 2, 3, etc.), from left to right in Arabic numerals. The generations are indicated in Roman numerals (I, II, III, etc.), from top to bottom on the left, with the earliest generation labelled I.

The proband is indicated by an arrow with the letter P, the consultand by an arrow alone. (N.B. earlier practice was to indicate the proband by an arrow without the P.)

Only conventional symbols should be used, but it is admissible (and recommended) to annotate diagrams with more complex information. If there are details that could cause embarrassment (e.g. illegitimacy or extra-marital paternity) these should be recorded as supplementary notes.

Include the contact address and telephone number of the consultand on supplementary notes. Add the same details for each additional individual that needs to be contacted.

The compiler of the family tree should record the date it was compiled and append his or her name or initials.

The practical approach

1 Start your drawing in the middle of the page;
2 Aim to collect details on three (or more) generations.
3 Ask specifically about:
 (a) consanguinity of partners;
 (b) miscarriages;
 (c) terminated pregnancies;
 (d) stillbirths;
 (e) neonatal and infant deaths;
 (f) handicapped or malformed children;
 (g) multiple partnerships;
 (h) deceased relatives.
4 Be aware of potentially sensitive issues such as adoption and wrongly ascribed paternity.
5 To simplify the diagram unrelated marriage partners may be omitted, but a note should be made whether their phenotype is normal or unknown.
6 Sibs of similar phenotype may be represented as one symbol, with a number to indicate how many are in that category.

The details below should be inserted beside each symbol, whether that individual is alive or dead. Personal details of normal individuals should also be specified. The ethnic background of the family should be recorded if different from that of the main population.

Details for each individual:
1 Full name (including maiden name).
2 Date of birth.
3 Date and cause of death.
4 Any specific medical diagnosis.

The stage of a pregnancy at the time of compilation of the pedigree can be indicated as number of weeks, or the date of the mother's last menstrual period (LMP) noted.

Use of pedigrees

A good family pedigree can reveal the mode of inheritance of the disease and can be used to predict the genetic risk in several instances (see Chapter 48). These include:
1 the current pregnancy;
2 the risk for future offspring of those parents (**recurrence risk**);
3 the risk of disease among offspring of close relatives;
4 the probability of adult disease, in cases of diseases of late onset.

48 Risk assessment

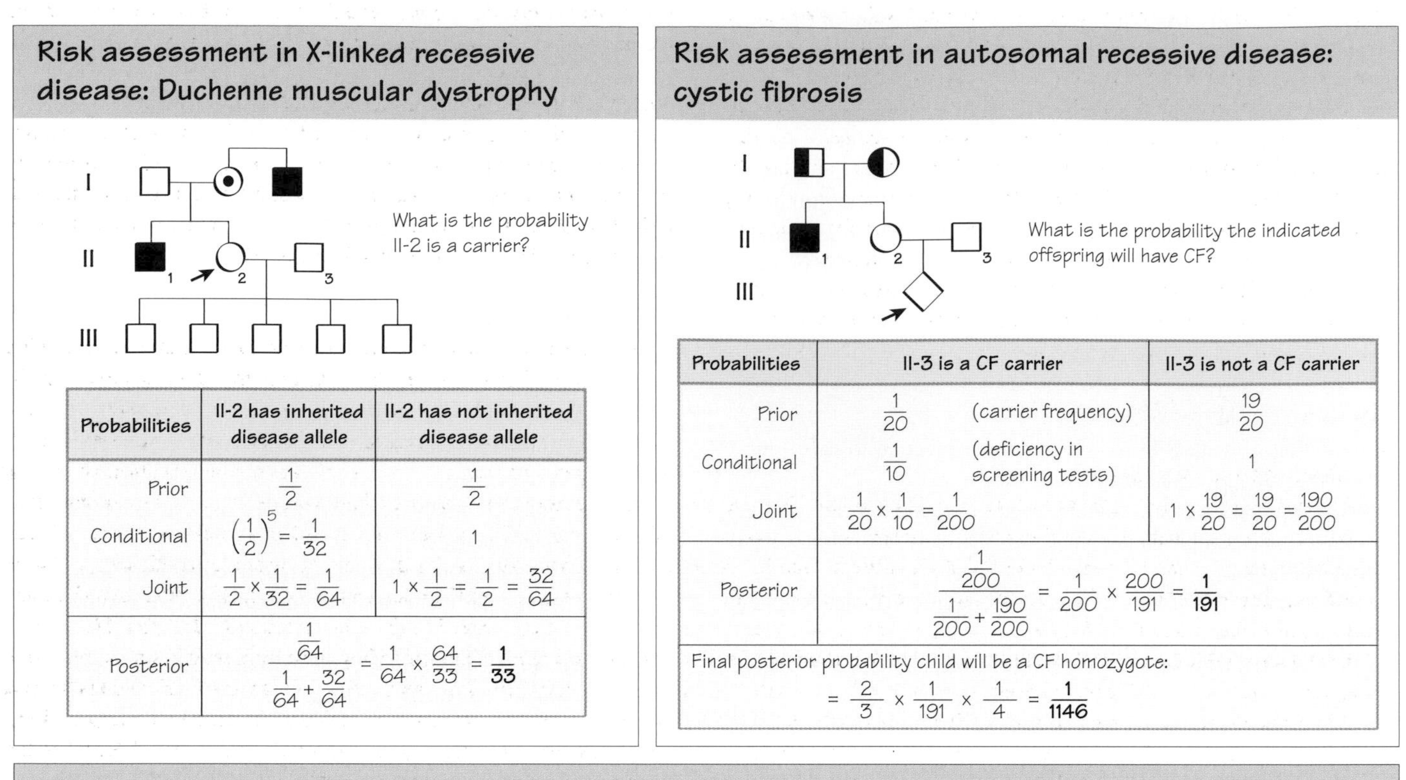

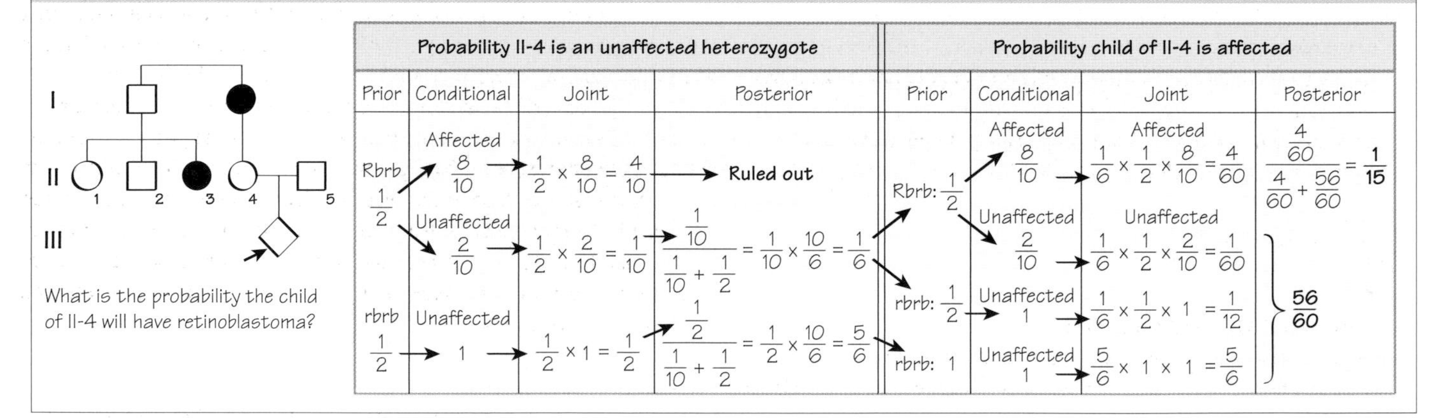

Overview

A major part of the burden of a genetic disorder is the risk of recurrence in the family. A prime goal of assessment therefore is to estimate the risk of transmission by the same couple to later children and by affected and unaffected family members to their children. The simple application of Mendelian theory can often provide a rough guide, but such estimates generally need to be refined by inclusion of other considerations such as penetrance (see Chapters 20 and 33). This is most readily achieved by application of Bayes' theorem.

Risk assessment

A combination of several factors is used to determine the basic risk of transmission of a genetic disorder:

1 Diagnosis. A correct diagnosis is critical for the accurate assessment of genetic risks. Correct diagnosis may indicate not only the mode of inheritance, but also suggest appropriate carrier and/or prenatal diagnostic tests.

2 Family history. Even in the absence of a diagnosis, assessment of the family history may reveal the pattern of transmission and provide clues to penetrance (see Chapter 47).

3 Ethnic background. Certain ethnic groups are known to be at increased risk for specific genetic traits (see Chapters 32, 34 and Table 46.1), so providing guidance for assessment of carrier status and prenatal diagnosis.

Bayes' theorem

Bayes' theorem is a mathematical approach that allows refinement of estimates of risk by taking into account all other knowledge relating to that situation. For example, the '**prior probability**' of the birth of an affected child can be derived in a straightforward fashion from classic Mendelian theory. However, if that parental partnership has already produced several unaffected offspring, this allows adjustment in terms of '**conditional probability**'. Multiplying the prior and conditional probabilities gives the '**joint probability**' of that outcome. A parallel calculation is performed with respect to the alternative outcome of the baby being healthy. The '**relative likelihood**' of a diseased child being born is then calculated as the joint probability of the first outcome, divided by the *sum* of the joint probabilities of *both* outcomes.

A benefit of using Bayes' theorem in such contexts is that it allows incorporation of a variety of modifying factors, such as age-related onset of disease, incomplete penetrance and results of genetic testing.

Application of Bayes' theorem

X-linked recessive disease

Consider a woman with both a brother and uncle with X-linked Duchenne muscular dystrophy (see figure 'Risk assessment in X-linked recessive disease: Duchenne muscular dystrophy'); since her mother is an obligate carrier she has a 50% chance also of being a carrier. This corresponds to the 'prior probability' of her being a carrier. However, if she has had five unaffected sons we can use this fact to recalculate the 'conditional probability' of her carrier status.

From the pedigree, the prior probability of this woman being a carrier is 1/2 and the conditional probability she would have five unaffected sons, given that she *is* a carrier, is $(1/2)^5 = 1/32$. The prior probability of her *not* being a carrier is also 1/2, and, if so, the conditional probability of her having five normal sons would be 1. The product of the prior and conditional probabilities (i.e. the joint probabilities) are 1/64 and 1/2 respectively.

The relative likelihood (also known as the '**posterior probability**') of her being a carrier, is then calculated as the joint probability of her being a carrier divided by the sum of the two joint probabilities.

In mathematical terms this is:

$$\frac{1/64}{(1/64 + 1/2)} = 1/33$$

Autosomal recessive disease

The risk of recessive disease depends on coincidence of three circumstances: mother being a carrier, father being a carrier and child inheriting both disease alleles.

Consider a phenotypically normal woman whose brother has cystic fibrosis (CF) (see figure 'Risk assessment in autosomal recessive disease: cystic fibrosis'). She is married to a white-skinned Northern European and wishes to know the chance their planned child will have CF. The carrier risk for CF among Northern Europeans is around 1/20 and there are laboratory DNA tests for 90% of all CF mutations. The tests on him yield negative results, making his posterior probability of being a carrier 1/191 (see figure 'Risk assessment in autosomal recessive disease: cystic fibrosis').

In matings between two heterozygotes we expect normal homozygotes, heterozygotes and mutant homozygotes in the ratio 1 : 2 : 1. Since this woman is unaffected, she is either a normal homozygote (CF/CF; initial probability 0.25) or a heterozygote (CF/cf; initial probability 0.5). Her probability of being a carrier is therefore $0.5/(0.5 + 0.25) = 2/3$. The relative likelihood of their having a child with CF is therefore $2/3 \times 1/191 \times 1/4 = 1/1146$.

This example is given to illustrate application of the theory: in a real situation of course the woman would usually also be tested, so reducing the range of possibilities and refining the estimate of risk.

Autosomal dominant of incomplete penetrance

Familial retinoblastoma is transmitted as a dominant of penetrance (P = 0.8) (see Chapter 40). As shown in the figure 'Risk assessment in autosomal dominant disease of incomplete penetrance: familial retinoblastoma', the posterior probability of the child of an unaffected suspected carrier (Rb/rb) being affected is 1/15.

Isolated cases

When a disease condition occurs with no family history, discerning the pattern of inheritance is difficult. Patterns of inheritance can be obscured by small sibship size and failure of some genotypes to survive to term. There can also be diagnostic difficulties due to non-penetrance, variable gene expression, or lack of accurate information on absent family members. An AD disorder could be due to a new mutation or false paternity. For an isolated case of congenital deafness risk can be based on the knowledge that 70% of cases are genetic and, of these, 2/3 are recessive. On the assumption it probably is both inherited and recessive, recurrence risk is then calculated as $7/10 \times 2/3 \times 1/4 = 1/9$.

Consider the case of a single boy being born with X-linked recessive Duchenne musuclar dystrophy (DMD). The parents ask what is the risk another son would have the same condition. There are three interpretations:

1 The mother is a heterozygous carrier of the disease allele; when the prior probability of recurrence would be 0.5.

2 A new mutation arose during the meiotic events that produced the ovum from which the boy is derived; recurrence risk is negligible.

3 The mother is a gonadal mosaic for a mutation that occurred during her own embryonic development; in this case recurrence risk relates to the proportion of her ova that carries the mutant X chromosome.

As a guide, among mothers of isolated DMD cases, 2/3 are carriers, in 25–30% there is a new mutation, while 5–10% are gonadal mosaics.

It is sometimes possible to deduce the probable mode of inheritance by comparison with other families with identical symptoms. However, it should be remembered that many conditions are genetically heterogeneous. In such cases ethnic background can be informative. Conversely, members of the same family may display variant manifestation of the same condition.

Empiric risks

If risks are not readily calculable, as in cases with chromosome imbalance and multifactorial disease, we refer to tables of **empiric risks**, i.e. observed incidences (see Chapters 31 and 32). The risk of Down syndrome is about 10% if the mother carries a 14;21 translocation, 2.5% when carried by the father. Risk of recurrence of a new translocation is low (< 1%).

The relative risk of developing an HLA-associated disease can be determined from the formula:

$$\frac{\text{no. of patients with the marker allele} \times \text{no. of controls without the marker allele}}{\text{no. of controls with the marker allele} \times \text{no. of patients without the marker allele}}$$

(see Table 43.1).

49 Dysmorphology

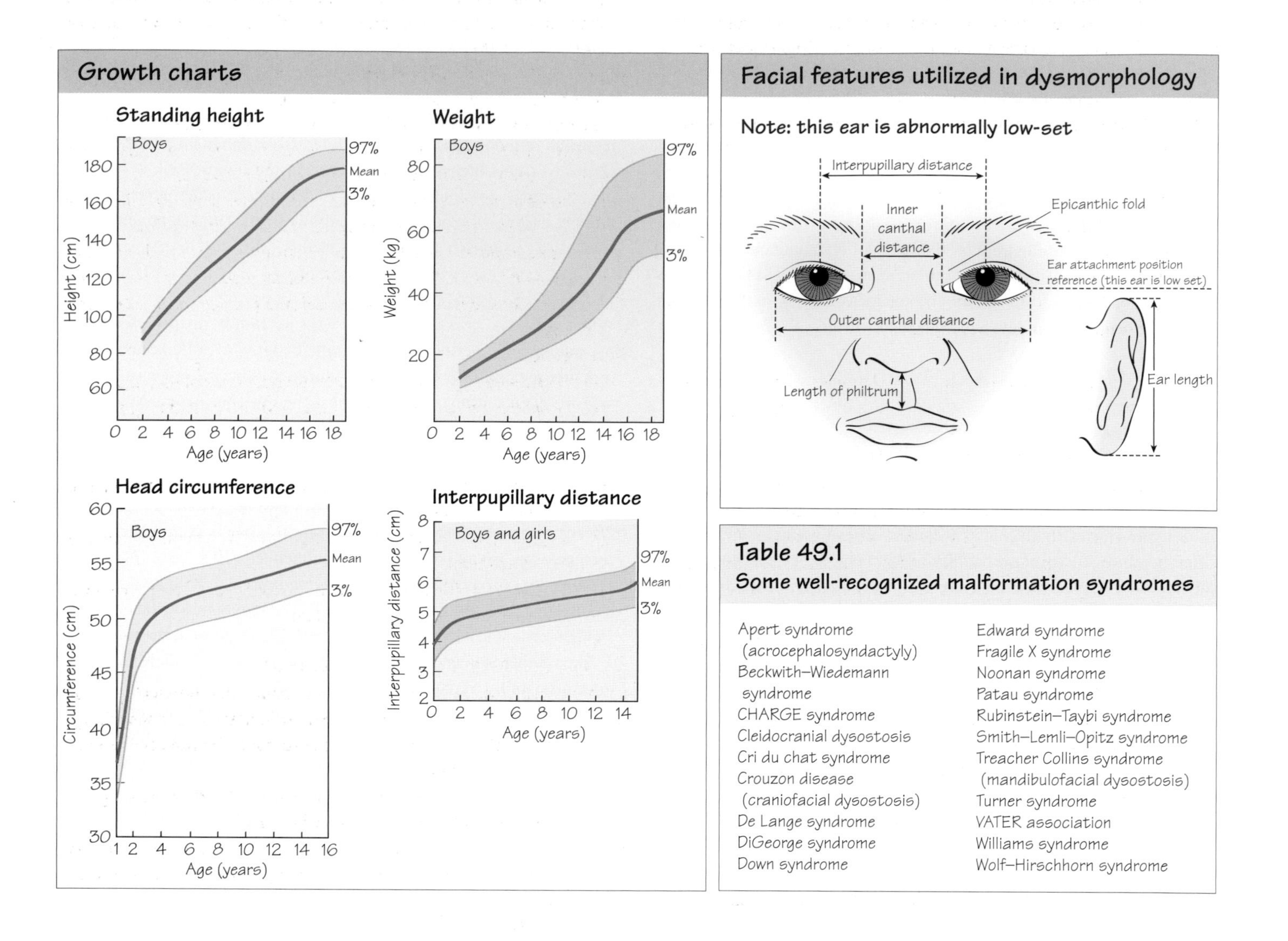

Table 49.1
Some well-recognized malformation syndromes

Apert syndrome (acrocephalosyndactyly)	Edward syndrome
Beckwith–Wiedemann syndrome	Fragile X syndrome
CHARGE syndrome	Noonan syndrome
Cleidocranial dysostosis	Patau syndrome
Cri du chat syndrome	Rubinstein–Taybi syndrome
Crouzon disease (craniofacial dysostosis)	Smith–Lemli–Opitz syndrome
De Lange syndrome	Treacher Collins syndrome (mandibulofacial dysostosis)
DiGeorge syndrome	Turner syndrome
Down syndrome	VATER association
	Williams syndrome
	Wolf–Hirschhorn syndrome

Overview

Anatomical features are considered **dysmorphic** if their measures or structures lie outside the normal range. **Dysmorphology** is the discipline concerned with their identification, delineation, diagnosis and management.

Quantitative characters vary with age and sex, but measures of different features in a normal subject should all lie within the same part of their respective ranges. An exceptional measure reflects abnormality. Since some dysmorphic features relate to age, re-examination at a later date can be helpful.

Two to four per cent of newborn babies have a physical anomaly and currently over 2000 dysmorphic diagnoses are listed. Multiple dysmorphic features enable identification of known syndromes. For example **fetal alcohol syndrome**, present in 1/300–1/1000 children, is indicated by the combination of growth deficiency, microcephaly, short palpebral fissures, a smooth philtrum and a thin upper lip (see Chapter 31).

Classification of abnormal developmental features

A variety of congenital anomalies have been delineated, the understanding of which is important in providing counselling to families (see Chapters 29 and 30). These are classified as follows:

- **malformations**, e.g. polydactyly;
- **deformations**, e.g. moulding of the fetal head due to uterine fibroids;
- **disruptions**, e.g. amputation of a limb due to entrapment by an amniotic band;
- **dysplasias**, e.g. neuronal **heterotopia** (i.e. presence of normal tissue at abnormal sites) in the brain.

Malformations may also be classified in terms of occurrence of features.

- **Isolated malformation**, e.g. extra digit on one hand.
- **Sequence**, e.g. cleft palate in infant with under-development of the jaw (**Pierre–Robin sequence**), in which upward displacement of the tongue in a very small mouth interferes with palatal closure (see Chapter 31).

• **Association**: tendency of multiple malformations to occur together non-randomly, usually for unknown reasons, e.g. **VATER** and **VACTERL associations** (see Chapter 28).
• **Syndrome**: a set of abnormal phenotypic features that frequently occur together due to a basic underlying cause, e.g. Down syndrome.

Assessment of development

Childhood development is monitored with regard to eight interconnected aspects:
1 hearing;
2 vision;
3 gross motor skills;
4 fine motor skills;
5 comprehension of language;
6 linguistic self expression;
7 behaviour and emotional development;
8 social skills.
Assessment involves checks on rate of development, qualitative scope of development in that aspect, and final level of achievement.

Clinically important growth parameters

Human growth charts show mean values and ranges plotted against age. Individuals who lie outside the third and 97th centiles are considered abnormal. Suboptimal growth and weight gain in infants and toddlers come within the term '**failure to thrive**' and their assessment requires careful physical examination, photographic records and history taking.

The following measurements may be taken if there are specific concerns about disproportionate growth.
1 Standing height:
(a) overall height;
(b) lower segment: floor to upper border of pubis;
(c) upper segment: overall height minus lower segment.
2 Sitting height.
3 Linear growth, i.e. change in body length over time.
4 Arm span.
5 Weight.
6 Head circumference: maximum occipitofrontal circumference is an indirect measure of brain size:
(a) **microcephaly** can reflect poor brain growth or premature fusion of skull sutures;
(b) **macrocephaly** may indicate high intra-cranial fluid pressure.
7 Eyes:
(a) **hypertelorism** is a feature of nearly 400 syndromes, describing abnormally widely spaced orbits;
(b) **hypotelorism** refers to abnormally closely spaced orbits, found in some 40 syndromes;
(c) **telecanthus** refers to an increase in the distance between the inner canthi with normal inter-orbital distance and is a feature of around 90 syndromes;
(d) **blepharophimosis** is reduction in the length of the palpebral fissures and features in over 100 syndromes;
(e) **epicanthic folds** are skin folds over the inner canthi;
(f) **upwards slant** of the eyes means that the inner canthi are lower than the outer, as in Down syndrome (see Chapter 24);
(g) **downwards slant** describes eyes with the inner canthi higher than the outer, as in Cri du chat syndrome (see Chapter 27).
8 Ears: Maximum ear length and ear position are recorded. Ears are described as low-set if the upper border of their attachment is below a line through the outer canthi and the occipital protuberance at the back of the skull.
9 Head shape:
(a) **brachycephaly** describes short anteroposterior skull length;
(b) **dolichocephaly** refers to long anteroposterior skull length.
10 Testicular volume.
11 Limbs:
(a) **syndactyly** indicates digital fusion, osseous (**synphalangism**), or cutaneous (**webbing**);
(b) **polydactyly** describes extra digits on the **pre-axial** (radial/tibial), or **post-axial** (ulnar/fibular) side;
(c) **clinodactyly** describes an incurved digit, most often the fifth finger (see Down syndrome, Chapter 24).

Diagnosis in dysmorphology

Correct classification of congenital anomalies has implications for diagnosis and hence for management, prognosis and counselling. Tissue samples should be taken from malformed stillbirths and fetuses for laboratory investigation.

A systematic approach to diagnosis would involve the following:
• **Family pedigree construction** (see Chapter 47).
• **Pregnancy history**. Record drug exposure (e.g. treatment for maternal epilepsy), excess alcohol intake, maternal physiological disorders such as diabetes, and infection (see Chapter 29).
• **Physical examination.**
• **Laboratory investigations**, e.g. chromosome analysis, skeletal survey or brain imaging.
• **Differential diagnosis**. Illustrated texts and computerized databases can be used for reference (see Appendix).
• **Conclusion**. Currently in perhaps 50% of cases a secure diagnosis cannot be reached.

50 Chromosome analysis

G-banding and labelling of chromosomes

Chromosome 7 is shown at resolutions of 450, 550 and 850 bands per haploid set. The indicated band is designated 7q31.32

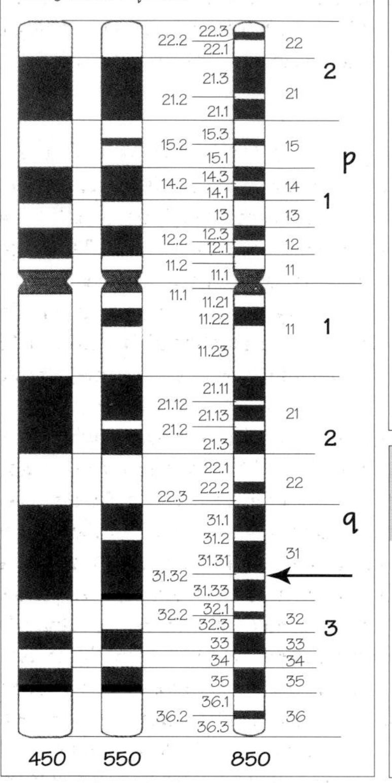

Three chromosome forms (alternative representation, at metaphase)

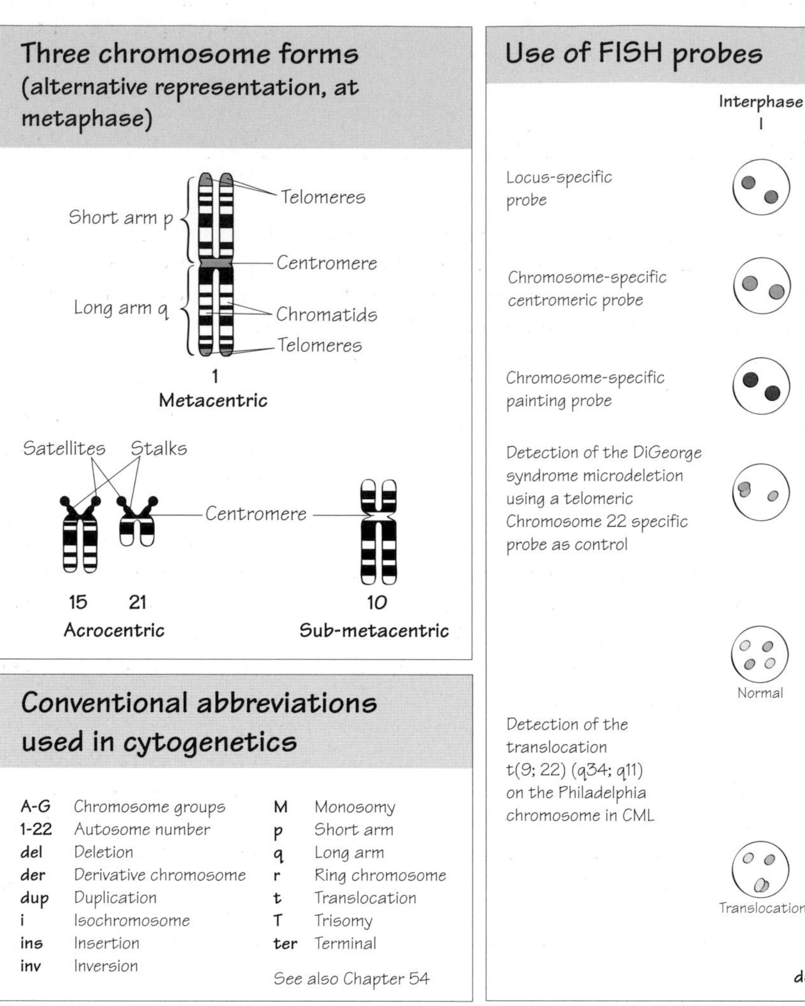

Conventional abbreviations used in cytogenetics

A-G	Chromosome groups	M	Monosomy
1-22	Autosome number	p	Short arm
del	Deletion	q	Long arm
der	Derivative chromosome	r	Ring chromosome
dup	Duplication	t	Translocation
i	Isochromosome	T	Trisomy
ins	Insertion	ter	Terminal
inv	Inversion		

See also Chapter 54

Use of FISH probes

	Interphase	Metaphase
Locus-specific probe		
Chromosome-specific centromeric probe		
Chromosome-specific painting probe		
Detection of the DiGeorge syndrome microdeletion using a telomeric Chromosome 22 specific probe as control		Deletion
Detection of the translocation t(9; 22) (q34; q11) on the Philadelphia chromosome in CML	Normal Translocation	22 9 der22 der9

Overview

The study of number and structure of chromosomes is called **cytogenetics**. Traditionally it is performed on compacted chromosomes at a magnification of about 1000×, providing resolution to around 3 million base pairs, or one narrow chromosome band (see Chapter 3). By incorporation of molecular techniques this can be reduced to 2 kb (2000 bp).

Conventional cytogenetics uses mitotic chromosomes. The chorion (**syncytiotrophoblast**) and bone marrow normally contain sufficient dividing cells for examination, but most tissues require culturing *in vitro*, with an overall time schedule of about 10 days. **Molecular cytogenetics**, utilizing DNA probes, can be applied directly to interphase nuclei.

Preparation of a karyotype

A visual karyotype is prepared by arresting dividing cells at metaphase with a spindle inhibitor such as *colchicine* (see Chapter 9), spreading the cells on a glass slide and staining with Giemsa stain. Traditionally a photographic positive is then made and the chromosomes cut out and assembled on a card, in pairs in order of size, sometimes in conventional groups A–E (see Chapter 54). In modern practice, this step is replaced by digital imaging. Chromosomes 1, 3, 16, 19 and 20, with the centromere in the middle, are known as **metacentric**; 13, 14, 15, 21, 22 and Y, with the centromere near one end, are **acrocentric**. The rest are **submetacentric**. The short arm is symbolized 'p' (for petite) and the long arm 'q'.

Karyotype formulae are described in Chapter 24. Positions of genes along chromosome arms are defined by **region** number (from the centromere outwards), **band**, **sub-band** and **sub-sub-band** numbers, e.g. 12q24.32 refers to Chromosome 12, long arm, region 2, band 4, sub-band 3, sub-sub-band 2. **High resolution banding** involves fixation before the chromosomes are fully compacted.

C-banding stains heterochromatin, **NOR staining** reveals the **N**ucleolar **O**rganizer **R**egions on the satellite stalks of the acrocentrics.

Fluorescent *in situ* hybridization (FISH)

FISH enables the specific localization of genes and the direct visualization of abnormalities at the molecular level. With chromosome-specific probes it allows rapid diagnosis or exclusion of trisomy in amniotic fluid cells.

Table 50.1 Single-gene disorders with cytogenetic effects.

Disorder	Inheritance	Cytogenetic effect
Ataxia telangiectasia	AR	Chromatid damage due to defective DNA repair; 7, 14 rearrangements
Bloom syndrome	AR	High frequency of sister chromatid exchange
Fanconi anaemia	AR	Chromosome breakage and translocation
Fragile X syndrome	XR	Chromosome breakage at Xq27.3
Roberts syndrome	AR	Premature separation of centromeres at metaphase
Xeroderma pigmentosum	AR	Defective repair of ultraviolet damage, sister chromatid exchange

In a typical application, a labelled probe is denatured by heating, added to a metaphase chromosome spread on a microscope slide and incubated overnight to permit sequence-specific hybridization. Surplus probe is then washed off and the bound probe located by overlaying the spread with a solution of fluorescent '**reporter molecule**'. Unbound reporter is washed off and a counterstain applied to reveal the chromosomes. Bound reporter, and hence the site of the gene of interest, is then located by its fluorescence under ultraviolet light.

Use of unique sequence probes

Microdeletions

Submicroscopic deletions can be detected with fluorescent probes directed against one or more unique sequences within the deleted interval. **Microdeletion probes** are used in diagnosis of **DiGeorge/VCFS** at 22q11; **Wolf–Hirschhorn** at 4p16.3, **Prader–Willi** and **Angelman**, **Williams** and **Smith–Magenis syndrome**, etc. (see Chapter 27).

Translocations

FISH probes directed at the *BCR* and *abl* sequences can be used to reveal the Philadelphia chromosome (see Chapter 26) as two fluorescent signals on the derivative Chromosome 22; in normal cells the signals are on separate chromosomes. FISH probes to regions near the telomeres can be useful in identifying subtelomeric rearrangements that result in unbalanced karyotypes which may lead to mental retardation.

Sex chromosome rearrangements

In some phenotypic males lacking a Y chromosome, an SRY probe reveals the site to which the male-determining *SRY* locus (see Chapters 13 and 22) has been translocated from its normal site at Yp11, often to the X.

Chromosome painting

When unique sequence probes for one chromosome are pooled and labelled with the same fluorochrome this creates a '**chromosome paint**' that identifies that specific chromosome or its fragments after translocation (see book cover).

In **reverse painting**, a battery of probes is made from an *abnormal* chromosome and hybridized to normal metaphase spreads, so allowing the derivation of the abnormal chromosome to be deduced. Such probes are created by assembling many copies of the abnormal chromosome using a **fluorescence activated chromosome sorter** (see Chapter 37).

Primed *in situ* hybridization

The primed *in situ* hybridization (PRINZ) technique involves setting up a polymerase chain reaction (PCR) *in situ* on a chromosome spread. Primers are added that define a specific genetic locus, resulting in a layer of target DNA at the site of interest. If a fluorescent base analogue is incorporated during the PCR reaction the sequence is rendered visible in one step.

Comparative genome hybridization (CGH)

CGH can be used to detect partial monosomies or trisomies, chromosome deletions and amplifications. It is based on making test DNA and control DNA compete at hybridizing to the same target. The target can be either a metaphase spread, or an array of tiny samples of DNA clones on a glass slide. It is especially valuable in cancer genetics to detect regions of allele loss and gene amplification and also for detecting subtelomeric deletions in patients with unexplained mental retardation.

In **standard CGH**, tumour or test DNA is labelled with green fluorescent dye and control DNA with red. The two samples are mixed, hybridized competitively to metaphase chromosomes and photographed using a fluorescence microscope. Regions duplicated in the tumour cells hybridize with excess green labelled DNA; regions deleted in the tumour cells light up as red, while unchanged regions appear yellow. The ratio of red to green FISH signal is automatically plotted along the length of each chromosome emphasizing regions where it deviates significantly from the 1 : 1 expectation. This is especially useful for inferring the state of progression of a cancer. The current limits of resolution are 10 Mb (10 million bases) for losses and 2 Mb for gains.

In **array CGH** DNA sequences rather than chromosomal band locations are identified, utilizing micro-arrays of DNA spotted onto glass slides (see Chapter 57). Each spot consists of cloned DNA from a defined chromosomal region. It is possible to create arrays that cover the entire human genome and carry out rapid robotic scans for micro-deletions and micro-duplications.

Multiplex PCR screening for aneuploidy

(see Chapter 57)

Indications for chromosome analysis

The following are situations in which cytogenetic investigation is advised.

1 Suspected chromosome abnormality.
2 Multiple congenital anomalies and/or developmental retardation.
3 Disorders of sexual function.
4 Undiagnosed mental retardation.
5 Certain malignancies.
6 Infertility or multiple miscarriage.
7 Stillbirth and neonatal death.

51 Biochemical diagnosis

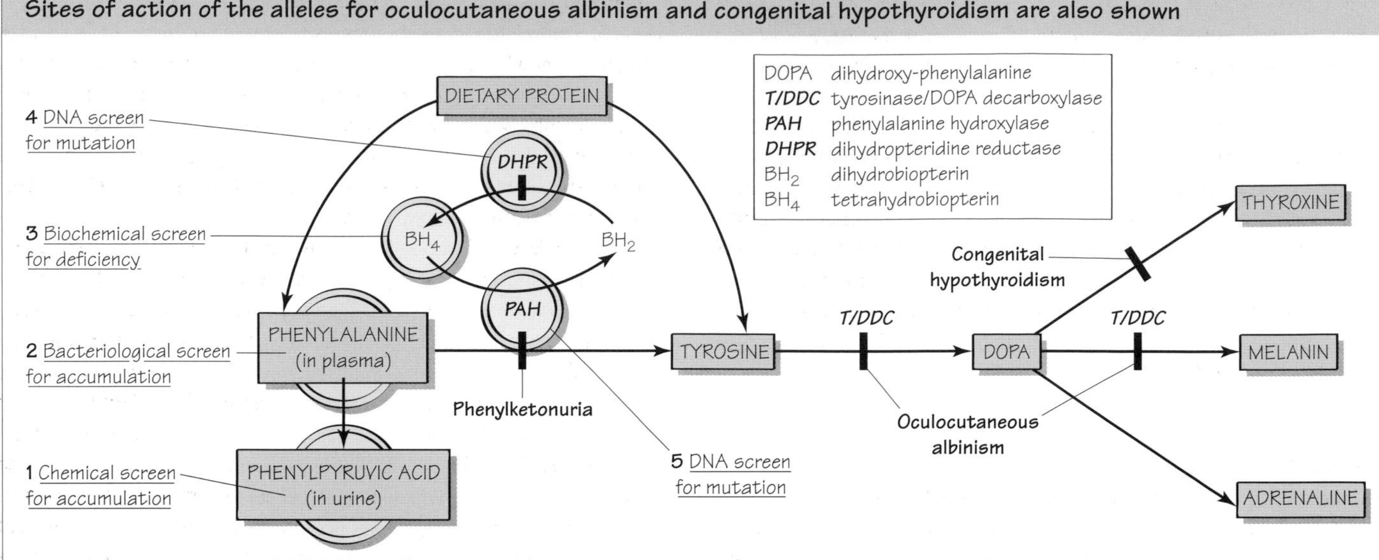

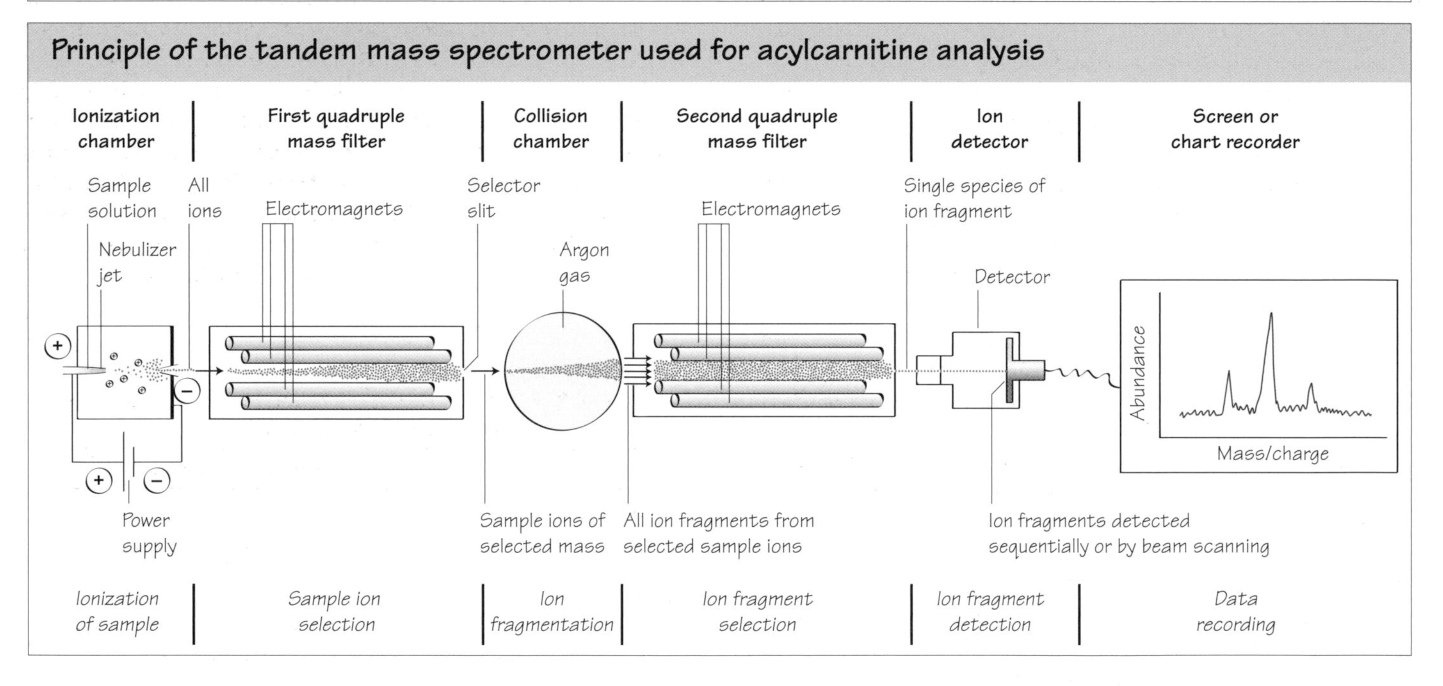

Overview

'Inborn errors of metabolism' result, directly or indirectly, mainly from either accumulation of an enzyme substrate to abnormal levels, or deficiency of the product of an enzyme reaction (see Chapter 44). An example of the latter is **oculocutaneous albinism**, in which deficiency of **tyrosinase** (**DOPA decarboxylase**) prevents synthesis of melanin pigment (see Chapter 18). Accumulated substrates can be toxic, notable examples being phenylalanine or its derivatives, methylmalonic acid and ammonia. Diagnosis of such conditions is usually by assay of accumulated metabolites, or alternatively by enzyme assay, but more recently direct detection of mutations at the DNA level, have come into favour.

Prenatal diagnosis is possible for many inborn errors. Analyses are performed on cultured amniocytes collected by mid-trimester amniocentesis, or more commonly now by biochemical or DNA testing on 12–14 week chorionic villus samples (see Chapter 53). Newborn screening and early diagnosis are performed routinely in most developed countries and recently the exceptionally rapid technique of **tandem mass spectrometry** (**MS/MS**) has come to prominence for metabolic and haematological disorders (see below).

Inborn errors of metabolism

The prototypical biochemical defect is **phenylketonuria** (**PKU**; see figure and Chapter 19) caused by a block in the conversion of phenylalanine to tyrosine. In most individuals this arises due to a fault in the gene coding for **phenylalanine hydroxylase** (PAH). Rarely (1–3%), it may instead be due to deficiency of one of the enzymes involved in the synthesis of **tetrahydrobiopterin** (BH_4), which serves as a cofactor in the reaction, for example **dihydropteridine reductase**, DHPR. Either way, phenylalanine and its derivatives, mainly phenylpyruvic acid, can build up to toxic levels, with ensuing irreversible damage to the CNS. The deficiency of tyrosine also depresses production of downstream products including melanin, resulting in hypopigmentation, and **DOPA** (**dihydroxy-phenylalanine**) possibly contributing to hormonal and neurological dysfunction.

The figure illustrates five levels at which the likelihood of a baby developing the disease can be assessed: (**1**) a chemical or biochemical screen of the urine; (**2**) a bacteria-based screen of the plasma; (**3**) a biochemical screen for BH_4 deficiency; (**4**) a DNA screen for DHPR mutation; and (**5**) a DNA screen for PAH mutation. Until DNA screening became available the disorder had to be screened for postnatally, as phenylalanine does not accumulate until after birth. Fortunately, dietary restriction of phenylalanine avoids most of the complications of the disorder (see Chapter 19).

Approaches to diagnosis

Detection of metabolites

Detection of metabolites is the time-honoured diagnostic approach. This offers an inexpensive, sensitive and specific means of diagnosis, and is the basis for most newborn screening methods where low cost and sensitivity are critical.

A limitation of metabolite detection is that for some disorders they accumulate only episodically. An example is **methylmalonic acidemia** (see Chapter 45) in which mild enzyme deficiency produces episodic crises between which, blood and urine studies can be unrevealing.

The technology for metabolite detection has undergone significant evolution. In the case of PKU, newborn screening was initially based on the green colour response when ferric chloride ($FeCl_3$) is sprinkled onto the baby's wet nappy (diaper) (No. 1 in figure). Following this came Guthrie's **bacterial inhibition assay** (No. 2 in figure). Heelprick blood samples impregnated onto discs of filter paper are placed on a lawn of bacteria that cannot grow in the absence of supplemental phenylalanine. A halo of bacterial growth surrounding a disc indicates high concentration of phenylalanine.

Quantitative analysis of amino acids and organic acids can be carried out by standard biochemical techniques such as **column chromatography, gas chromatography** or, recently, **tandem mass spectrometry**.

Enzyme assay

Enzyme activity can be assayed *in vitro* using either synthetic or natural substrates. This approach is commonly used to diagnose lysosomal storage disorders, where metabolites are trapped within lysosomes and inaccessible to direct assay (see Chapter 45). It is, for example, used for screening for **hexosaminidase A** deficiency in white blood cells of carriers of Tay–Sachs disease (see Chapters 19 and 45).

Enzyme assay offers the advantage over substrate quantification that heterozygotes are also identifiable, although in some cases there is overlap between their levels and those in normal homozygotes.

DNA diagnosis

There are now many techniques for analysis of DNA (see Chapters 55–58). The advantages of the DNA approach include the ability to test very early in development and on any nucleated cell type, obviating the need to sample tissues that express the enzyme concerned or accumulate relevant metabolites. It is also highly specific, particularly in detecting clinically unaffected carriers, and is finding increasing use in **carrier detection schemes**, such as for **Canavan** and **Gaucher diseases** in the Ashkenazi Jewish population (see Chapter 45).

Tandem mass spectrometry (MS/MS)

Tandem mass spectrometry enables very rapid and simultaneous diagnosis of around 40 disorders of body chemistry from heel-prick blood samples of newborn babies (Table 51.1). It is especially valuable for the disorders of mitochondrial fatty acid β-oxidation associated with **sudden infant death syndrome**, cyclic vomiting and maternal complications of pregnancy. A general feature of these conditions is a decreased level of **carnitine** and an increased ratio of an **acylcarnitine** to free carnitine in the blood plasma.

In a basic MS/MS analysis, as for the acylcarnitines, the preparation is atomized by passage through a fine jet and exposed to an electric field which gives the resulting droplets an extra positive charge (see figure). The ions are then directed through selector slits and into the first quadrupole magnetic 'filter', where oscillating electromagnetic fields sort and select the ions by their mass : charge ratio. Selected ions are then transmitted into a 'collision cell' for fragmention by collision with argon molecules. The ion fragments are passed through a second quadrupole filter, which carries out a second sorting on the basis of mass : charge ratio, to impact on a detector that converts the charges of individual species of ion fragment to electric currents. A molecular profile of the sample is displayed on a chart or computer screen, with each key metabolite represented as a peak in the 'mass spectrum'.

Diseases detectable by MS/MS include the amino acidaemias, organic acidaemias and fatty acid disorders (see Table 51.1), particularly diagnosing disorders of fatty acid oxidation involving acyl group transport across mitochondrial membranes (**MCAD** deficiency; see Chapter 44), as these involve the highly polar carnitines. The first episode of hypoketotic hypoglycaemia in MCAD deficiency is fatal in 30–50% of patients; but MS/MS allows *presymptomatic* detection.

Table 51.1 Some disorders detectable by tandem mass spectrometry. (From ACMG/ASHG statement. (2000) Tandem mass spectrometry in newborn screening. *Genetics in Medicine* **2**(4).)

Disorder	Diagnostic metabolite
Amino acidemias	
Phenylketonuria	Phenylalanine, tyrosine
Maple syrup urine disease	Leucine, isoleucine
Homocystinuria	Methionine
Citrullinemia	Citrulline
Hepatorenal tyrosinemia	Methionine, tyrosine
Organic acidemias	
Propionic acidemia	Acylcarnitine
Methylmalonic acidemia	Acylcarnitine
Isovaleric acidemia	Isovalerylcarnitine
Glutaric acidemia (Type 1)	Glutarylcarnitine
Fatty acid disorders	
SCAD* deficiency	Acylcarnitine
MCAD* deficiency	Acylcarnitine
VLCAD* deficiency	Acylcarnitine
Glutaric acidemia (Type 2)	Glutarylcarnitine

*SCAD, MCAD, VLCAD: short, medium and very long chain acyl CoA dehydrogenases (see Chapter 44).

52 Reproductive genetic counselling

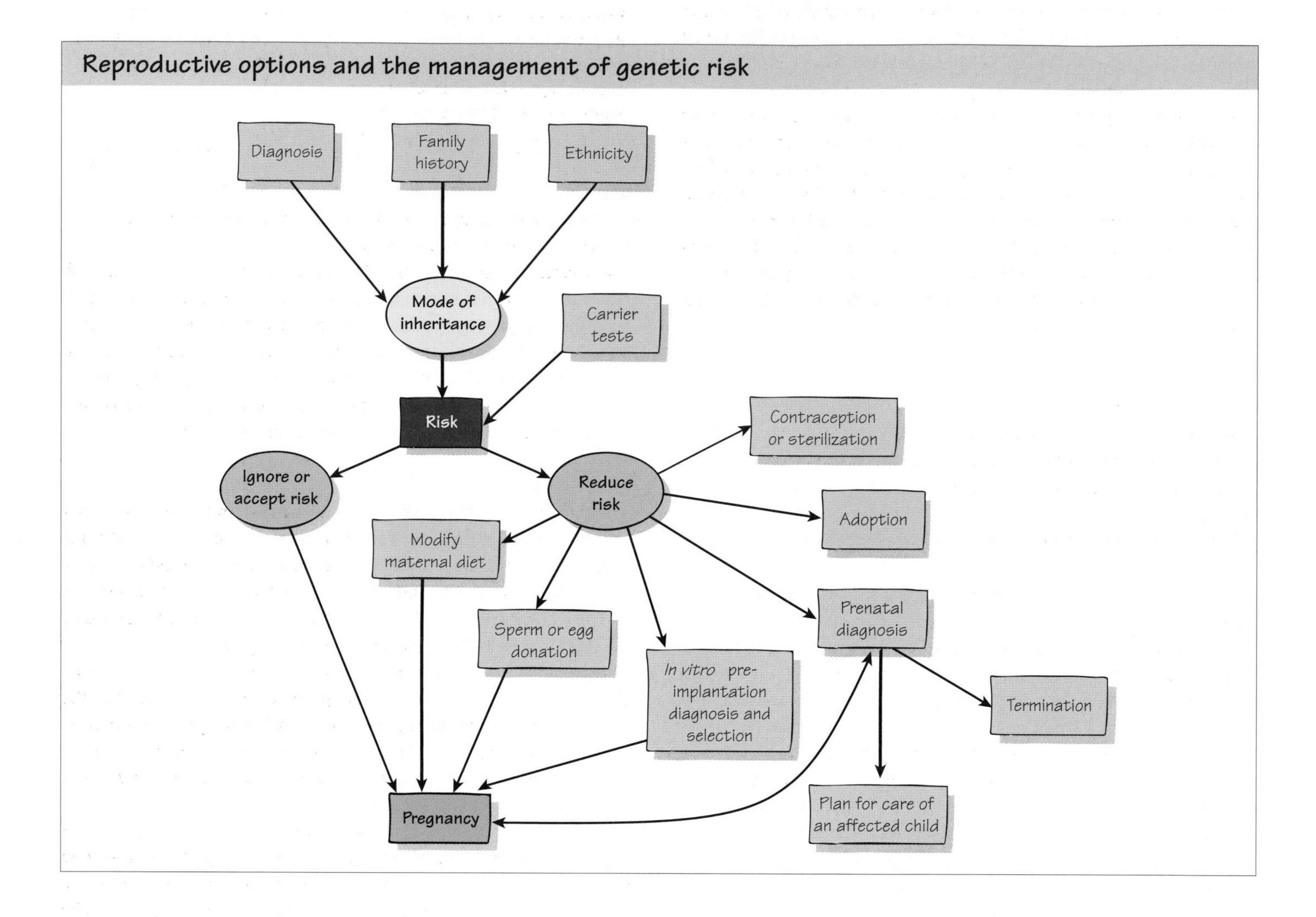

Overview

Genetic counselling is provided by practitioners with specialist training both in the principles of genetics and in the processes of communication with patients and families. In essence it involves accurate assessment of the genetic risk associated with reproduction by the couple concerned (see Chapter 48), communication of this risk to the consultand(s) and, if necessary, the offer of advice on reproductive options.

A major tenet of genetic counselling is to be non-directive, i.e. the personal opinions of the counsellor should not bias the information provided, or create pressure toward a specific management decision. The non-directive approach applies particularly to decisions on prenatal diagnosis, as there is wide divergence of opinion regarding termination of pregnancy. In Britain, legal grounds for termination include 'a substantial risk that if a child were born it would suffer from such physical or mental abnormality as to be seriously handicapped' (UK Abortion Act, 1967).

The psychological approach

Genetic counselling normally begins with the compilation of a family pedigree. The interview at which this is drawn serves four main purposes:

• Establishment of rapport between counsellor and consultand(s).

• Elucidation of the mode of inheritance of the relevant trait in that family.

• Collection of information on family relationships, with identification of others at risk.

• Identification of the consultands' concerns and perceptions of the disease.

As a counsellor you should observe several pointers.

1 Introduce yourself and maintain a warm approach.

2 When dealing with children provide a toy to occupy them while you speak with the parents.

3 Never *assume* relationship such as paternity or maternity.

4 Be aware that members of the family who have died may not be mentioned unless you specifically ask about them and that their memory may cause distress.

5 Take information from both sides of the family. This may not only reveal additional information, but avoids the possible feeling that guilt or blame is directed at one person.

6 While recording the family history watch for clues, such as agitation and the tone of interaction between family members.

The counselling process

The counselling process can be considered under four headings.

1 Genetic contribution. An understanding of the genetic component of the disorder requires integration of clinical diagnosis, family history and the results of laboratory testing. The affected individual and/or other family members should be made aware of the significance of the diagnosis and how genetic factors lead to risk of recurrence.

2 Natural history of the disorder. The patient and family must be educated in the disorder and the medical problems to be expected. It is often helpful for them to meet with parents and physicians who care for patients with similar problems.

3 Management. Management of genetic disorders includes anticipatory guidance, recognizing possible complications and how these can be prevented or ameliorated; surveillance for treatable or preventable complications and management of risk. The latter includes genetic testing to elucidate carrier risk and education on reproductive options and treatment. Some couples want reassuring advice on caring for an affected child, rather than termination.

Table 52.1 Reproductive hazards in the population at large.

Condition	Risk	Risk (%)
Spontaneous miscarriage	1/6	17
Perinatal death	1/30–100	1–3
Neonatal death	1/150	0.7
Major congenital malformation	1/33	3
Minor congenital malformation	1/7	14
Serious mental or physical handicap	1/50	2

4 Support. The genetic counsellor should offer both emotional and logistical support in helping the family make reproductive decisions and cope with genetic risk and its associated emotional burdens. It is difficult for most people to see these in perspective, but an appreciation of the magnitude of reproductive risks in general may be gained by reference to Table 52.1. Any risk over 1/10 is a high risk; one of less than 1/20 is considered by some authorities as low.

Reproductive options

An estimate of risk of disease for a child to be born to the couple concerned is derived from an understanding of the ethnic background of the family, the deduced mode of inheritance of the condition and the results of laboratory tests. Depending on the magnitude of the perceived risk and/or the outlook of the family, the couple may decide to ignore or accept that risk, or take steps to reduce it (see figure).

The latter course could involve *modification of maternal diet or lifestyle*, or *aiming for prenatal diagnosis at a later stage*, with the option of termination. Other options could include *pre-implantation diagnosis*, *artificial insemination by donor*, *egg donation*, *in vitro fertilization with embryo selection*, and *contraception or sterilization, combined with adoption of a healthy child*.

In some cases *intra-cytoplasmic sperm injection* (*ICSI*) may be advised. The main indication for this is male subfertility due to low sperm count, poor sperm motility, abnormal sperm morphology, Y deletion, or physical obstruction or absence of the vas deferens. The latter, CBAVD, is associated with cystic fibrosis carrier status (see Chapter 19). Low sperm count, etc., are frequently associated with Klinefelter syndrome and 13:14 translocation (see Chapters 24 and 25).

There is a small (1.6%) increase in chromosome abnormalities in babies conceived by ICSI; the karyotype of the sperm donor should be checked, especially for submicroscopic deletions of the Y.

It should be remembered that males conceived by ICSI with sperm from a naturally infertile man are likely also to be infertile.

X-linked disease

In some cultures, avoidance of X-linked recessive disease is achieved by termination of all male fetuses carried by heterozygous mothers. Where appropriate prenatal diagnosis is available only the affected 50% of male pregnancies may be terminated. With *in vitro* fertilization and pre-implantation molecular diagnosis, embryo genotypes can be identified and selection imposed. Intervention prior to implantation is acceptable to some branches of Judaism and Islam, although abortion is forbidden. The Roman Catholic Church however disapproves of *in vitro* fertilization, pregnancy termination, sterilization and contraception.

53 Prenatal sampling

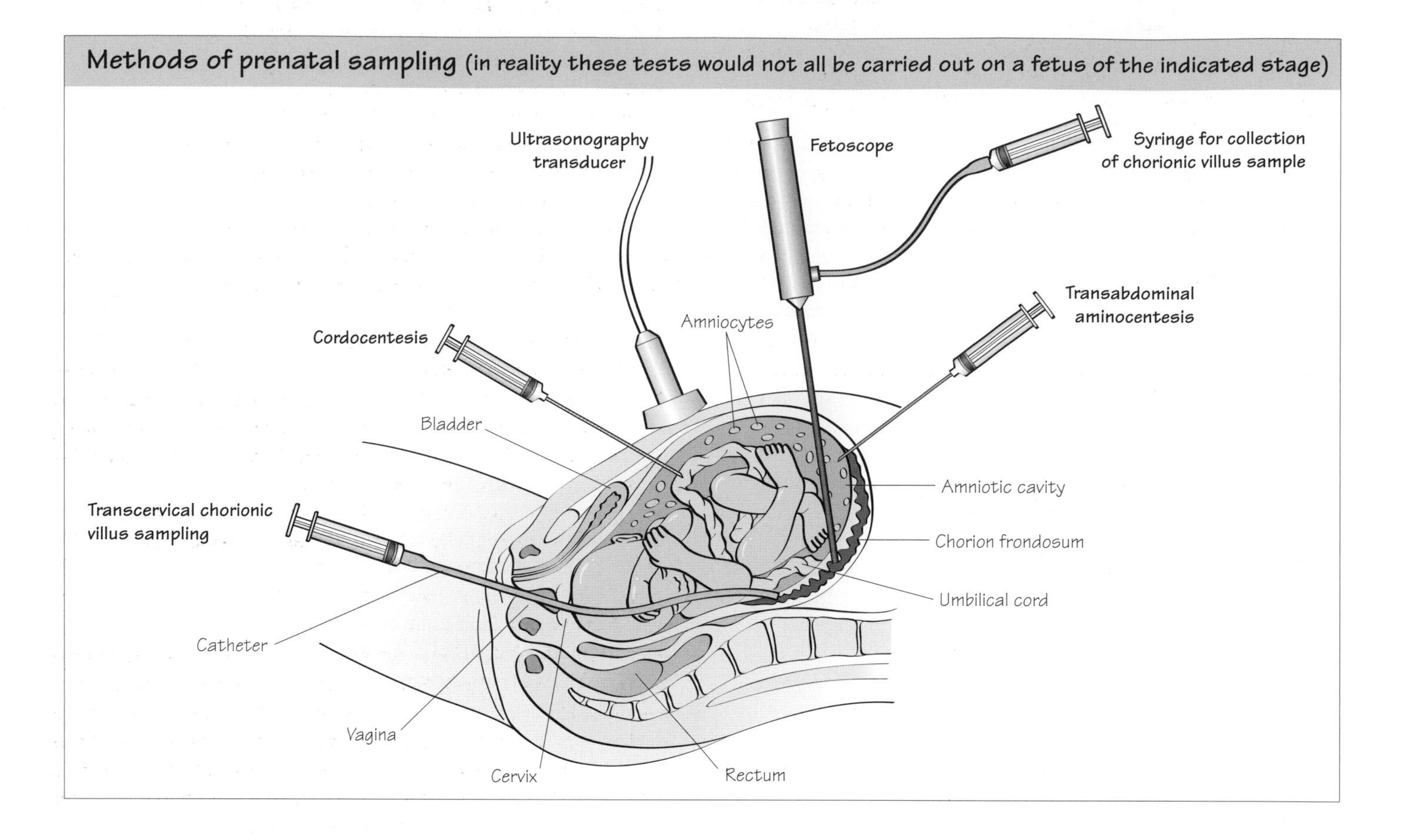

Overview

The term '**prenatal diagnosis**' refers to the diagnosis of genetic disorders in established pregnancies. Such information can guide the family in reproductive decision-making, which may involve terminating the pregnancy, or facilitate planning of appropriate medical, surgical or psychological support. Timing, safety and accuracy are critical.

In North America and Western Europe most pregnant women aged over 35 years are offered a dating scan at about 12 weeks and a fetal physical anomaly scan at 18–20 weeks. If there is to be a termination this is preferable in the first trimester (up to 13 weeks), as it can then be performed by surgery under general anaesthesia, whereas for mid-trimester termination the woman must undergo labour and delivery. There is a generally applied 24-week limit for pregnancy termination in Britain, but the law permits termination for severe abnormalities up to 40 weeks.

Potential benefits of prenatal testing include:

- Reassurance when results are normal.
- Provision of estimates of risk for couples who would otherwise not begin a pregnancy.
- Psychological preparation for the arrival of an affected baby.
- Advance warning for the medical care team.
- Provision of risk information for couples for whom termination is an option.

It should be emphasized that the great majority of prenatal diagnoses yield *normal* test results.

Non-invasive procedures

Ultrasound scanning

In **ultrasound scanning**, echoes reflected from organ boundaries are converted to images on a monitor. This identifies around 300 different malformations, with only a 1% risk of miscarriage.

Anencephaly can be detected at 10–12 weeks, but for most abnormalities the optimum is 18–20 weeks, when the neural tube defects (NTDs), severe skeletal dysplasias, cleft lip and palate, microphthalmia and structural abnormalities of the brain, abdominal organs and heart are usually detectable (Table 53.1). By the third trimester hydrocephalus, microcephaly and duodenal atresia are also detectable.

Obstetric indications for ultrasonography include confirmation of viable or multiple pregnancy, assessment of fetal age and growth, location of the placenta and assessment of amniotic fluid volume. Ultrasonography is an integral aspect of invasive techniques such as **amniocentesis**, **chorionic villus** and **fetal blood sampling**.

X-rays

Because of the risk of mutagenic injury X-rays are preferably avoided altogether during pregnancy (see Chapter 38), although they are sometimes used to assess fetal skeletal dysplasia.

Magnetic resonance imaging (MRI)

New, fast MRI techniques permit prenatal imaging, useful in the diagnosis of internal anomalies such as brain malformation.

Table 53.1 Some major disorders detectable by ultrasound in the second trimester.

CNS	*Skeleton*	*Multi-system disorders*
Anencephaly	Achondroplasia	Growth retardation
Encephalocoele	Osteogenesis imperfecta	Hydrops
Holoprosencephaly	Thanatrophic dysplasia	Oligohydramnios
Hydrocephalus	Polyhydramnios	
Abdomen and pelvis	*Chest*	*Head and face*
Omphalocoele	Congenital heart disease	CL ± P
Renal agenesis	Diaphragmatic hernia	Microphthalmia
Gastroschisis		
Gastrointestinal atresia		
Renal cysts		
Hydronephrosis		

CL ± P, cleft lip with or without palate.

Table 53.2 Prenatal sampling and associated risks.

Stage	Optimal time	Risk of miscarriage	Availability
Pre-implantation			
Embryo biopsy	6–10 cell stage	Unknown, presumed safe	Limited
First trimester (0–13 weeks)			
Chorionic villus sampling			
Transcervical	9–12 weeks	0.5–2.0%	Specialized
Transabdominal	9–13 weeks	0.5–2.0%	Specialized
Maternal circulation	From 6 weeks	Safe	Specialized
Second trimester (14–26 weeks)			
Placental biopsy, transabdominal	14–40 weeks	0.5–2.0%	Specialized
Ultrasonography	16–18 weeks	Safe	Widely available
Amniocentesis	16–18 weeks	0.5	Widely available
Cordocentesis	18–40 weeks	1%	Specialized
Fetoscopy	18–20 weeks	3%	Widely available
Fetal tissue biopsy	18–20 weeks	3%	Very specialized

When culture of embryonic tissue is necessary diagnosis is delayed by 2–4 weeks.

Screening of maternal blood

Maternal serum can provide useful indicators, e.g. of α-fetoprotein (**AFP**), chorionic gonadotrophin (**hCG**) and **unconjugated oestriol** (**UE3**) in relation to Down and Edward syndromes (see Chapters 24, 60). Elevated levels of AFP are associated especially with NTDs (see Chapters 28, 60). Fetal nucleated erythrocytes and trophoblasts isolated from maternal blood by newly developed immunological techniques can also reveal aneuploidy and the Rhesus status of the fetus.

Invasive procedures

The accepted guideline for invasive testing is that the risk of a seriously abnormal fetus must be at least as great as that of miscarriage from the procedure. **Conditions considered serious include those that lead inevitably to stillbirth or early death, or to children with severe multiple or progressive handicap.** The chief indications for prenatal diagnosis are:

1 Maternal age > 35 years at term.
2 Previous child with *de novo* chromosome abnormality.
3 Presence of a recognized chromosome anomaly.
4 Family history of detectable genetic defect.
5 Family history of an X-linked disorder.
6 Elevated serum AFP or family history of NTD.
7 Parental consanguinity in families with recessive disease.
8 Maternal illness, medication, or teratogen exposure.
9 Abnormal amniotic fluid volume.
10 Parents known to be carriers of certain disorders.

Induction of Rhesus iso-immunization by invasive procedures in Rh^- mothers is prevented by administration of anti-D immunoglobulin.

Chorionic villus sampling (CVS)

In CVS a **syncytiotrophoblast** biopsy is aspirated via a catheter through the cervix at 10–12 weeks, or by transabdominal puncture at any time up to term, both guided by ultrasonography. The early timing allows diagnosis by about 12 weeks, but there is an associated risk 0.5–2.0% above the spontaneous abortion rate of 7%.

Since syncytiotrophoblast nuclei divide rapidly, karyotyping is possible without culturing, but cultured material provides more reliable results.

Amniocentesis

Amniocentesis is especially valuable at 16–18 weeks for estimating AFP concentration and acetylcholinesterase activity in pregnancies at risk of NTDs. After prior localization of the placenta by ultrasound, a needle is inserted aseptically through the mother's abdominal wall and into the amniotic cavity, and a 10–20 mL sample is withdrawn. This carries a 0.5% risk of causing miscarriage, in addition to the natural risk of 2.5% at 16 weeks, or 7% when AFP levels are high.

Cordocentesis

From Week 18 onwards a fetal blood sample can be taken by inserting a fine needle transabdominally into the umbilical cord. This is carried out with guidance by fetoscopy (with a 3% extra risk of miscarriage) or ultrasonography (with a 1% extra risk).

Fetoscopy

Fetoscopy involves viewing the fetus through an **endoscope**. The optimum stage is 18–20 weeks and it carries a risk of fetal loss of 3%. Fetoscopy enables biopsy collection for prenatal diagnosis of serious skin and liver disorders, but its most common application is in the investigation of fetal bladder obstruction (see the Potter sequence, Chapter 28).

Pre-implantation genetic diagnosis

In the context of *in vitro* fertilization, one or two cells are collected at the 6–10 cell stage for direct examination by FISH or PCR (see Chapters 50 and 57), enabling selection of healthy embryos for implantation. (Culturing of these cells would contravene the UK Human Fertilization and Embryology Act, 1990.)

Problems of prenatal sampling

True fetal **mosaicism** is found in around 0.25% of fetuses, indicated by discrepant primary cultures. About 1% have **confined placental mosaicism. Maternal cell contamination** is a problem in long-term CV cultures.

54 Clinical application of linkage

Linkage analysis in an autosomal dominant disorder

The two alleles at the disease locus are labelled '+' for wildtype and '–' for disease; alleles at marker locus 'A' are labelled '1' and '2'. At the right, the map of the region is shown, as well as the consequence of recombination. Unborn child III-4 has probably (99%) not inherited the '–' allele, but there remains a 1% chance that recombination occurred during formation of its paternal pronucleus.

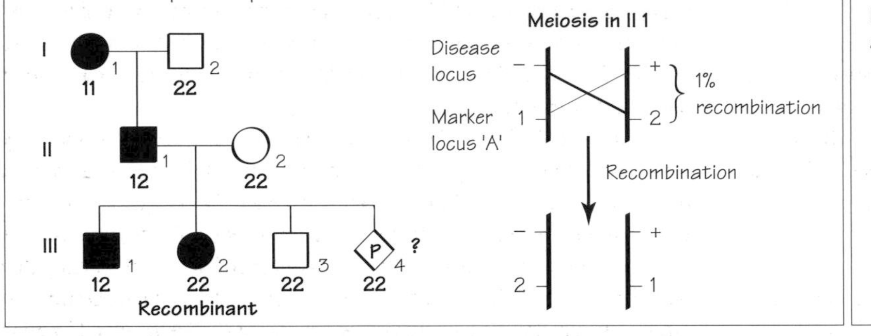

Linkage analysis in an autosomal recessive disorder

Both parents are heterozygous, having alleles '1' and '2' at a polymorphic marker closely linked to the disease allele. The affected child has inherited allele '1' from both parents so, assuming no recombination, this is the allele in coupling with the disease allele in both parents. The second child can be offered testing; if she has genotype '11' she is likely to be affected, '22' unaffected and '12' heterozygous.

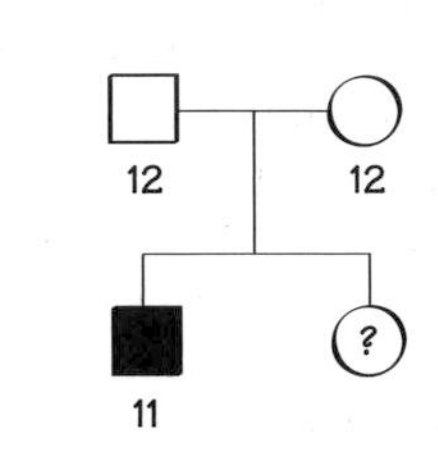

The G-banded human karyotype (chromosomes are shown at the 550 band level of resolution)

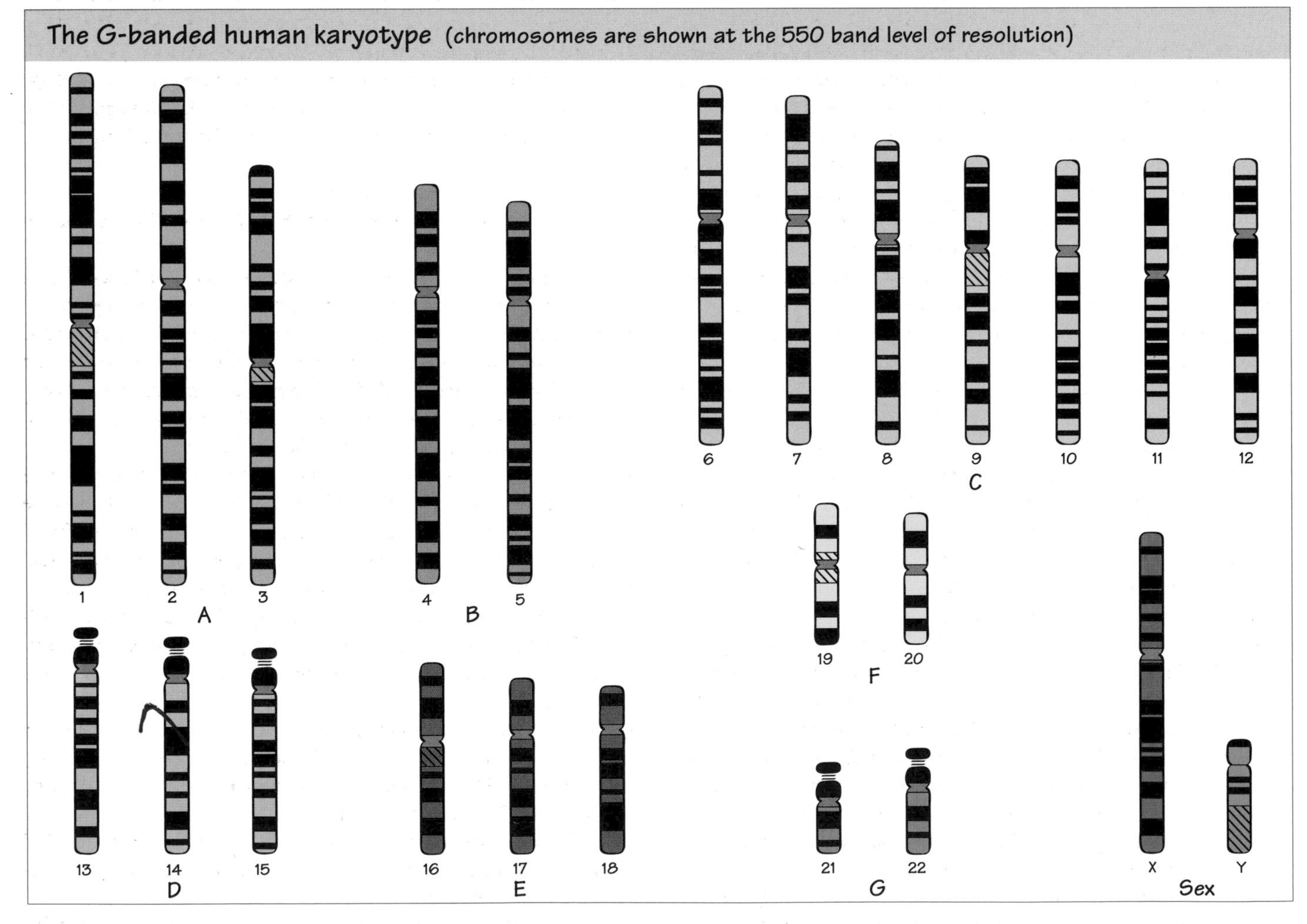

Overview

If we know the mode of transmission of a monogenic disorder, we can use Mendelian reasoning to predict the probability certain individuals will have affected children (see Chapters 15–23). Such predictions are, however, never precise. The mapping of the human genome (see Chapters 36 and 37) enables a powerful supplementary approach based on tracking disease alleles by means of closely linked polymorphic markers. Use of linkage analysis is limited by the possibility of genetic recombination and the need to collect samples from many family members, but it offers two major advantages: disease genes need not be identified, and we need have no molecular understanding of the genes concerned.

Principle

The linkage approach depends on the concept that genes are organized in the same linear order in (virtually) every person. If a polymorphic locus is revealed to be closely linked to a disease locus, that linkage is true for (almost) all individuals. If a carrier of genetic disease is heterozygous for the polymorphism and the coupling phase of marker and disease alleles can be determined (see Chapter 36), then alleles at the polymorphic locus can be used as markers for the disease.

Intragenic neutral polymorphisms can also be used in an adaptation of this approach and in such cases we assume zero recombination.

The polymorphisms most valuable as genetic markers are RFLPs, microsatellites and VNTRs (see Chapters 56 and 58). When linkage phase has been established in a family, the marker locus can be assayed in the at-risk individual to determine whether he or she has inherited the chromosome segment containing the disease allele, or alternatively its homologue carrying the normal allele. Since this approach requires no direct examination, or indeed knowledge, of the disease-causing mutation or its product, it can be considered a form of **indirect diagnosis**.

Disadvantages of the linkage approach are that the marker gene may not show sufficient heterozygosity in that family and that recombination can occur between disease and marker genes within the family. These problems can in practice often be overcome by using several markers located either side of the disease locus.

Autosomal dominant traits

In the dominant pedigree (see figure 'Linkage analysis in an autosomal dominant disorder'), the affected individual, II-1, is heterozygous for both the disease gene and for alleles '1' and '2' at locus 'A.' The 'A' locus is known from studies in other families to be closely linked to the disease gene, with a 1% rate of recombination between them. Individual II-1 has inherited both the disease allele and marker allele '1' from his diseased mother, so in this individual marker allele '1' is located on the same chromosome as the disease allele. His partner (II-2) is homozygous for the '2' allele at the marker locus. We can trace the inheritance of the disease allele in their children by determining whether marker allele '1' or '2' was inherited from the father. Child III-1 has inherited allele '1' and is affected, while III-3 has inherited '2' and is unaffected. Child III-2 is an exception as she inherited the '2' allele from her father, yet is affected. This is due to recombination, the probability of which is known from other studies to be 1%. If the unborn child, III-4, is a '22' homozygote, the probability he or she will be affected is only 1%, despite the existence of a recombinant sib. If necessary, additional polymorphic flanking markers can be used to confirm such deductions and increase the accuracy of analysis.

Autosomal recessive traits

Linkage-based diagnosis can also be performed with recessive traits to follow transmission of alleles from each parent to affected or unaffected children (see figure 'Linkage analysis in an autosomal recessive disorder'). In such cases one must use the situation in an affected child to infer coupling phases in the parents.

X-linked traits

The same analysis can be done for X-linked traits, tracking the inheritance of the two X chromosomes from a heterozygous female. If the grandparental generation is not available for study, one can infer coupling phase from affected children, with the caveat that one or more might be recombinants. This caveat introduces some uncertainty, and thus decreases analytical power, but it is still better than the estimate of 50% based on the equal probability of inheriting one or the other chromosome homologue.

Linkage analysis was the mainstay of diagnosis at a time when many disease genes were mapped, but few were cloned. It is less often used today, but is still helpful in instances where the disease gene is mapped but not identified, or where there is a wide diversity of mutations and the gene is large so that molecular analysis is impractical. Until recently this was the case with the **dystrophin** gene responsible for **Duchenne** and **Becker muscular dystrophies** (see Chapter 57). The dystrophin gene has 79 exons and 2/3 of disease alleles have intragenic deletions. Most of the remaining 1/3 have more subtle mutations such as single base pair changes, which may be anywhere within the gene. In these, linkage analysis using polymorphic markers remains a powerful approach to carrier testing and prenatal diagnosis (see also Chapters 56 and 57).

Pitfalls in interpretation

There are a number of potential pitfalls in interpretation of linkage-based tests:

• The clinical diagnosis in the family must be firmly established, since linkage testing alone will not confirm or refute the original diagnosis.

• Different genetic loci are sometimes responsible for clinically indistinguishable disorders. This is the case for **tuberous sclerosis**, where **TSC1** (Chromosome 9) and **TSC2** (Chromosome 16) produce the same condition. Such **genetic heterogeneity** must be taken into account and in some cases may prohibit the use of linkage analysis.

• There must be polymorphic markers near the disease locus and these must be heterozygous in an individual heterozygous for the disease allele from whom transmission is being tracked. The high density of the gene map makes this likely, but before diagnostic testing is offered, the family must be studied individually to determine which markers are informative. Specific alleles in coupling with the disease allele will differ between families, though where linkage disequilibrium occurs, one particular allele may be non-randomly associated with disease (see Chapters 36, 43).

• Linkage analysis is a family-based test and multiple family members must be available and willing to participate in the study. This may present problems with severe recessive disorders if the proband is deceased and his or her DNA is not available.

• Finally, the outcome of a linkage analysis remains only a statistical probability; genetic recombination may always occur and can potentially lead to misdiagnosis.

These issues must be explained to a family that requests testing and this can present a formidable challenge in counselling.

55 DNA sequencing

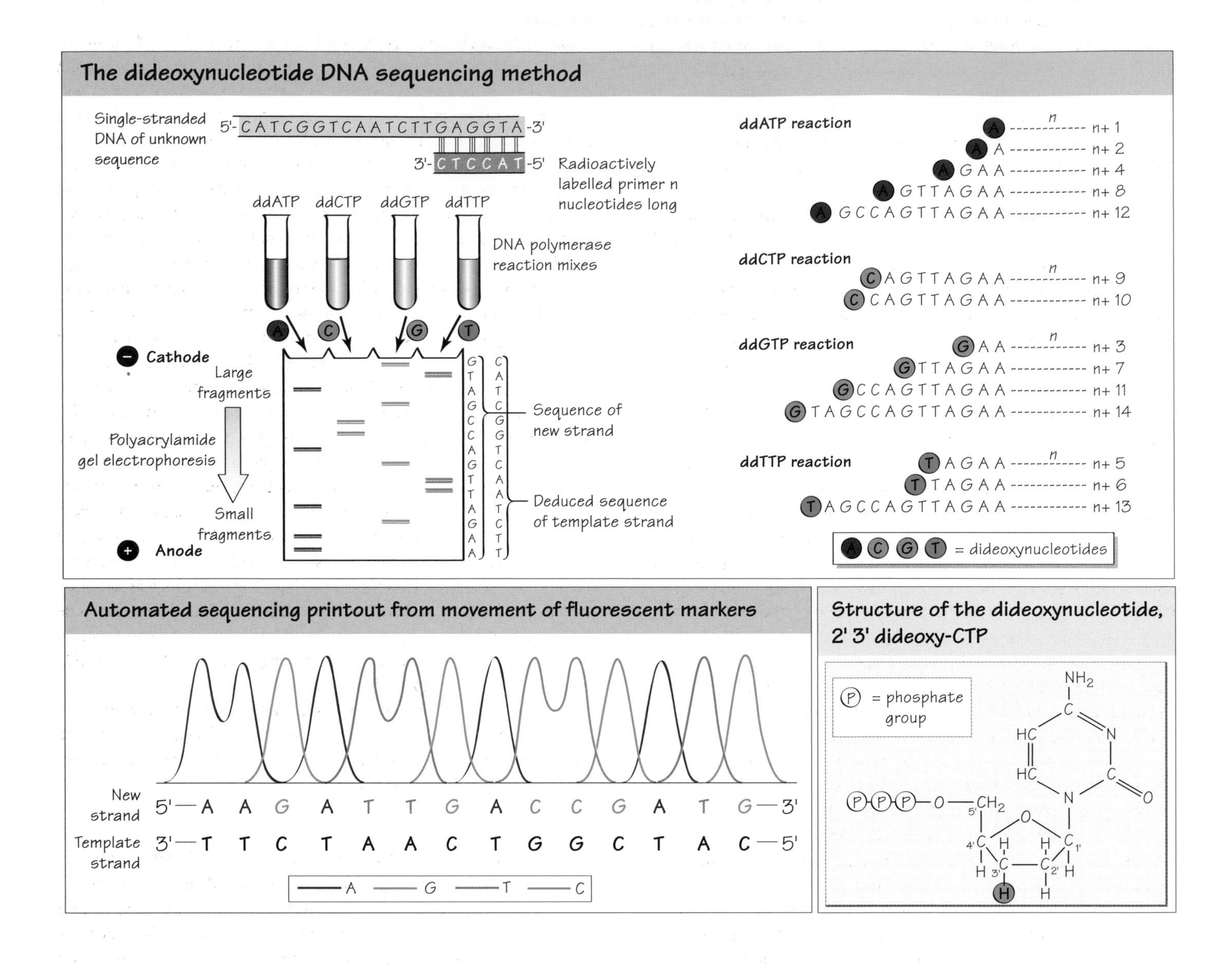

Overview

A complete description of most mutations requires knowledge of the base sequence of the DNA at the site of error. Currently most DNA sequencing is carried out by the enzymic method of Sanger and co-workers; the end result is a ladder of bands from which the base sequence can be read directly, or a row of peaks on a graph.

The dideoxy-DNA sequencing method

For this method the DNA to be sequenced is prepared in multiple copies of one 'template' strand. DNA polymerase is then used to synthesize multiple new complementary strands.

The enzymic reaction requires a primer complementary to the 3′ end of the sequence, DNA polymerase, co-factors, etc. and base-specific **dideoxynucleotides** (ddATP, ddTTP, ddCTP and ddGTP), in addition to the normal deoxynucleotide precursors (dATP, etc.). The dideoxynucleotides lack the hydroxyl group present on the 3′ carbon atoms of deoxynucleotides that in DNA forms the link to the adjacent nucleotide. They are incorporated into growing DNA as normal, but chain extension is blocked beyond them by the lack of the 3′ hydroxyl group. A radioactive label is incorporated either into these ddNTPs or into the primer.

Four parallel base-specific reactions are conducted using a mix of all four normal nucleotide precursors, one with a radioactive label, plus a small proportion of *one* of the four dideoxy-derivatives. If the concentration of the latter is low compared to that of its normal analogue, chain termination occurs randomly at each of the many positions containing that specific base. Each base-specific reaction generates many fragments of different lengths, with variable 3′ termini but a common 5′ end, corresponding to the primer.

In the original method the DNA fragments were then separated by electrophoresis through polyacrylamide gel, in which they migrate at speeds inversely proportional to their lengths. Following electrophoresis the gel was dried out and an autoradiographic (or X-ray) film placed in contact with it. After suitable exposure the film was developed to produce a pattern of dark bands. The sequence was then read off by simple inspection of the autoradiograph, providing the 5′-to-3′ sequence of the new strand complementary to the original template.

This process has now been automated by attaching four differently coloured fluorescent markers to the four ddNTPs, instead of a radioactive label. The DNA synthesis is performed in one vessel and the fluor-labelled reaction products are electrophoresed together through a capillary glass tube. As they migrate past a window they are excited by a beam of laser light and emit coloured fluorescence. This is captured by a digital camera, translated into an electric signal and represented as a graph, with the four dideoxynucleotides shown as peaks of different colours. The position of a mutation is then located by comparison of mutant and normal sequences. These adaptations allow sequencing to proceed at a rate of up to a million bases per day.

Diagnostic applications

DNA sequencing can be used in diagnostic testing, when the aim is to identify *specific* pathogenic mutations. To determine whether a known mutation, or the normal sequence, is present involves sequencing the region of the gene for a short stretch around the mutant site. In an individual heterozygous for a single base substitution two different bases would be found at that site, one representing each DNA strand.

Heterozygous insertions or deletions produce a complex pattern of two superimposed sequences, one mutant and one normal. To elucidate this it may be necessary to clone and sequence the two DNA duplexes separately.

DNA sequencing can also be used to scan large regions of a gene for mutations. This offers the advantage that the specific mutation does not need to be known in advance as it can in principle detect a wide variety of types of mutation. However, several precautions must be observed in the interpretation of sequence variants detected in this way. First, not finding a mutation does not necessarily mean no mutation is present: there may be mutations outside the structural gene, perhaps in regulatory regions. Also, certain types of structural rearrangements, such as deletion of an entire gene, can remain undetected by sequencing. It should also be recognized that not all sequence variants disrupt gene function, as is necessary for it to constitute a pathogenic mutation.

Evidence that a variant is pathogenic might include inference from its likely impact on the gene product; for example, mutations that cause frameshifts are more likely to disrupt function than single base substitutions (see Chapter 39). Demonstration that a mutation is present only in affected individuals and segregates in families together with disease is highly suggestive that that is the gene causing the disorder, or else is in close linkage with it. Another important clue is recapitulation of the mutant phenotype in an animal model based on a known mutation.

Direct sequencing is currently not the method of choice for most diagnostic laboratories, when the goal is to identify the presence of a limited repertoire of mutations. This is the case, for example, with the β-globin mutation responsible for sickle cell anaemia. Since only one mutation is being sought, it is easier and less expensive to use methods of direct mutation analysis, such as the polymerase chain reaction (PCR) followed by restriction enzyme digestion or oligonucleotide hybridization (see Chapters 56 and 57).

Direct sequencing is, however, used commonly in the identification of mutations in the *BRCA1* and *BRCA2* genes (see Chapter 41). Here the mutant sites are highly diverse and widely scattered, making it necessary to scan the gene sequences in full.

Real-time PCR

Even in analysis of the CFTR (cystic fibrosis; see Chapter 19) gene, where more than 1300 mutations have been described, direct sequencing of the entire gene is usually too expensive. Furthermore, sequencing increases sensitivity by only about 10% over analysis of a limited number of relatively common known mutations by techniques like dot-blot oligonucleotide hybridization (see Chapter 56).

However, once the DNA sequence of a mutation is known probes can be constructed specific to that mutation and this opens up additional opportunities. For example, oligonucleotides are designed corresponding to sequences on either side of each of the common mutations causative of cystic fibrosis. For each mutation the 'probes' corresponding to the two sides are labelled with one component of a **fluorescence resonance energy transfer** (**FRET**) molecule. Many copies of each of the 15 exons of the CFTR gene are generated by multiplex PCR (see Chapter 57) and challenged with these special probes. When the two probes corresponding to a mutant exon bind in close proximity, the two halves of the FRET combine and become capable of fluorescing. Emission of fluorescent light of a specific colour then indicates a specific CF mutation. This method is known as '**real-time PCR**'.

56 Southern blotting

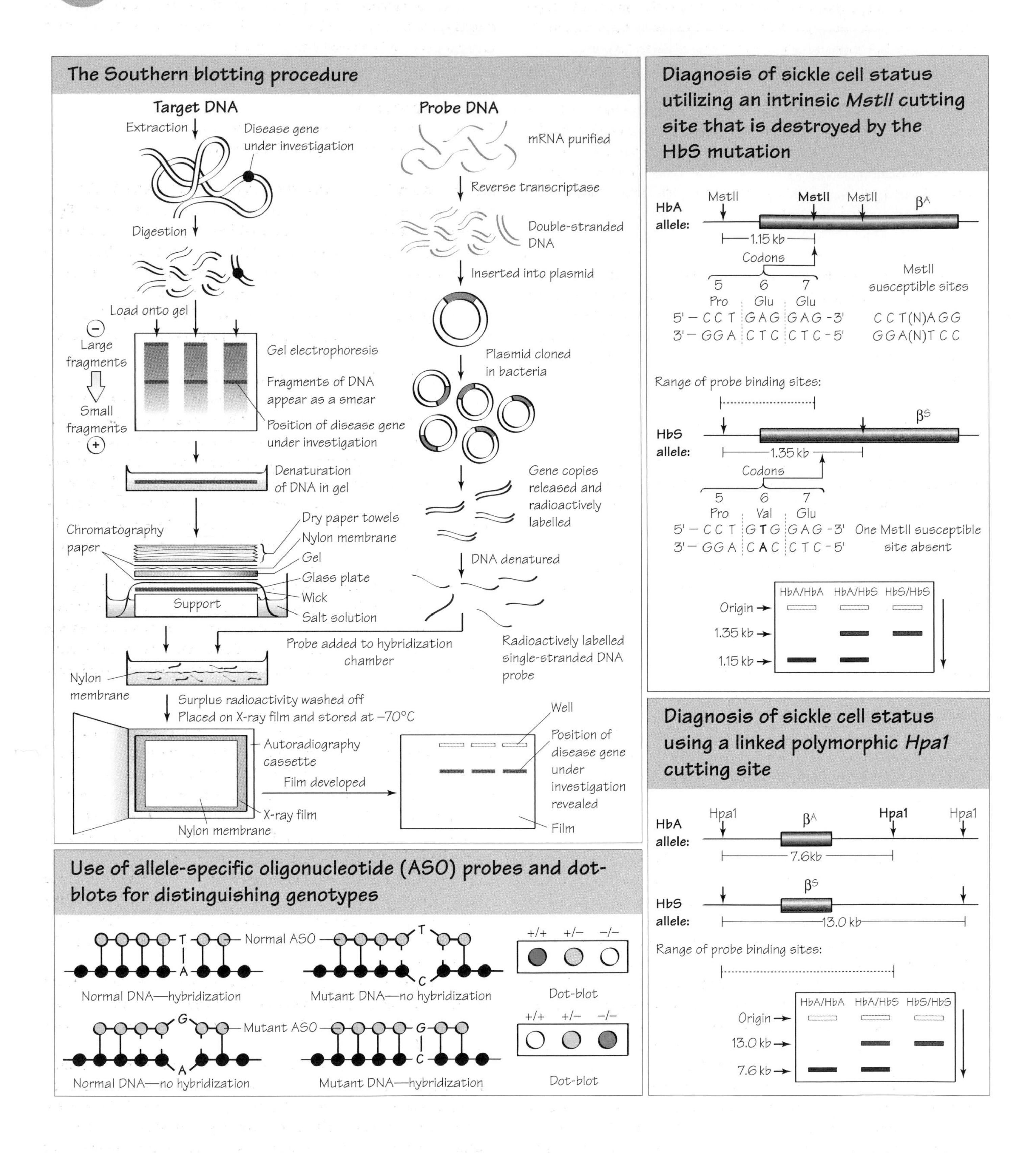

Overview

A set of highly specialized molecular techniques collectively known as 'Southern blotting', was one of the earliest effective molecular diagnostic approaches. Although largely superseded now, the components of the original method are applied in many other techniques, so it is instructive to present them in some detail. The choice of method to carry out a practical genetic investigation depends primarily on whether it is to test for a *known* sequence change, or to look for *any* mutation in a particular gene. Other issues are the size and structure of the gene, the equipment and skills available, the sensitivity required and the cost.

Four concepts are necessary to understand the Southern blotting procedure: **DNA probes**, **restriction endonucleases**, gel electrophoresis and DNA polymorphism.

DNA probes

A DNA probe is a short section (0.3–5.0 kb, or longer) of double-stranded DNA corresponding to part of the locus of interest. It can be prepared, for example, from the **cDNA** (copy DNA) copy of a purified mRNA, generated with the enzyme **reverse transcriptase**, then radioactively labelled and 'denatured' into single strands. Alternatively, cloned segments of genomic DNA can be used.

Restriction endonucleases and DNA polymorphism

Restriction endonucleases are bacterial enzymes that cut double-stranded DNA at specific sequences. Such sites occur throughout the genome and the sections of DNA that result from enzyme cutting are called **restriction fragments**. Variation in the length of restriction fragments, due to polymorphism at potential cutting sites, is called **restriction fragment length polymorphism** (**RFLP**). These variant cutting sites provide valuable markers for disease genes that can be exploited in linkage studies (see Chapter 54).

Gel electrophoresis

A gel is a three-dimensional mesh with pores of different sizes. They are cast as slabs of **agarose** or **polyacrylamide**, with a row of wells at one end for insertion of samples. During electrophoresis the gel is subjected to an electric current, when negatively charged DNA fragments are repelled by the negative terminal, or cathode, and migrate toward the **anode**. The smallest fragments run fastest, with the others behind them in order of size.

Southern blotting

The usual source of DNA is white blood cells, but for prenatal diagnosis samples may be taken from chorion villus, or amniotic fluid cell cultures (see Chapter 53). The DNA is digested with restriction enzymes, inserted into a well of the gel and the electric current applied.

Since these gels are too fragile for manipulation, the electrophoretically fractionated DNA is denatured and transferred to a more durable support, usually a nylon membrane, by the Southern blotting technique (see figure). This in effect produces a print of the DNA array in the gel, with all its bands in perfect register. The DNA is then bound to the membrane by exposure to UV light and incubated in a solution containing the denatured radioactive probe. The probe 'hybridizes' with its complementary sequence in the sample. Unbound probe DNA is washed away and the position of the bound radioactivity is located by autoradiography. This involves placing the nylon membrane face down on an X-ray film and storage at –70°C for several hours or days. When the film is developed, black bands appear, indicating the location, and hence the length, of the restriction fragment containing the gene of interest.

Modern approaches use digital systems that detect the radioactivity directly, conferring the advantage of instantaneous results. In some instances non-radioactive labels are used.

Methodological variants

Northern blotting

This variant is used to identify mRNA species in a mixture subjected to electrophoresis and probing in a similar way.

Dot blots and allele-specific oligonucleotides (ASOs)

When both normal and mutant sequences are known, very short '**oligonucleotide**' probes can be synthesized biochemically to match each one. These are hybridized to '**dot-blots**' of denatured DNA applied directly to a nylon membrane, allowing rapid identification of homozygotes and heterozygotes, and distinction between alleles.

This approach offers an inexpensive and rapid method of diagnosis, but it is limited by the need for prior knowledge of mutant sequences.

Pulsed field gel electrophoresis (PFGE)

Standard agarose gel electrophoresis efficiently separates DNA fragments only up to 30 kb in length. PFGE allows resolution of DNA fragments ranging in size from 20 000 to several million base pairs.

White blood cells are embedded in agarose blocks which are exposed to proteolytic enzymes that digest away cellular materials, leaving the chromosomes intact. They are then exposed to 'rare cutter' restriction endonucleases which create very long pieces of DNA defined by the susceptible sequences at each end. These are separated electrophoretically in agarose gel, but every so often the direction of the current is changed by 90°. The DNA fragments are therefore repeatedly required to change conformation, and the time taken for them to reorient themselves is strictly size dependent. Consequently, they end up in reverse order of size along the diagonal. This allows examination and separation of very large genes, like dystrophin and multigenic functional units.

Diagnostic applications

One application involves selection of a restriction endonuclease for which the recognition site corresponds with either the mutant or normal version of the sequence in question. DNA is cut with the enzyme and the fragments are analysed using as a probe a DNA sequence near the site of mutation. If the mutation disrupts a normal cutting site, that segment of DNA will remain intact. Presence or absence of the mutation can then be determined by comparing fragment sizes.

An example is sickle cell disease (see figure in Chapter 39). In the normal β-globin allele the sixth codon is cut by the enzyme MstII, but the HbS mutation destroys that site and a longer DNA fragment is produced. In most cases polymorphic cutting sites are identified outside the disease genes (see figure).

In most laboratories polymerase chain reaction (PCR) has replaced Southern analysis for detection of specific alterations in base sequence (see Chapter 57), but it still finds application where larger rearrangements are involved.

Very long triplet repeat expansions (see Chapters 21 and 39) cannot be reliably amplified by PCR, but Southern analysis can reveal the expanded allele by its reduced mobility. In Fragile X disease the unexpressed, expanded allele is invariably methylated; differential diagnosis can therefore be performed with a restriction endonuclease that cleaves only *non*-methylated DNA.

57 The polymerase chain reaction

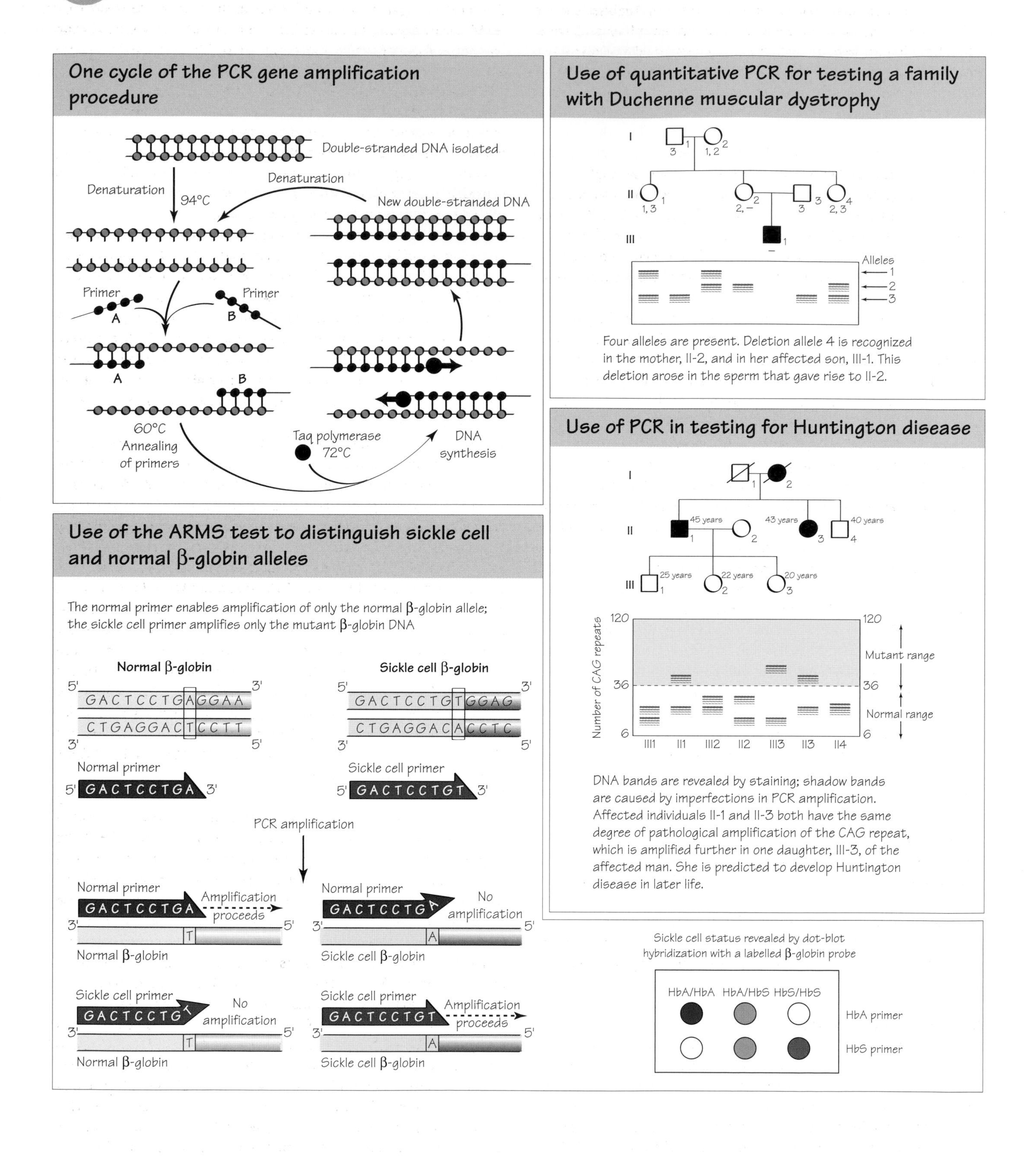

Overview

The **polymerase chain reaction** (**PCR**) has utterly revolutionized the diagnosis and molecular analysis of genetic disease. Analyses can be performed on samples as minute as a single nucleus obtained from a preimplantation embryo, a mouthwash, hair root, or other source. It is performed in a few hours and is cheaper than any other method. *PCR-based techniques have therefore become the most widely used methods of genetic analysis.*

The polymerase chain reaction

The reaction uses *Taq* DNA polymerase and operates on single-strand DNA, replacing the missing strand in much the same way as in DNA replication (see Chapter 5). *Taq* polymerase is isolated from *Thermus aquaticus*, a hot-spring bacterium and can withstand temperatures up to 95°C. It requires a start point of duplex DNA, which is provided by single-strand **primers** annealed one at each end of the sequence to be duplicated.

To carry out the reaction the DNA sample is first heated to 94°C to 'melt' the hydrogen bonds joining the two polynucleotide strands. The temperature is reduced to ~60° and short oligonucleotide primers are added. These are usually 15–30 nucleotides long and designed to match and anneal to complementary conserved stretches flanking the chosen sequence. In the third step, carried out at 72°, the polymerase moves down the DNA strand, away from the primers and synthesizes a complementary strand, so re-creating a double-stranded molecule.

This set of three steps can be considered as one 'cycle', which is repeated by careful temperature control in the presence of excess primers. Each cycle takes only a few minutes and the amount of DNA doubles every time. After 30 cycles over 100 000 000 copies of the original sequence are created. The process is normally performed automatically in a programmed thermocycler.

PCR can also be used to amplify RNA sequences, if they are first copied into cDNA replicates by means of reverse transcriptase.

Comparative advantages of PCR

- **Sensitivity:** PCR is applicable to single-genome quantities of DNA.
- **Speed:** the procedure is very fast (3–48 hours).
- **Safety:** no radioactivity is involved.
- **Molecular product:** the product is suitable for further analysis by established molecular techniques.
- **Resolution**: the process can be applied to even badly degraded DNA.

Disadvantages of PCR

- **Size of template:** long sequences cannot be amplified.
- **Prior knowledge:** the base sequences of flanking regions must be known.
- **Contamination:** absolute purity of the sample is essential.
- **Infidelity of replication:** there is no 'proof-reading', or error correction, so that mutations that occasionally arise during the process are also propagated.

Diagnostic applications

The value of PCR in diagnosis lies in its ability to provide large quantities of specific gene sequences that can be subjected to further analysis. Primers are used that flank one specific region of a gene, or alternatively multiple regions such as several exons. Applications include the following:

1 Diagnosis of triplet repeat disorders (e.g. Duchenne muscular dystropy and Huntington disease; see figure and Chapters 21 and 39).

2 Direct sequencing of the gene(s) (see Chapter 55).

3 Restriction endonuclease digestion. This approach can be applied when a *specific* mutation is being sought. An endonuclease is chosen that has a recognition sequence spanning the mutant site (see Chapter 56). The enzyme will then either cut or not cut the DNA, depending on whether the mutation is present. Analysis of fragment sizes by agarose gel electrophoresis then indicates the genotype.

4 Single strand conformation polymorphism (SSCP). PCR-amplified DNA is denatured and electrophoresed without renaturation, when mutant strands are detectable by their abnormal speeds of migration.

5 Allele-specific oligonucleotide (ASO) dot blots. This method, described in Chapter 56, is commonly used where analysis involves detection of a single mutation (e.g. sickle cell disease) or a limited range of *common* disease alleles (e.g. cystic fibrosis).

6 The amplification refractory mutation system (ARMS) depends on specificity of binding of PCR primers to template DNA (see figure). A primer is designed with a 3′ end corresponding to either a mutant, or the wild-type sequence. The primer will bind only with its exact complement, so a wild-type primer permits amplification of only wild-type DNA, mutant primer only mutant DNA. Two separate PCR reactions, with either mutant or wild-type primer, together with another primer elsewhere in the gene, can be used to determine heterozygosity or homozygosity of either sequence. This approach also has been used to identify CFTR mutations.

7 Multiplex PCR. In multiplex PCR amplification is carried out on many exons in the same reaction mix. It is particularly valuable for Duchenne muscular dystropy, with any of many possible deletions in the very long dystrophin gene (see Chapter 22). The PCR products are designed to be all of different lengths, so they can be separated by agarose gel electrophoresis on the basis of size and scanned simultaneously, when deletion of an exon is indicated by a missing band.

8 Multiplex amplifiable probe hybridization (MAPH). A problem with multiplex PCR is differential amplification of individual exons; MAPH is a more reliable variant. Genomic DNA from the patient is bound onto a nylon filter and a mixture of perhaps 40 DNA probes, each specific to one exon, is hybridized to it. The probes are all of different lengths and each carries common primer sequences at its ends. After careful washing, the filter is placed in a PCR reaction mix that amplifies all the bound probes uniformly. If an exon is deleted from the genomic DNA its absence is reliably indicated by release of the amplified DNA followed by gel electrophoresis.

9 DNA micro-arrays. This approach also exploits the extraordinary miniaturization and accuracy of inkjet printing and the speed of computer-based analysis. It involves synthesizing custom-designed 20–25 bp oligonucleotide sequences of normal and known (or expected) single-base substitutions of a gene. For example, ASOs could be created corresponding to each of the 1300+ known cystic fibrosis mutations. These would be spotted onto a 1 cm^2 nitrocellulose-coated glass surface constituting a '**DNA chip**'. The spotting is done by robotic gridding devices which place hundreds of thousands of samples at positions defined by linear coordinates. The test DNA is fluorescently labelled and hybridized to the array, and the pattern of binding analysed by computer.

10 Chromosomal diagnosis. Rapid screening for aneuploidy is carried out by multiplex PCR amplification of microsatellites specific to Chromosomes 13, 18 and 21, followed by quantitative assay for each chromosome.

11 Mass spectrometry. Mass spectrometry (see Chapter 51) provides an exceptionally rapid means of analysing PCR amplified DNA. This is proving of great value in screening the CFTR and Apolipoprotein-E genes of major importance in Alzheimer disease (see Chapter 32).

12 Real-time PCR (see Chapter 55).

58 DNA profiling

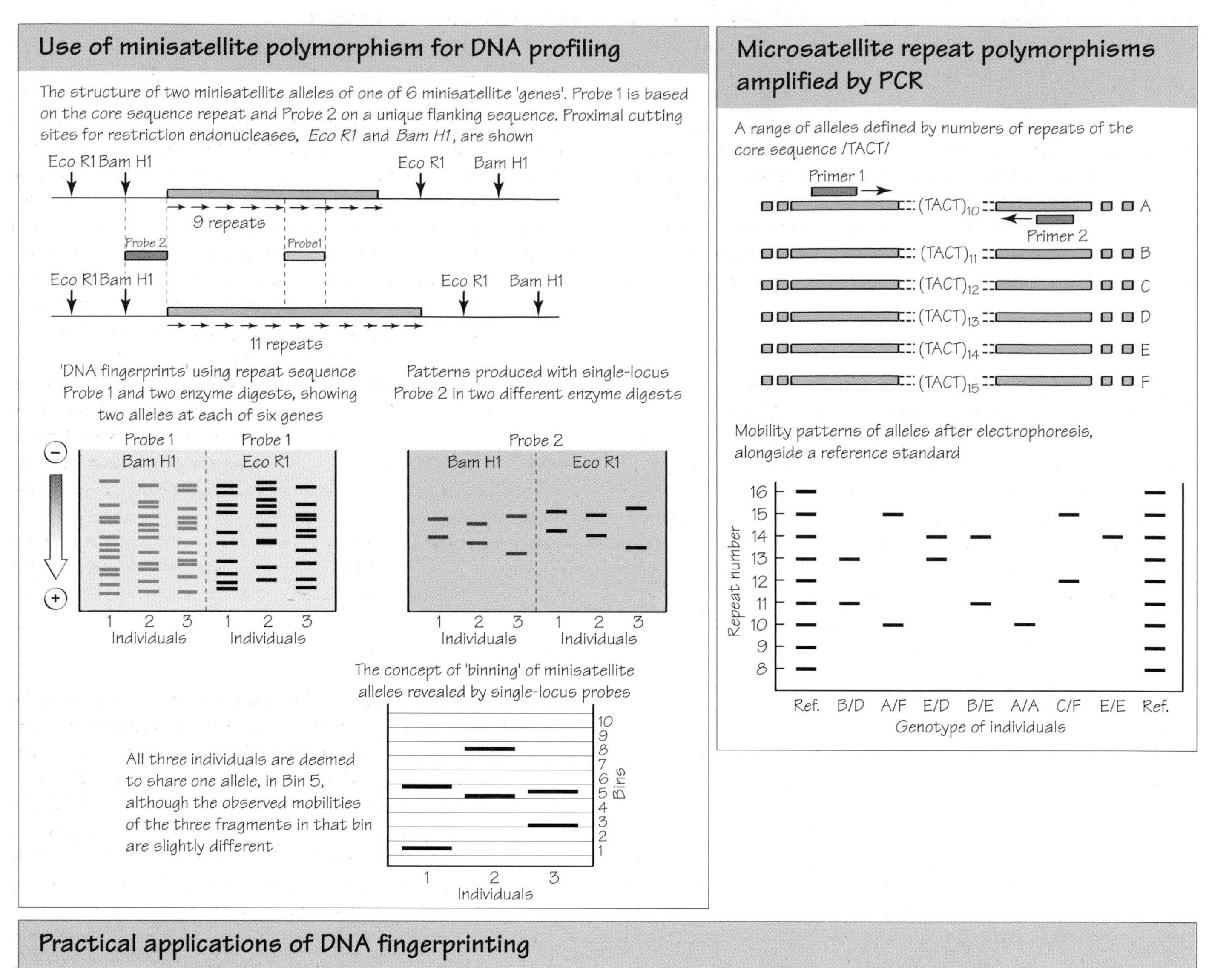

Practical applications of DNA fingerprinting

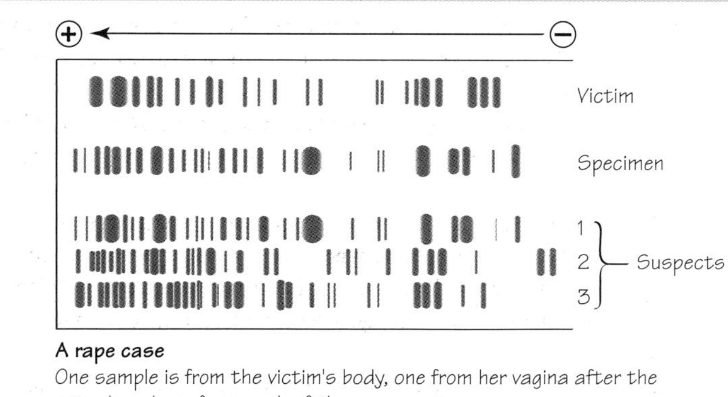

A rape case

One sample is from the victim's body, one from her vagina after the attack and one from each of three suspects.
Suspect 1 was found guilty

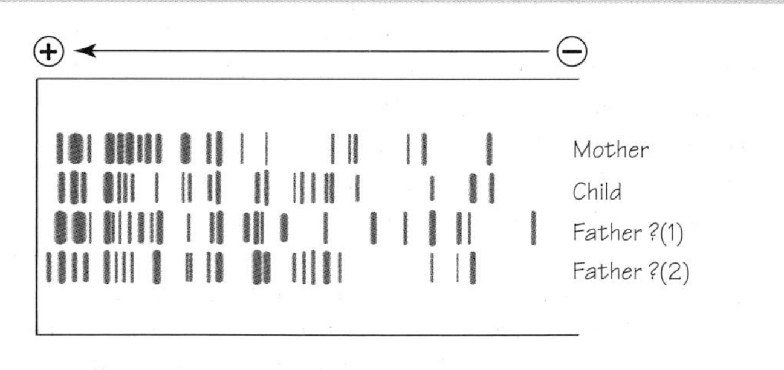

A paternity case

DNA fingerprints from a mother, her child and two men. Every band in the child is traceable either to the mother or to putative father 2

Overview

DNA profiling is the characterization of an individual genome by DNA analysis. It includes **DNA fingerprinting**, use of **single locus probes**, microsatellite, Y-chromosome, mitochondrial and ethnic polymorphisms. It is of enormous value for identifying the father in paternity disputes, for confirming family membership in immigration cases and for identifying the perpetrators and victims of crime from traces of biological material.

As explained in Chapter 4, our genomes contain a large quantity of highly repetitive DNA called '**microsatellite DNA**', when the sequence is short (1–4 bp), and '**minisatellite DNA**', when the sequence is longer (5–64 bp). Microsatellite DNA is scattered throughout the chromosomes and provides useful markers for disease genes (see Chapter 54). Minisatellite DNA is concentrated near the centromeres and telomeres and is particularly valuable for DNA profiling, but both are exploited in this respect.

Application of Southern blotting

DNA fingerprinting with minisatellite markers

The Southern blotting approach to DNA analysis (see Chapter 56) depends on the creation of **restriction fragment length polymorphisms** (**RFLPs**) due to polymorphism at restriction endonuclease cutting sites. DNA fingerprinting also depends on fragment length polymorphism, but due to variation instead in the length of repetitious sequences *between* cutting sites. These are also known as **VNTRs**, or **variable number tandem repeats**.

The original probe used in fingerprinting was directed against the repeated minisatellite **core sequence /GGGCAGGAXG/** (where X is any nucleotide) within the myoblobin gene. Tandem repeats of two to several hundred copies of this sequence are present in the human genome at over 1000 sites, although only 8–17 are of practical value in fingerprinting.

If a sample of human DNA is digested with a restriction enzyme for which there are many cutting sites (a '**frequent cutter**'), multiple fragments are produced of many sizes and of great variation between individuals. Those fragments that contain repeats of the core sequence can be visualized on Southern blots by the core sequence probe, as a ladder of bands (see figure). The chances of any two unrelated individuals having the same pattern are estimated at $< 1/10^{11}$. The only exceptions are members of genetic clones, such as MZ twins. These patterns are known as '**DNA fingerprints**' (see figure).

The statistical evaluation of multilocus fingerprint evidence in forensic casework rests on the proportion (x) of bands which on average are shared by unrelated people. 'x' is estimated as 0.14 for both the most commonly used probes, irrespective of ethnicity. A conservative estimate of 0.25 is normally used to prevent over-interpretation and to allow for possible relationship between the suspect and guilty party.

Assuming statistical independence of (i.e. no linkage between) all bands then the chance that n bands in individual A are matched by bands of precisely similar electrophoretic mobility in B is x to the power n.

In paternity disputes germline mutation can lead to invalid exclusion of a putative father. In fact 27% of offspring show one band not present in either parent, 1.2% show two, and an estimated < 0.3% show three new bands.

Repetitious regions containing multiples of other core sequences can be exploited to produce different fingerprints, using the same enzyme digest and appropriate probes. Alternatively, the same DNA sample can be digested with a different restriction enzyme and examined with the same probe or others.

Use of single locus probes

If a fingerprinting blot is examined with a probe complementary to a sequence *flanking* one hypervariable region a much simplified pattern is revealed, derived from just that one locus (see figure). Each such probe should reveal a maximum of two bands in any person, representing the two alleles and on average 70% of people are heterozygous at any such locus.

Statistical proof of identity requires examination of 4–10 such loci and if the population frequency of each 'allele' is known, it is possible to make exact calculations of probability. However, exact numbers of repeats are not always known and fragment band positions do not always correspond precisely. So for statistical purposes the DNA track is divided into a number of 'bins' and bands are deemed to match if they fall within the same bin. Although 'binning' introduces inaccuracies it is necessary to estimate the population frequencies of fragments of specific lengths. This is always done conservatively, so that the statistical weight of evidence is biased in favour of the defendant. Appropriate ethnic databases also have to be set up and when applying Hardy–Weinberg reasoning (see Chapter 35) due allowance must be made for possible population stratification based on, for example, ethnicity, religion or social class.

The Southern blotting approach to genetic profiling described above requires the DNA of about a million cells. For these reasons of scale and problems in the identification of alleles, that method is becoming obsolete.

Application of polymerase chain reaction (PCR)

PCR amplification (see Chapter 57) dramatically increases the potential range of forensic analysis to minute samples and degraded material and enables precise identification of alleles. It can be applied to minisatellite polymorphisms by use of primers based on unique sequences flanking the tandem repeat arrays. However, the introduction of PCR also brings formidable problems of sample contamination (see Chapter 57).

The most common microsatellites are runs of A, AC or AG. In PCR applications they have the advantage over minisatellites in that discrete 'alleles' can be defined unambiguously by the precise number of repeats, calibrated by the mobility of standards. This avoids the requirement for some aspects of statistical proof and makes it easier to relate experimental findings to allele frequencies. The combination of data on 10–15 unlinked, highly polymorphic loci from any individual is usually unique and definitive.

Recently (2006) a computer-based analysis, called '**DNA boost**' was devised that allows discrimination of individual DNA profiles in mixed samples.

Y-chromosome and mitochondrial DNA polymorphisms are especially useful in some circumstances, such as deducing relationships to people who are deceased, because of their sex-specific modes of transmission and the fact that their genomes are transmitted complete (see Chapter 22).

Human DNA is distinguishable from non-human by testing for hybridization with a probe directed at the human-specific *Alu* repeat. Probes have also been designed for population-specific polymorphisms that indicate ethnic origins.

59 Management of genetic disease

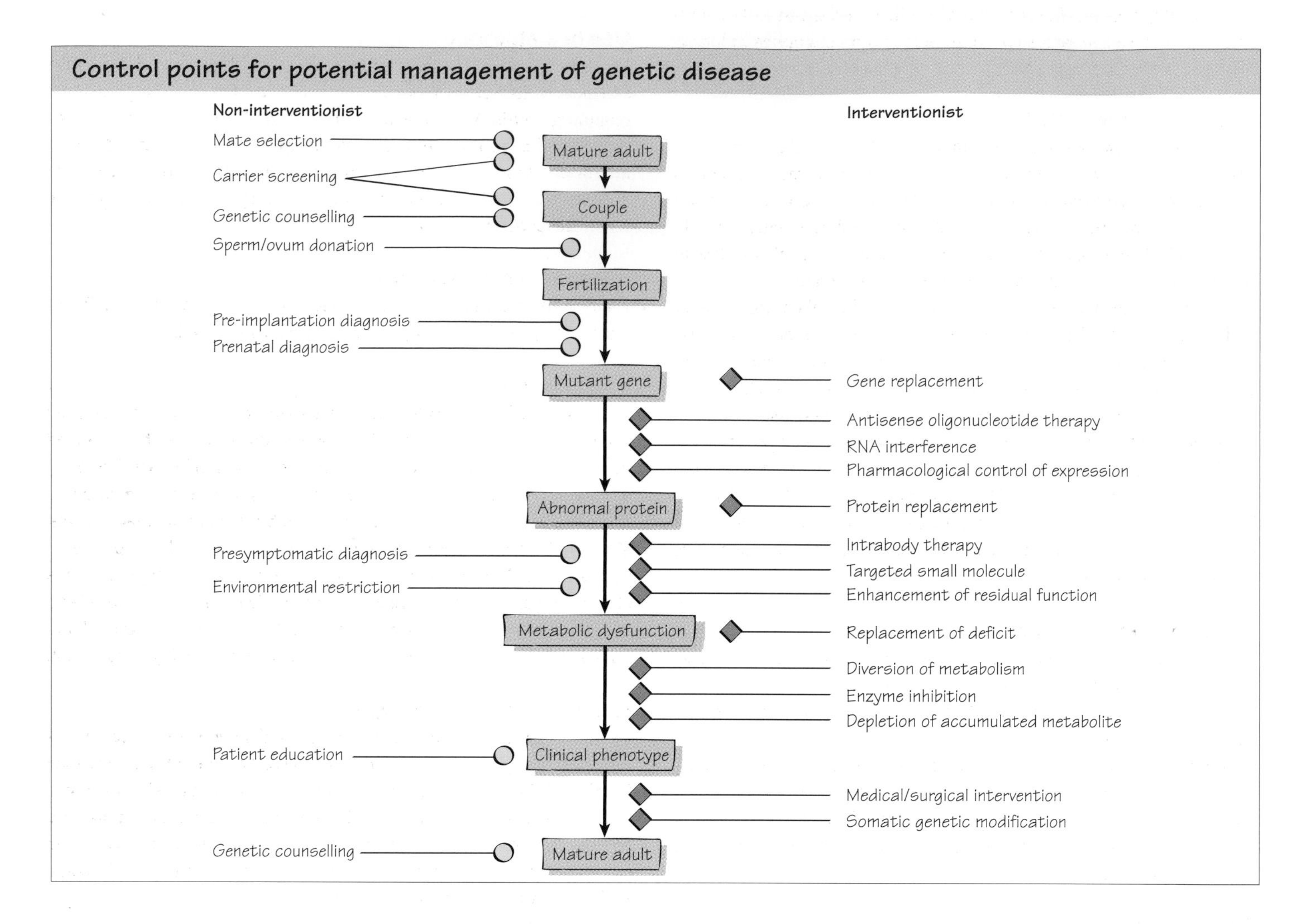

Overview

There are many potential ways to reduce the impact of genetic disease that offer possibilities for clinical management. These include non-interventionist strategies as well as medical intervention. An early intervention was to protect Rh^+ fetuses from immune attack by Rh^- mothers. Among North American caucasians, approximately 13% of all matings are Rh^- incompatible, but Rh sensitization of mothers following the birth of an Rh^+ baby is prevented by her injection with anti-Rh antibodies to destroy fetal erythrocytes before she can mount an immune response. Non-interventionist approaches would include the education and guidance of individuals or couples, and early diagnosis. Technologies are now available for robotic screening of DNA samples for hundreds of thousands of mutations in a single operation.

Correction of defects may require postnatal or even prenatal surgery, physiological adjustment, the switching on or off of genes, replacement of gene products and use of drugs to reduce the effects of genetic errors.

Genetics is also providing new insights into pathogenesis, enabling development of new pharmacological therapies and inspiring entirely novel approaches involving control, replacement or modification of defective genes. Several methods are available to introduce genes into cells, including incubation with 'naked' DNA, or DNA enclosed within artificial lipoprotein vesicles called **liposomes**. In **receptor-mediated endocytosis** a complex is made of the DNA construct and specific polypeptide ligands for which the cell has receptors on its surface. Other approaches utilize **retroviruses**, which have their own means for introducing genes into chromosomes. '**Gene therapy**' offers exciting prospects, although there is very real concern that chromosomal integration of vectors might disrupt other genes, causing side effects as bad as or worse than the original disease.

Correction of gross phenotype

Surgical correction of cleft lip with or without palate (CL ± P), cleft palate, pyloric stenosis and congenital heart defects accounts for the treatment of 20–30% of all infants with major genetically determined disorders. Spina bifida has been successfully treated by prenatal surgery.

Correction of metabolic dysfunction

Environmental restriction

Environmental restriction includes avoidance of tobacco smoke by those with emphysema due to α_1-antitrypsin deficiency; of skin diving and high altitude flying by sickle cell heterozygotes; of sunlight by patients with albinism, porphyria and xeroderma pigmentosa and of X-rays by those with a DNA repair disorder.

A diet low in phenylalanine is most effective in ensuring normal brain development in children with phenylketonuria, and early exclusion of galactose and lactose prevents serious complications in babies homozygous for galactosaemia.

Replacement of deficit

The lysosomal storage disorders include defects in the delivery of enzymes into the lysosomes. These are normally targeted by enzymes carrying mannose-6-phosphate residues that bind specifically to lysosomal surface receptors. There was dramatic recession of organomegaly in type 1 Gaucher disease after intravenous infusion of β-glucosidase to which mannose phosphate had been artificially attached.

Pluripotent haematopoietic stem cells can be taken from donor umbilical cord blood and transfused into the fetus before generation of immune tolerance. This technique could potentially cure severe combined immune deficiency (SCID) (see Chapter 43), alpha- and beta-thalassaemias, sickle cell disease, Fanconi anaemia and adenosine deaminase (ADA) deficiency as well as the lysosomal storage disorders.

'*Ex vivo*' gene therapy of haemophilia involves treatment of a patient's own fibroblasts with DNA coding for Factor VIII or IX, followed by their re-inocculation into the peritoneal cavity. Another approach to haemophilia is by intramuscular injection of adeno-associated virus expressing Factor VIII.

Diversion of metabolism

This includes stimulation of alternative pathways, as in correction of ornithine/urea cycle disorders (see Chapter 45), and enhancement of expression of the normal allele in heterozygotes for familial hypercholesterolaemia.

Administration of **dexamethasone** to the mother from 4–5 weeks' gestation can suppress androgen production and virilization of little girls with congenital adrenal hyperplasia (see Chapter 23). Maternal intake of biotin will correct biotin-responsive **multiple carboxylase deficiency** in the unborn baby.

Enzyme inhibition

Competitive inhibition of rate-controlling enzymes has proved effective, e.g. in familial hypercholesterolaemia (Chapter 17).

Enhancement of enzyme function

This can sometimes be achieved by administration of a cofactor, such as vitamin B_6 for homocystinuria.

Depletion of accumulated metabolite

An example is renal dialysis and use of phenylacetate and benzoate to avoid the complications of defective kidney function.

Modulation of gene expression

Hydroxyurea administered to sickle cell patients can restimulate synthesis of fetal haemoglobin ($\alpha 2\gamma 2$). One experimental approach to Duchenne muscular dystrophy is to up-regulate transcription of the homologous **utrophin** gene.

Antisense oligonucleotide (ASO) therapy

ASOs delivered into cells by liposomes can inhibit gene expression at translation. The principle is sequence-specific binding of antisense oligonucleotide to the target mRNA. ASOs can also force exonskipping and convert out-of-frame deletions of dystrophin, causative of Duchenne muscular dystropy, to in-frame deletions that cause the milder Becker muscular dystrophy.

Intrabody therapy

Intrabodies are genetically engineered intracellular antibodies. One involves fusion of components of the dimeric enzyme, **caspase 3**, to immunoglobulin V regions specific to each of the two halves of the BCR-Abl fusion protein in chronic myelogenous leukaemia (CML). Intrabodies bind in pairs to the two parts of the fusion protein, allowing the caspase to dimerize and trigger apoptosis specifically of leukaemic cells (see Chapter 27, 50).

Targeted small molecules

Gleevec (or *imatinib*) is another product designed to bind to the BCR-Abl fusion protein. *Gleevec* acts as a tyrosine kinase inhibitor.

RNA interference

In **RNA interference** (**RNAi**), selected species of mRNA are destroyed using artificial **small interfering RNAs** (**siRNAs**). Double-stranded RNA precursors, delivered in drug form or by plasmid or viral vectors, are processed by the cell's own enzymes to produce double-stranded siRNAs about 22 nucleotides long. These bind to and activate natural **RNA induced silencing complexes** (**RISCs**) with the capacity to recognize mRNA containing the homologous 22-base sequence. This cleaves the target mRNA, reducing it to undetectable levels. SiRNAs can move between cells, so that artificial RNA duplexes introduced into one part of an embryo can cause specific messenger 'silencing' throughout.

Gene replacement therapy

The ultimate approach to therapy of genetic disorders is replacement of the defective gene, but such attempts have had mixed success. One involves inhalation of disabled cold virus (**adenovirus**) carrying a copy of the normal CFTR allele, but this has proved only temporarily effective in treatment of cystic fibrosis. Replacement of the ADA gene in bone marrow cells of children with SCID led to leukaemia in some patients and so has now been withdrawn.

Pharmacogenomics

'Genomics' refers to the study and application of knowledge about the genome, pharmacogenomics with the stratification of diseases to guide selection of appropriately designed drugs and prescription of drug dosages compatible with individual metabolic rates. Microarrays are created corresponding to hundreds or thousands of cloned alleles (see Chapter 57). The amount of mRNA from a patient's tissue that hybridizes to the different clones then defines that tissue's gene expression profile. Automated analysis of genome-wide single-nucleotide polymorphisms makes it possible to identify genes involved in drug metabolism or transport, and receptors that may govern efficacy, side-effects or toxicity.

DNA microarrays can also be used to create unique genetic profiles of cancers, enabling design of individualized therapy regimens. The drug *Herceptin* targets over-expression of **HER2/neu** protein, as in about a third of breast cancer patients. Tumour expression profiling allows restriction of this expensive drug to those patients that could benefit.

Another anti-cancer measure involves injecting a *Herpes*-virus-based vector expressing thymidine kinase directly into brain tumours, which makes those cells uniquely susceptible to the normally non-toxic anti-*Herpes* drug, *Ganciclovir*.

60 Avoidance and prevention of disease

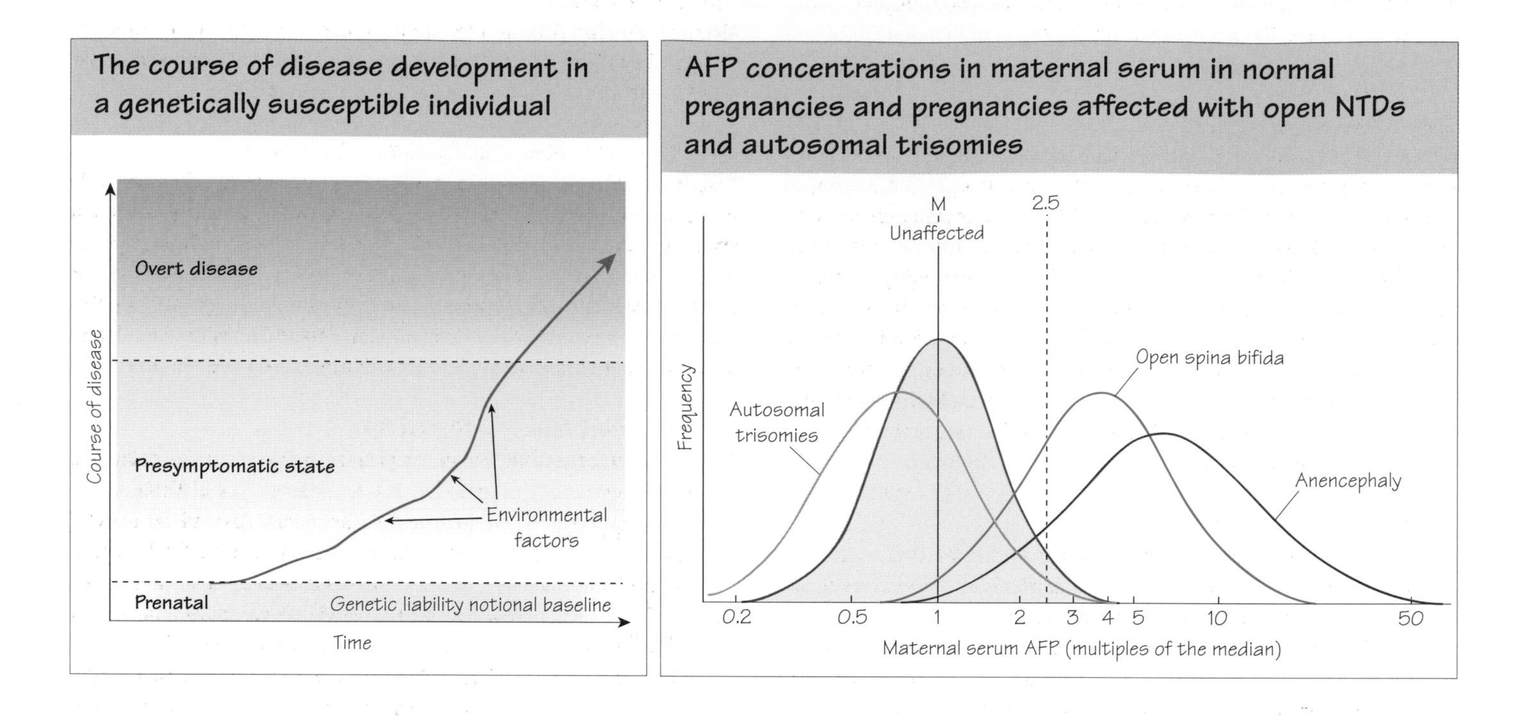

Overview

Each of us inherits genes that contribute some degree of liability toward many disorders. In the case of monogenic diseases, one or a pair of defective alleles alone confers sufficient liability to cause disease. In other instances genetic liability is expressed merely as a susceptibility and manifestation of disease requires the passage of time and/or accumulation of specific environmental exposures (see figure). **Preventive** (or **preventative**) **genetics** is based on testing for factors that contribute to genetic liability. This identifies persons at risk, enabling them to be educated about individually hazardous environmental factors and providing opportunities for modification of lifestyles (see Chapter 32). In some cases proactive treatment can be offered to reduce risks, or surveillance to ensure early diagnosis and the prompt institution of therapy. In the UK antenatal or neonatal screening programmes for cystic fibrosis, thalassaemia and sickle cell disease have been instigated at many centres.

There are three classes of heterozygous carrier for which population screening might be appropriate:

- autosomal recessive diseases of high incidence;
- relatively common X-linked disorders;
- autosomal dominant disorders of late onset.

A genetic disease is suitable for population screening if it is clearly defined, of appreciable frequency, and early diagnosis is advantageous. The test should be easily performed, be non-invasive and yield few false positives or false negatives. Screening should be widely available, morally acceptable and preferably show a net cost benefit. Appropriate information and counselling should also be available. Testing a child for a disorder of adult onset, or for carrier status, should be postponed until the child is of an age to appreciate the issues and to give informed consent.

Preimplantation diagnosis

Preimplantation diagnosis is valuable as an adjunct to *in vitro* fertilization and for couples who rule out termination.

Blastomere sampling One or two blastomeres are taken from embryos at the 6–8 cell stage. The DNA is tested by fluorescent *in situ* hybridization (FISH) for aneuploidy or amplified by polymerase chain reaction (PCR) and analysed for a specific known genetic mutation. Since PCR amplification sometimes fails for technical reasons, use of two blastomeres is recommended. Three-day sampling allows time to implant a healthy embryo.

Blastocyst sampling Sampling of trophectoderm at the 100-cell stage reduces the PCR failure rate, but introduces the risk of maternal contamination (see Chapter 11).

Polar body sampling This is of most value in testing for aneuploidy, or when the *mother* is heterozygous for a disease allele. In the latter case, either polar body is examined, on the theory that if it contains the disease allele, the ovum does not (see Chapter 10).

Prenatal screening

Neural tube defects

Ninety to ninety-five per cent of neural tube defect (NTD) births occur in the absence of a family history of NTDs. They are detectable at 16 weeks by assay of α-fetoprotein (AFP) concentration in amniotic fluid and in many cases also in maternal serum. However, in maternal serum there is overlap between unaffected and NTD pregnancies, so an arbitrary concentration is identified below which no further action is taken. A cut-off at 2.5 multiples of the normal median identifies > 90% of fetuses with anencephaly and ~80% of those with open NTDs (see figure).

Over 20 years, maternal serum screening with dietary improvements and pre-conceptional folic acid supplementation, have yielded a 25-fold decrease in NTDs in England and Wales.

Down syndrome

The combination of maternal age and abnormal concentrations of four biochemicals in a mother's serum can identify most pregnancies with Down syndrome. At 16 weeks, concentrations of AFP and **unconjugated oestriol** tend to be reduced in the blood of women pregnant with babies with Down syndrome, whereas that of **human chorionic gonadotrophin (hCG)** is raised. The 'triple test', combining the three, identifies 60% of pregnancies with Down syndrome. Inclusion of **inhibin A**, increased in pregnancies with Down syndrome, raises this to 75%. Incorporation of the ultrasonographic observation of **increased fetal nuchal transparency** (abnormal accumulation of fluid behind the baby's neck) at 12 weeks, with confirmation by cytogenetic testing, detects 80% of babies with Down syndrome.

Neonatal screening

If neonatal screening is to be undertaken, the consultative follow-up should be prompt and involve definitive diagnosis, prompt initiation of management and appropriate genetic counselling.

Phenylketonuria (PKU), **galactosaemia** and **congenital hypothyroidism** all cause mental retardation, but can be screened for in newborns and prophylactic regimens imposed. Screening for phenylketonuria is routine in most developed countries, galactosaemia screening is less common. Congenital hypothyroidism is not usually genetic, but screening is nevertheless routine in many countries.

The test for galactosaemia is similar to the Guthrie test for PKU (see Chapter 51), with confirmation by enzyme assay. Screening for hypothyroidism involves assay of thyroxine and thyroid stimulating hormone.

Cystic fibrosis (CF)

Currently neonatal diagnosis of CF is based on immunological quantification of trypsinogen in the blood (a consequence of blockage of the pancreatic ducts *in utero*) supplemented by DNA analysis (see Chapter 57). Up to 80% of heterozygotes of northern European or Ashkenazi Jewish ancestry are detectable by tests for the ΔF508 allele and a further 10% by multiplex tests for several rarer alleles, depending on ethnicity. Early antibiotic- and physio-therapy improve long-term prognoses.

Sickle cell disease

Several techniques have been used for diagnosis of sickle cell anaemia, including electrophoresis of haemoglobin, demonstration of red cell sickling at low oxygen tensions and a range of DNA tests (see Chapters 56 and 57). Many babies die of pneumococcal infection, but prophylactic treatment can be given by administration of oral penicillin.

Thalassaemia

Populations for which thalassaemia carrier screening programmes might prove, or have proved advantageous include China and East Asia (for alpha-thalassaemia), the Indian subcontinent and Mediterranean countries (for beta-thalassaemia). In Cyprus, screening led to a 95% decline in babies with beta-thalassaemia in 10 years. Similar programmes in Greece and Italy have created a better than 50% reduction. Early diagnosis makes it possible to optimize transfusion and iron-chelation therapy at an early stage.

Tay–Sachs disease

Carrier screening followed by prenatal diagnosis and termination has reduced Tay–Sachs disease by 95% among American Ashkenazi Jews (see Chapter 45).

Screening for adult-onset disease

Late-onset diseases for which screening may be advised include **Huntington disease**, **myotonic dystrophy**, **retinitis pigmentosa** and **spinal cerebellar ataxia**. Early diagnosis of these can allow psychological, emotional and financial preparation. Predictive testing for inherited cancer predisposition, such as **familial adenomatous polyposis** and **breast/ovarian cancer**, can ensure inclusion in clinical surveillance programmes and the possibility of prophylactic surgery.

Occupational screening

In the workplace, genetic screening is done to monitor genetic damage due to exposure to ionizing radiation (see Chapter 38 and Table 59.1), or for susceptibility to environmental chemicals. Around 50 genetic traits are related to specific environmental agents (Table 59.2). These include **G6PD deficiency**, for which oxidants such as ozone and nitrogen dioxide are contra-indicated and the **sickle cell trait**, carriers of which are highly susceptible to carbon monoxide and cyanide.

Alpha1-antitrypsin (α1-AT) deficiency (AR) is as common as cystic fibrosis in Caucasians, but virtually absent in Chinese and Japanese.

Table 60.1 Estimated new genetic abnormalities in one-million live births in a population exposed to low-dose radiation equivalent to 1 rad of X-rays.

Category	No. of cases
Aberrant chromosomes	38
Autosomal dominant and X-linked	20
Recessive lesions	30
Multifactorial diseases	5

Numbers based on atomic bomb survival statistics and animal experiments.

Table 60.2 Genetic conditions that create health risks with specific environmental agents.

Genetic susceptibility	Environmental agent	Resultant condition
G6PD deficiency	Fava beans, mothballs	Haemolytic crisis
Hypercholesterolaemia	Saturated fats	Atherosclerosis
Gluten sensitivity	Wheat protein	Coeliac disease
Defective Na/K pump	Common salt	Hypertension
Lactose intolerance	Milk sugar	Colic and diarrhoea
Deficient ADH	Alcohol	Alcoholism
Deficient ALDH	Alcohol	Flushing response
Hyperoxaluria	Oxalates*	Kidney stones
Haemochromatosis	Iron food supplement	Iron overload
α_1-antitrypsin deficiency	Tobacco smoke	Emphysema
Atopic diathesis	Pollen	Hay fever

ADH, alcohol dehydrogenase; ALDH, acetaldehyde dehydrogenase.
* e.g. in spinach and rhubarb.

Homozygotes typically develop lung emphysema in middle age, especially tobacco smokers, in whom life expectancy in the USA is reduced from 62 to 40 years. Homozygotes can be identified by dot-blots with ASO probes (see Chapter 56).

Limitations of genetic testing

1 Somatic mosaicism and operator error mean that genetic tests are never 100% reliable.
2 DNA testing can reveal mutations that are not necessarily expressed as disease because, for example, they may occur in an unimportant part of the gene, or the mutant allele is incompletely penetrant.
3 Genetic testing may not detect all the disease alleles of a specific gene.
4 Genetic testing can introduce unwanted social and ethical problems.

Genetic registers

Genetic registers are records of local families with genetic disease. Entry to a register should be entirely voluntary and it is essential that confidentiality is never breached. Their primary purpose is to maintain two-way contact between the clinical genetics unit and relevant family members. This ensures families do not feel excluded from a source of support and allows investigation to be offered as appropriate.

They are most valuable for relatively common conditions of late onset, with potentially serious effects that are amenable to prevention or treatment. However, there are negative implications, including invasion of privacy, implied compulsion, the 'right not to know' about one's deficiencies, possible stigmatization and possible leakage of confidential data.

Prophylactic surgery

Prophylactic surgery may be appropriate for some late-acting cancer-predisposing alleles of high penetrance. These include familial adenomatous polyposis coli, breast and ovarian cancer, and thyroid cancer due to the MEN2B allele (see Chapter 41). The anti-oestrogen drug ***Tamoxifen*** is an option for women carrying the BRCA1 or BRCA2 alleles (see Chapter 41), who should avoid oral contraception and hormone replacement therapy. For patients at high risk of colon cancer, non-digestible starch can slow polyposis and the anti-inflammatory ***Sulindac*** can reduce rectal and duodenal adenomas.

Therapeutic cloning

Embryonic stem cells offer the possibility of therapy for many conditions, e.g. as a source of dopamine-producing neurons capable of correcting Parkinson disease.

61 Ethical and social issues in clinical genetics

Overview

Ethics is the science of morals and human duty. It deals with the rules by which we should conduct our lives. In clinical ethics avoidance of conflict requires endorsement of high moral values, such as mutual respect, honesty and compassion, by both clinician and client. Ethicists talk about additional values such as beneficence and justice (see below). Occasionally there can be disagreement, or accepted values may face unexpected challenges and it is then that ethical problems can arise. For example, abortion of an affected pregnancy pits the right of choice of the parent against the right to life of the unborn child. The opportunity to terminate creates a major ethical dilemma. Optimal outcomes require that medical staff and families work constructively together to identify, analyse and resolve such dilemmas.

The Darwinian perspective

Every species shows phenotypic variation due partly to genetic variation between individuals. In accordance with Darwin's 'Theory of Evolution through Natural Selection', the assembly of alleles within the human species derives from selection by hazards faced by our ancestors and by ourselves earlier in life. Natural selection ensures that the genes of unfit or reproductively unsuccessful members of wild species are unlikely to be represented in subsequent generations, with consequent improvement in the average fitness of its members. New gene variants and combinations are constantly created by mutation and reassortment at meiosis and mating and, with the passage of generations, those that are favourable increase in frequency while the unfavourable decline. The outcome is that members of naturally selected populations are largely healthy, well adapted and fully capable of reproduction.

Goals of medicine include the restoration, maintenance, or improvement of quality of life and extension of lifespan. It helps patients survive life-threatening disease and assists reproduction of the infertile, i.e. it reduces or negates natural selection. In so doing it necessarily allows increase in the population frequency of harmful alleles. In the long term, therefore, the practice of traditional medicine is 'dysgenic', increasing the burden of harmful alleles (the 'genetic load') our species has to carry (see Chapter 35).

By contrast, medical practices that involve healthy embryo selection (see Chapter 52) reverse the dysgenic influence and go some way toward reducing our genetic load. However, deliberate application of measures *with the aim of* changing the population frequencies of disease alleles leads us into the realm of 'eugenics', which history has taught is a dangerous path to tread (see below).

An historical perspective

The first great exposition of the ethical basis of medicine was the fifth century BC Hippocratic Oath. It notably includes the pledge: 'the regimen I adopt shall be for the benefit of my patients according to my ability and judgement, and not for their hurt or for any wrong'. This still forms the basis of the graduation ceremony in many medical schools, although dropped by others. It strongly condemns the practice of pregnancy termination currently permitted in some societies.

In the nineteenth-century Francis Galton, inspired by the evolutionary ideas of his cousin, Charles Darwin, coined the word 'eugenics' (the prefix 'eu-' denoting 'good') to describe scientific endeavours aimed at increasing the proportion of persons with better-than-average genetic endowment, through selective mating. The central idea is that human evolution could be guided toward a better future if human reproduction were to come under social guidance.

'Negative eugenics' is primarily directed toward reduction in the incidence of hereditary disease, whereas 'positive eugenics' favours aims to increase the frequency of superior endowments. Most medical practitioners view reduction of disease incidence as desirable but, because of unpredictable outcomes or on religious grounds, are more cautious about 'genetic enhancement'.

Notwithstanding, most medical geneticists become distinctly uncomfortable if their practices are described as eugenic, as they view their mission as straightforward improvement of the quality of life for individuals. Furthermore, the word 'eugenics' has been irredeemably besmirched by its use in the past to justify genocidal policies and extermination atrocities, especially in Nazi Germany. To avoid misinterpretation, we believe use of the word 'eugenics' in general discussion is therefore probably best avoided.

Screening and termination of affected pregnancies are sometimes advocated as more cost-effective than caring for the affected individuals. This argument is deplored by most clinical geneticists, who generally think in terms of avoidance of health problems for individuals or families, rather than the overall health of the population.

The religious perspective

Bioethical principles derive from the societal values of the culture in which they originate. Western medical ethics derived from Judeo-Christian and classical Greek humanitarian principles sees all individuals as having equal rights, irrespective of ethnicity, social standing or caste, sex, religion or wealth. It however generally seems to appreciate the lives of young persons as more valuable than those of the elderly. These concepts are not necessarily recognized by members of other cultures, but Western society generally considers that they represent best practice in most medical circumstances. Should they cause conflict in any instance, attempts should be made to accommodate client values.

Contemporary Western society places a value on the gender-balanced family, but others, notably in northern India and China, have a preference for sons. The World Health Organization proposes that only disease-related criteria should be used for prenatal gender selection. Different groups view matters of genetic intervention very differently. For example, some individuals of Islamic and Jewish traditions oppose abortion, but find pre-implantation gender selection acceptable. The Roman Catholic Church condemns both abortion and *in-vitro* fertilization, restricting the reproductive options available.

Application of ethical principles

Important principles for the counsellor to bear in mind are:

1 One person cannot be the object of another person's 'right'.

2 Both biological parents should normally have a say in the fate of their offspring.

Some couples with what many would consider a deficiency, such as deafness or very short stature, express the wish that they would like children resembling themselves. The definition of 'deficiency' in itself is problematic, but it is a matter of serious debate whether or not medical techniques should be used deliberately to select or create such a baby, in order to satisfy parental wishes.

Texts on medical ethics generally recognize four overriding principles: (i) *respect for patient autonomy*; (ii) *beneficence* (i.e. 'being of benefit'); (iii) *non-maleficence* (i.e. avoidance of doing harm); and (iv) *justice*.

The ethical problems of clinical genetics are mainly those common throughout medicine: of conveying difficult information with adequate care; ensuring genuinely informed consent to tests and treatment; preserving confidentiality; and identifying the best available treatments. Distinctive additional problems arise with genetic tests in that they can reveal information about individuals who are not tested and about diseases of late onset. This presents ethical challenges to health professionals, the family and society at large.

A crucial distinction is between services available for pre-existing concerns of individuals or families, and population screening offered pro-actively to citizens who have not sought the test. Typical scenarios in the first category could involve, for example, a family seeking an explanation for a serious developmental problem in their child, a person wishing to know their risk of developing a degenerative condition, or a couple wanting to know the risk their child could develop a condition shown by an existing family member. By contrast, where the issue is of population screening, the professional, or the medical community, is actively promoting a specific course of action – that the client or patient should undergo an investigation. The offer of screening in itself may generate concerns and imply that compliance is being recommended, definitely so in newborn screening for inborn errors of metabolism.

Non-directiveness in genetic counselling

The counsellor's involvement should be both non-judgemental and non-directive. Allowing the client to reach his or her own decision has important psychological benefits for the client, but it also benefits the counsellor.

1 It helps him or her avoid emotional involvement with that decision.
2 It ensures legal responsibility for the decision lies with the client.
3 It avoids the possible implication that the counsellor is following an eugenic agenda.

The British Mental Capacity Act (2005) provides a statutory framework to empower and protect vulnerable people unable to make decisions on their own behalf.

Conflicts of interest between family members

Consider the case of a man aged 20 years whose grandfather died of Huntington disease. He wants to marry and start a family, but wishes to clarify his genetic status first. His at-risk father, aged 40 years, seems healthy, but recognizes that if his son tests positive, he himself will soon show signs of disease. Such knowledge can be very distressing and can even precipitate suicide. Should their clinician make testing available to the son, if in doing so it may have adverse consequences for the father?

This is a dilemma that requires careful consideration of the rights of all parties and usually involves many different professionals and multiple counselling sessions. Current practice in some centres in the UK supports the principle that generally, the right of (adult) offspring to know should take precedence over that of their parents *not* to know. Others simply decline such tests.

Genetic testing of children

Genetic testing of a child is appropriate: (a) if the child may have a genetic disorder requiring immediate diagnosis and management (e.g. phenylketonuria, PKU); (b) for prediction of a condition that may later manifest itself and which either requires surveillance (e.g. Duchenne muscular dystrophy); or (c) can be treated at an early stage (e.g. some types of familial cancer). It is usually considered inappropriate to test children for untreatable conditions of adult onset: identification of a child as a disease gene carrier can have subtle, undesirable influences on their sense of self and well-being. Such tests are usually best deferred until the child is of an age to make his or her own informed choice.

Genetic screening

Prediction of future disability can be highly accurate but, in those who test positive, uncertainty as to *whether* an individual will develop the disease becomes replaced by worry over *when* or *how* it will manifest. Negative consequences of carrier status include the emotional impact of that knowledge, concerns about health, the burden of reproductive decisions, and potential stigmatization and discrimination in personal relationships.

In cascade screening within a family, consent forms may be passed on to family members who have not been fully informed and may reveal information about family members without their consent. There can also be unexpected responses by family members given favourable predictions, such as guilt when other family members are not so favoured. Family ties strengthened from sharing concerns about the disease may weaken for those no longer personally so involved.

Additional problems in genetic counselling

Additional problems for the counsellor or client include:

1 Facility with language.
2 Issues of power between husband and wife.
3 Religious stances and associated cultural values.
4 The sex and personal presentation of the medical contact.
5 A tradition of consanguineous marriage (especially in some South Asian and Middle Eastern groups).
6 Cultural stereotyping.
7 Thoughtlessly disturbing or offensive terms, like 'CATCH 22' and 'CRASH syndrome'.

Areas of ethical challenge arising from new reproductive technologies

The Ethical, Legal and Social Implications (ELSI) Program makes recommendations about how new information arising from the Human Genome Project (see Chapter 36) may be handled safely. Controversial issues that may be relevant to such considerations include the following:

1 Gamete donation.
2 Use of frozen sperm from a dead man.
3 Creation of 'saviour siblings' for tissue donation.
4 Implantation of embryos in postmenopausal women.
5 Human embryo cloning.
6 Gene therapy and patenting.
7 Creation of interspecific human hybrids.
8 Mitochondrial replacement therapy.
9 Stem cell research.
10 Life insurance and health insurance.
11 The stage at which new individuals acquire human rights.
12 Molecular definition of race.

Self-assessment case studies: questions

Case 1: Unbalanced translocation

You are called to see Betsy, a 12-hour-old girl in the neonatal intensive care unit, for evaluation of multiple congenital anomalies. Betsy was born after a 37-week gestation complicated by intrauterine growth retardation. An ultrasound scan performed in the third trimester was otherwise normal. Birth weight was 1.5 kg (this is below the third centile). Multiple anomalies were noted soon after birth, including microcephaly, club feet, high, narrow palate, low-set posteriorly rotated ears, fifth finger clinodactyly, and hypotonia. Both parents are phenotypically normal. The nursery resident asks if you would do interphase FISH studies because she has heard that rapid results can be obtained with this method. You suggest instead that a full karyotype analysis be done.

1 *Why would interphase FISH not be the ideal test to perform in this case?*

Five days later you get a call from the cytogenetics laboratory with the results: 46,XX,add(14p).

2 *How would you interpret this karyotype? Is it balanced or unbalanced?*

The laboratory agrees to pursue additional FISH studies to better define the chromosomal abnormality. Based on their findings, they issue a report with the following karyotype: 46,XX,der(14)t(14;17)(p11.2;p11.2).

3 *How does this new information change your interpretation?*

You explain the results to Betsy's parents and suggest that both of them have chromosomal studies. Her father is found to have the following karyotype: 46,XY,t(14;17)(p11.2;p11.2).

4 *Betsy's father's karyotype is abnormal, but he is phenotypically normal. How would you explain this?*

5 *How does this finding explain the karyotype in Betsy?*

6 *Betsy's mother has had two miscarriages prior to Betsy's birth. Do these findings have relevance to those miscarriages as well?*

Two years have passed. Betsy has had a difficult time, with major feeding problems and developmental delay. Her parents are interested in having additional children.

7 *How would you counsel them regarding their recurrence risk of similar problems? What options are available to them to manage this risk?*

Case 2: A metabolic problem

You get a call from the newborn screening laboratory about one of your patients, a girl named Sophia. You learn that her newborn plasma screen test was abnormal, revealing a high level of phenylalanine. You have not met Sophia or her parents yet – one of your partners was on call when she was discharged from the hospital. Now you call her parents to arrange for them to come into the office for a repeat blood sampling, and also set them up to meet with a metabolic disease specialist the next day.

1 *Why is it urgent to follow up on the abnormal metabolic screening test?*

Sophia is seen in the Metabolism Clinic, and her parents meet with several members of the team. They are told that Sophia's phenylalanine level was 26 mg/dL (normal is < 2 mg/dL). She is started on special formula food without phenylalanine, and blood and urine are obtained for tetrahydrobiopterin analysis.

2 *What is the underlying basis for phenylketonuria (PKU)?*

3 *What is the purpose of the tetrahydrobiopterin analysis?*

The tetrahydrobiopterin analysis is negative and Sophia's parents gradually become familiar with the low phenylalanine diet. At the second visit to Metabolism Clinic they ask to speak with a genetic counsellor. They have learned that PKU is a genetic disorder, but are puzzled that they could have an affected child in spite of the fact that neither parent has ever heard of a relative with the condition.

4 *How would you explain the lack of family history, and how would you counsel Sophia's parents about their risk of having another affected child?*

Sophia's parents ask whether it is possible to obtain prenatal testing if they have another child.

5 *What would be involved in providing prenatal testing?*

Sophia is now 14 years old; she has remained on her special diet all these years, but is becoming increasingly independent and rebellious. Her parents ask for a counsellor to speak with Sophia, to discuss the need to remain on the low phenylalanine diet.

6 *Is there a stage in life when the low phenylalanine diet can be relaxed?*

7 *What are the special issues that are faced by a woman with PKU as she reaches childbearing age?*

Case 3: A child with skin spots

James is a 3-year-old boy referred for evaluation of skin spots. His mother had noticed them when he was about 2 months old, but the spots have become more numerous and distinct over the past 2 years. At first the paediatrician dismissed these as 'birthmarks', but James's mother insisted that an evaluation be done as she began to do research on her own as to what they might be. On examination, James is found to have 10 café-au-lait spots ranging in size from 5 mm to over 2 cm. His physical exam is otherwise unremarkable, with no skin-fold freckling or other skin lesions, though his head circumference is in the 95th centile (i.e. large, but within the normal range). You suspect a diagnosis of neurofibromatosis type 1 (NF1).

1 *Based on the information provided, can a definitive diagnosis of NF1 be established?*

A complete family history is taken, and it is learned that no one else in the family has ever had multiple café-au-lait spots or any other signs of NF1. You examine both of James's parents, and neither has café-au-lait spots.

2 *Does the lack of family history reduce your suspicion that James might have NF1?*

You arrange for genetic testing of the NF1 gene from a blood sample. A missense mutation (i.e. a base substitution) is found in the coding sequence. This mutation has never been seen before, either in affected or unaffected individuals. Most NF1 mutations are truncating mutations that lead to premature termination of translation, so the pathogenicity of this mutation is uncertain.

3 *What kind of evidence would you require to determine whether this mutation is pathogenic or a benign variant?*

After further studies, it is concluded that the mutation could well be pathogenic. You follow James on an annual basis, and by 4 years of age he is manifesting skin-fold freckling, confirming the clinical diagnosis. He does not have any visible tumours, and ophthalmological follow-up has not revealed signs of optic glioma. There is some concern that James is experiencing learning disabilities. His parents are interested in having another child, and ask about their risks of a second child having NF1.

4 *How would you counsel James's parents regarding their recurrence risk?*

James is now 14 years old, and has been doing well since his diagnosis was established. He is getting special help in school for learning problems, but is making good progress. He is now beginning to manifest small tumours on his skin, which appear to be cutaneous neurofibromas.

5 *What is believed to be the mechanism for development of neurofibromas? Why does one see multiple individual tumours instead of development of tumours along every nerve?*

Ten more years pass and now James and his wife are considering having children. They ask whether prenatal testing is possible. They also inquire about the current state of treatment of NF1.

6 *How would you answer the questions about prenatal testing and treatment?*

Case 4: Muscle weakness

Luke is 4 years old and his parents are concerned that he is getting more and more clumsy rather than less and less as he gets older. At first their paediatrician was not concerned, but then, as Luke began having difficulty climbing stairs, the paediatrician referred him to you for neurological assessment. Examination reveals a healthy looking boy who has difficulty getting up off the floor without using his arms for support. He has mild weakness of the hip flexors and prominent calves. Blood is sent for determination of creatine phosphokinase (CPK) and the result is a staggering 25 000 U/L, normal levels being up to 170.

1 *What is the significance of the elevated CPK?*

Suspecting Duchenne muscular dystrophy, you send a blood sample for dystrophin gene deletion analysis. A few days later the test result comes back and reveals that Luke has a deletion of exons 44–47, which has resulted in juxtaposition of out-of-frame exons. You explain to Luke's parents that, unfortunately, the test reveals he has Duchenne rather than Becker dystrophy.

2 *What is the difference between Duchenne and Becker dystrophy, and how does the deletion test help to make the distinction between the two disorders?*

After considerable discussion with Luke's parents, it is decided to start him on treatment with prednisone, an anti-inflammatory corticosteroid. He is also introduced to a programme of physical therapy.

3 *What is the approach to management of Duchenne muscular dystrophy and what is the prognosis?*

A genetic counsellor explained the genetics of the disorder to Luke's parents the day the diagnosis was established. Luke has one sibling, an older sister. His parents are well and his mother has a brother and a sister, both of whom are well. Luke's mother has no maternal uncles. Luke's maternal aunt is particularly worried when she hears about Luke's condition because she has just learnt that she is pregnant.

4 *How would you counsel Luke's mother and maternal aunt?*

Dystrophin gene deletion testing is carried out on Luke's mother's DNA and that of his aunt, and both are found to carry the deletion.

5 *What can be offered to Luke's aunt in terms of prenatal testing?*

Luke's aunt's unborn baby turns out to be a girl, who is found to have inherited the deletion.

6 *Is a female dystrophin deletion carrier at risk of developing muscular dystrophy?*

Case 5: Cancer in the family

Ted is a 40-year-old man who is seeking counselling regarding genetic testing for breast cancer. He is concerned not for himself, but for his two daughters, who are 10 and 12 years old. Ted's sister has been diagnosed with breast cancer at age 36 years and recently had a bilateral mastectomy. His mother died of breast cancer when she was 40 years of age; he has two maternal aunts, one of whom is currently being treated for ovarian cancer at age 65 years, while the other is in good health.

1 *Would Ted's family history suggest an increased risk for hereditary breast cancer?*

Ted is told that testing would be possible, but that it would be preferable to test his sister first.

2 *What is the reason for testing Ted's sister before Ted is tested?*

Ted's sister is tested for mutation in the *BRCA1* and *BRCA2* genes. Several weeks later the results are returned, and she is found to carry a stop mutation in the *BRCA1* gene.

3 *Would you expect that this mutation would be pathogenic?*

4 *What advice would you give Ted's sister based on this result?*

Ted's sister has given her permission to communicate these results to Ted. Upon hearing of this, he explains that he is not concerned for himself, but is interested in having his daughters tested.

5 *Does Ted face any cancer-related risks if he is found to carry a BRCA1 mutation?*

6 *What would you advise regarding testing his daughters?*

Case 6: Targeted treatment

Mary is a 63-year-old woman referred for evaluation of fatigue and weight loss. She had been healthy until about 3 months ago, but now has little energy and has lost 15 pounds (6.8 kg). On examination she is noted to have a palpable spleen and slightly enlarged liver. Blood testing is done and she is found to have 22 000 white blood cells per cubic millimetre, and a mild anaemia. The blood smear shows myeloid cells at various stages of maturation. This explains the enlarged liver and spleen, which are probably similarly engorged with myeloid cells. A bone marrow aspirate is done, and chromosomal analysis reveals the presence of the Philadelphia chromosome.

1 *What is the Phildephila chromosome and what is its significance in this patient?*

Mary is diagnosed as having chronic myelogenous leukaemia (CML). After consideration of her options, it is decided to start her on treatment with *imatinib* (Gleevec).

2 *What is imatinib and how does it work?*

Mary has been on treatment for 2 months, and her white blood count has returned to normal. Cytogenetic studies indicate her cells no longer have the Philadelphia chromosome, though PCR analysis still reveals presence of the translocation.

3 *What do you think is the basis for PCR testing for the presence of the Philadelphia chromosome?*

4 *Why would PCR testing detect the translocation when cytogenetic analysis was negative?*

Mary has been doing well for 18 months, but recently she has begun to feel fatigued again. She is found once again to have increased white blood cells on her blood smear, and Philadelphia chromosome positive cells are once again found.

5 *Why does relapse occur in patients with CML after treatment with imatinib?*

Case 7: Alzheimer disease

Larry is a 54-year-old man whom you have been treating for mild hypertension for the past 4 years. His health is otherwise good, though he also has mild hypercholesterolemia, for which he was recently started on statin therapy to protect him from atherosclerosis by lowering his cholesterol. At a routine follow-up visit he asks about testing for

Alzheimer disease. His mother had been diagnosed as having presenile dementia several years ago, and recently died of the disorder. There is no other family history of which Larry is aware.

1 *Is Larry at high risk of developing Alzheimer disease based on this family history?*

Larry is told that there is no genetic testing that would be recommended at this time. He has no symptoms of Alzheimer disease and his examination is entirely normal. Not entirely satisfied, Larry goes on the internet that night and does some research on his own for genetic testing for Alzheimer disease. It doesn't take him long to find a lab that offers ApoE testing.

2 *What is the relationship of ApoE to Alzheimer disease?*

Larry calls the office the next day to ask if he can be tested for ApoE. You explain that this testing is not recommended as a screen for Alzheimer disease.

3 *How would you evaluate ApoE testing in terms of clinical accuracy, clinical validity and clinical utility?*

Returning to the internet, Larry finds a laboratory that will accept a cheek brushing sample (mouth swab) without a physician's referral. The internet advertisement notes that the laboratory is 'CLIA certified'. He contacts the laboratory, which provides a kit in the mail. His wife helps him do the cheek brushing, and the sample is sent off to the laboratory.

4 *Are there specific concerns about cheek brushing as a source of material for testing that would be different from blood?*

A month later, Larry gets a report in the mail saying that his ApoE genotype is ε2/ε4. Now he calls your office again to ask what this means. Is he going to get Alzheimer disease?

5 *How would you counsel Larry?*

Case 8: A sleepy infant

You are called to see Kirsten, a 1-day-old girl in the newborn intensive care unit. Kirsten was born after a 37 week pregnancy with birth weight of 2200 g (4 lb 13 oz). Her doctors are concerned because she seems to be unusually sleepy, with minimal responses to stimulation and very lethargic feeding. She is being fed by nasogastric tube and her vital signs are stable. Evaluation for infection has been negative, and she has no evidence of any metabolic derangement. On examination, she is breathing on her own and has no dysmorphic features. She is very lethargic and hypotonic, though there are no fasciculations (visible muscle flickering) and deep tendon reflexes can be elicited, which both argue against spinal muscular atrophy (see Chapter 19). The extreme lethargy and poor feeding are more typical of a central nervous system, rather than a neuromuscular cause for the hypotonia, though congenital myopathy or congenital myotonic dystrophy remain a possibility.

You suspect Prader–Willi syndrome and ask for chromosome analysis, FISH testing and DNA methylation testing.

1 *What role do these tests play in the genetic diagnosis of Prader–Willi syndrome?*

The chromosomes are normal female and the FISH test result is normal also. The methylation analysis, however, reveals only a maternal pattern. You suspect uniparental disomy.

2 *What kind of testing can you do to confirm your suspicion?*

DNA testing reveals that, indeed, Kirsten has two maternal copies of Chromosome 15 and no paternal copy.

3 *What is the mechanism whereby uniparental disomy causes Prader–Willi syndrome?*

You explain the results to Kirsten's parents, and the natural history of Prader–Willi syndrome. Kirsten's parents are both 39 years old. They ask whether they would be at risk of having another child with the disorder, and whether their healthy 6-year-old girl will be at risk of having affected children when she grows up.

4 *What is the recurrence risk of uniparental disomy in this family?*

5 *Is Kirsten's sister at risk of having an affected child?*

Kirsten's parents ask whether there are treatments available for children with Prader–Willi syndrome.

6 *What would you advise Kirsten's parents about the availability of treatments?*

Case 9: Advance warning

Bill and Rita are interested in starting a family. Bill is 29 and Rita 27 years old. They arrange an appointment with Rita's obstetrician-gynecologist to discuss pre-pregnancy issues. Bill's ancestors came from Germany and Rita's from Scotland. They are not aware of a family history of any specific genetic disorder and both are in good health. They are told that carrier testing for cystic fibrosis is available if they are concerned for their future offspring.

1 *What is the risk that Bill and Rita would have a child with cystic fibrosis?*

2 *How is cystic fibrosis carrier testing performed?*

Bill and Rita decide to go ahead with testing. A few weeks later they learn that Rita carries the ΔF508 mutation, but Bill's DNA contains no detectable mutation. The testing is estimated to reveal 88% of all pathogenic alleles.

3 *Are Bill and Rita at risk of having an affected child?*

4 *How does the ΔF508 mutation affect the function of the gene?*

Bill and Rita ask whether a carrier would be expected to manifest any signs of cystic fibrosis. They also ask whether it is possible to determine if a fetus has inherited cystic fibrosis.

5 *How would you answer these questions?*

Case 10: Enzyme replacement

Tom is a 41-year-old man who is seen in the Nephrology Clinic. He was diagnosed as having Fabry disease at 26 years of age (see figure in Chapter 45). At that time, he had suddenly developed left-sided weakness and diplopia (double vision), and was diagnosed as having had a mild stroke. He was also found to have mild proteinuria. Over the ensuing years he has noted that he does not sweat and has had some difficulty with overheating in hot weather. This has caused him to limit his activity on warm days. He has occasional chest palpitations but no chest pain. Every 6–8 weeks he has attacks of vomiting and diarrhoea, which resolve within a day. He also notices pain and some numbness and tingling in his fingertips and toes.

1 *How could the diagnosis of Fabry disease be confirmed?*

Tom has a brother and a sister. His brother is also known to be affected and is undergoing enzyme replacement therapy. His sister is well and has two sons, ages 9 and 11 years, who are in good health. Tom's mother is 65 years of age and is well. His father died of myocardial infarction at age 58 years. Tom's mother has a brother who is well, and she has two sisters who are also unaffected with Fabry disease. Tom has two daughters, ages 6 and 8 years, both of whom are well.

2 *What pattern of inheritance for Fabry disease is suggested by this family history?*

Tom is wondering whether he might also be a candidate for enzyme replacement therapy. His physical examination is notable for angiokeratoma on the palms of the hands and both knees. He has mild ankle oedema. Liver and spleen are not enlarged. He has mild weakness in his legs and some decreased sensation to light touch in the finger tips and toes. Laboratory studies reveal 2.68 g of protein/24 hours (normal is < 150 mg/24 hours) in the urine and a creatinine clearance of 81.5 mL/min (normal: 97–137 mL/min). Blood pressure is normal. Ophthalmological examination reveals bilateral corneal opacities and dilated conjunctival vessels, although his vision is normal. Some left ventricular hypertrophy is indicated by ECG and echocardiogram, but cardiac function is normal.

3 *What could be the pathophysiological mechanism by which these problems develop?*

It is determined that Tom is eligible for enzyme replacement therapy, and when his initial evaluation is completed he is begun on the protocol. This entails intravenous infusion of α-galactosidase every second week. He is re-evaluated 5 weeks later. His energy level has increased and he reports marked improvement in the pain in his fingers and toes. He has had no further episodes of vomiting or diarrhoea. Over the ensuing year, he is also noted to have reduced proteinuria. Gastrointestinal episodes are much less frequent than they had been in the past.

4 *How does infused enzyme reach the normal site of action of α-galactosidase within lysosomes?*

5 *What other lysosomal storage disorders are currently treated by enzyme replacement therapy?*

Self-assessment case studies: answers

Case 1: Unbalanced translocation

1 Interphase FISH provides the ability to determine aneuploidy for any of the chromosomes for which chromosome-specific probes are applied. In practice, this usually means Chromosomes 13, 18, 21, X and Y, since these are the chromosomes most likely to be responsible for aneuploidy in a liveborn child. Aneuploidy for other chromosomes and structural rearrangements would not be detected with the probes normally used. Therefore, interphase FISH is used to exclude major aneuploidy, but would not be useful in evaluation of a child where aneuploidy for those chromosomes is not clinically suspected.

2 The karyotype designation indicates that there is additional material on the short arm (p arm) of Chromosome 14, though the origin of that extra material is not specified. This would indicate partial trisomy for some genetic material, yet to be identified. The abnormality is unbalanced, indicative of the presence of extra chromosomal material, though at this point it remains to be determined where this extra material comes from. For details about nomenclature of chromosomal abnormalities, see *ISCN (2005) An International System for Human Cytogenetic Nomenclature*. Eds: Shaffer LG, Tommerup N. Basel: S. Karger, 2005.

3 The more detailed karyotype reveals the additional material is from the short arm of Chromosome 17, attached to the base of one Chromosome 14. The coincidence in breakpoints of the two chromosomes has no significance.

4 Although abnormal, the father's karyotype is balanced, with a reciprocal translocation between Chromosomes 14 and 17. This exchange resulted in transfer of the short arm of Chromosome 17 to the base of the short arm of Chromosome 14, and a small amount of material from Chromosome 14 to the base of the short arm of 17. No material was apparently lost or gained in this process, explaining why the father is phenotypically normal.

5 Betsy received the derivative 14 chromosome from her father (i.e. the copy of 14 with extra material derived from 17), as well as the normal Chromosome 17. This made her trisomic for most of the short arm of Chromosome 17 and monosomic for the short arm of Chromosome 14. Most of the short arm of Chromosome 14 encodes ribosomal RNA. Loss of this material is unlikely to be consequential, since other acrocentric chromosomes also carry ribosomal DNA. Trisomy of most of 17p, however, is likely to be clinically significant, given the large size of the region.

6 Although miscarriage is relatively common and may have been coincidental, the fact that Betsy's father is a balanced translocation carrier means that it is possible that an unbalanced chromosome complement was transmitted in either or both of these miscarried pregnancies. This would not be unusual for a couple where one partner is a balanced translocation carrier, since the father in this case faces a risk of creating sperm cells with unbalanced karyotypes (e.g. with the derivative 17 and the normal 14, making the zygote essentially monosomic for most of 17p). In some cases, chromosomal imbalance is so severe as to lead to miscarriage.

7 The couple faces an increased risk of having another child with genetic imbalance regarding Chromosomes 14 and 17. The exact magnitude of the risk is difficult to know, since this is a very rare chromosome rearrangement, and risk of unbalanced gametes varies with different rearrangements. The couple can be offered prenatal testing by chorionic villus sampling or amniocentesis to see if a future fetus has inherited an unbalanced karyotype, or *in vitro* fertilization with preimplantation diagnosis.

See Chapter 52 for further information.

Case 2: A metabolic problem

1 PKU is a disorder of amino acid metabolism in which there is a buildup of phenylalanine due to deficiency of activity of phenylalanine hydroxylase. Phenylalanine is cleared through the placenta *in utero*, and therefore does not begin to build up until after the first feed. Neurological damage begins to occur thereafter, provoking the urgency to restrict phenylalanine intake if the diagnosis is confirmed.

2 PKU is an inborn error of metabolism, most often due to mutation in the gene that encodes the enzyme phenylalanine hydroxylase required to convert phenylalanine to tyrosine (see Chapter 51). In the absence of enzyme activity, phenylalanine builds up to toxic levels, and also is converted to phenylpyruvic acid, which is also toxic. In addition, there is a deficiency of tyrosine, and its metabolites, including the neurotransmitter DOPA and the pigment melanin. The former may contribute to neurological problems and the latter results in hypopigmentation.

3 Although most affected individuals have a mutation in the gene that encodes phenylalanine hydroxylase, a small minority have a deficiency of tetrahydrobiopterin, due to mutation in one of several enzymes required to synthesize this coenzyme. Tetrahydrobiopterin is a cofactor required for conversion of phenylalanine to tyrosine.

4 PKU is inherited as an autosomal recessive trait. Both parents must be heterozygous carriers, and probably other members of their families are carriers as well. The carrier frequency in the Caucasian population is about 1/50, so the likelihood is low that other family members have also had a carrier partner. Sophia's parents, though, face a 25% recurrence risk with each pregnancy.

5 Prenatal testing is best done by molecular genetic analysis. This requires identification of the mutant alleles in the two parents, which now is possible to arrange on a routine clinical basis (see www.genetests.org). Once the mutations are identified, fetal tissue can be obtained by chorionic villus biopsy, or amniocentesis, and tested to determine if one or both mutations has been transmitted.

6 It used to be thought that phenylalanine restriction could be relaxed in late childhood, as the nervous system matures. It is now recognized that phenylalanine restriction needs to be continued for a lifetime, as there are continued neurological consequences of high phenylalanine levels.

7 Women with untreated PKU have high blood phenylalanine levels that will cross the placenta if they are pregnant. This exposes the fetus to toxic levels of the amino acid and results in low birth weight, congenital anomalies and abnormal neurological development. It is therefore critical that a woman maintains careful control of phenylalanine, beginning prior to conception and continuing throughout pregnancy.

See Chapters 19, 51, 60 for further information.

Case 3: A child with skin spots

1 A clinical diagnosis of NF1 requires that any two of the following features be present.

(a) Six or more café-au-lait spots larger than 5 mm in a prepubertal child.
(b) Skin-fold freckling (e.g. axillary or inguinal).
(c) Two or more neurofibromas or one plexiform neurofibroma.
(d) Iris hamartomas (Lisch nodules).
(e) Characteristic skeletal dysplasia (orbital or tibial dysplasia).
(f) Optic glioma.
(g) Affected first degree relative.

Based on the information provided, James fulfills one criterion (multiple café-au-lait spots), but not two, and therefore a definitive diagnosis cannot be established clinically. Many of the features, however, are age-dependent, so the diagnosis cannot be excluded at this point (see Chapter 20).

2 Approximately 50% of cases occur sporadically, without apparent family history of NF1. The lack of signs in the parents therefore does not exclude the diagnosis in James.

3 A missense mutation could be pathogenic, or might represent a benign variant. Given the fact that both parents are clinically unaffected and that the penetrance of known NF1 mutations is essentially 100%, the most powerful approach to determining the significance of the mutation would be to test both parents. If the mutation is not present in either of them, you can conclude that James has a new mutation, and this mutation would very likely be pathogenic. If the mutation is present in a parent, it would most likely be a benign variant, assuming no signs of the disorder in the parent. Other approaches would be to investigate more thoroughly if the mutation has ever been seen before in affected individuals, whether it segregates with the disease in families, whether it is seen in control individuals who are unaffected, and whether it affects the function of the gene product. The latter is difficult to do in a direct manner, but can be inferred from determination of whether the amino acid in question is conserved and by looking at the nature of the mutation in relation to the properties of the protein.

4 The penetrance of NF1 is usually considered to be essentially 100%, so if both parents are free of signs it is unlikely that they carry an *NF1* gene mutation. There is a possibility, though, of mosaicism, including germ line mosaicism. Therefore, one cannot counsel that recurrence is impossible, only that the risk is low. Since the mutation in the affected child is known, prenatal testing could be offered for a subsequent pregnancy.

5 The *NF1* gene behaves as a tumour suppressor. Therefore, the tumour cells (Schwann cells in the case of a neurofibroma) have both the germline mutation and an acquired mutation of the homologous *NF1* normal allele. These mutations of the normal allele occur after conception, and account for the fact that neurofibromas are multifocal growths, and not all derived from a single progenitor cell.

6 Assuming the pathogenic mutation is known, prenatal testing can be offered to detect the mutation, usually by chorionic villus sampling or amniocentesis. In some cases, single cell analysis is possible, enabling pre-implantation diagnosis. Such testing would determine if the *NF1* mutation was transmitted, but does not predict the severity of the disorder. Regarding treatment, there are several clinical trials currently under way, including some that test drugs which target specific aspects of the Ras signalling pathway known to be involved in the pathogenesis of NF1. The major current targets are neurofibromas and learning disabilities. It is expected that additional medication trials, targeted at a variety of clinical problems in NF1, will be launched in the coming years.

See Chapters 5, 20, 40 for further information.

Case 4: Muscle weakness

1 CPK is an intramuscular enzyme that leaks out of damaged cells and the grossly elevated level suggests ongoing muscle damage. The examination reveals proximal muscle weakness, prominent calves, and the difficulty getting up from a supine position referred to as the Gower sign. These features are all suggestive of Duchenne muscular dystrophy (see Chapter 22).

2 Duchenne and Becker dystrophy are both disorders in which there is gradual degeneration of muscle, but Duchenne tends to have earlier onset and more rapid progression. Both are due to mutation in the gene on the X chromosome that encodes the protein dystrophin. Duchenne tends to occur when there is complete absence of functional dystrophin, whereas Becker results from mutations that result in abnormal quantity or quality of dystrophin. The most common type of mutation is deletion that affects one or more exons. If the deletion results in juxtaposition of exons with different reading frames (i.e. introduces a 'frame shift'; see Chapter 39), a truncated dystrophin is produced, resulting in Duchenne dystrophy. If it juxtaposes exons 'in-frame', dystrophin will be produced, albeit missing some protein domains due to the missing exons, resulting in Becker muscular dystrophy.

3 There is no definitive treatment for Duchenne muscular dystrophy. The mainstay of management is physiotherapy, aimed at maintaining strength and mobility as long as possible. There is evidence that treatment with steroids slows progression of the disorder, and therefore its use is recommended, with careful monitoring for side-effects.

4 Duchenne muscular dystrophy is an X-linked recessive disorder, and therefore usually affects only males. Although there is no apparent family history of the disorder, there is a paucity of males in the mother's family who would have been at risk. Approximately 2/3 of the mothers of apparently sporadically-affected boys are carriers; half of these mothers carry new mutations, half inherited them from their mothers. Both Luke's mother and his maternal aunt are therefore at risk of being carriers.

5 Given that Luke's aunt is a carrier, prenatal testing can be offered. This can include sex determination (since it is almost always males who are affected) as well as dystrophin gene deletion analysis. Fetal cells obtained by amniocentesis or chorionic villus sampling may also be tested.

6 Duchenne muscular dystrophy typically affects males, but on rare occasions a female can be affected. This may be due to non-random X chromosome inactivation, or the occurrence of a single X chromosome as in Turner syndrome. Some female carriers display mild signs such as muscle cramping and a proportion will develop a dilated cardiomyopathy.

See Chapters 22, 39 for further information.

Case 5: Cancer in the family

1 This family history suggests increased risk of breast and ovarian cancer. Aside from having two first degree relatives affected with breast cancer at a young age, he also has a relative with ovarian cancer. The most common cause of hereditary breast and ovarian cancer is mutation in the *BRCA1* or *BRCA2* genes (see Chapter 41). Approximately 7–10% of cases of breast cancer have a genetic basis, and of this approximately 52% is accounted for by *BRCA1* mutation and 32% by *BRCA2* mutation. The hallmark of a genetic predisposition to cancer includes the occurrence of cancer at a young age compared to the general population risk. There are several computer programs that are used to estimate risk of hereditary breast and ovarian cancer. One, called BRCAPRO, estimates Ted's risk at around 30%. Testing is usually offered to individuals whose risk is 10% or higher.

2 Current approaches to mutation testing do not detect all possible mutations in the *BRCA1* or *BRCA2* genes. Therefore, a negative test does not rule out the possibility of having a mutation. If Ted is tested and is negative, it may be that he did not inherit a mutation or it may be that the family mutation cannot be detected. On the other hand, it is very likely that his sister did inherit a mutation if there is one in the family, so a negative test in her would suggest that either there is no BRCA1 or BRCA2 mutation explaining this family history, or the mutation is not detectable with current approaches to testing. If she is found to have a mutation, Ted can be offered definitive testing to determine whether he inherited the same mutation.

3 Given that the mutation is a stop, causing premature termination of translation of the protein, it is very likely to be pathogenic. The *BRCA* genes function as tumour suppressors, and the majority of pathogenic mutations lead to lack of expression of the gene product.

4 Having had a bilateral mastectomy, Ted's sister does not face significant further risk of breast cancer. She does face, however, a risk of ovarian cancer (a lifetime risk of 28–44%). Her options to manage this risk include oophorectomy or surveillance with transvaginal ultrasound and CA-125 blood testing.

5 Ted's risk of breast cancer is only minimally increased, though BRCA2 mutation is associated with an increased risk of breast cancer in males. There may be a slightly increased risk of prostate cancer in males with both *BRCA1* and *BRCA2* mutations.

6 If Ted is a *BRCA1* mutation carrier, his daughters would each be at 50% risk of inheriting the mutation, in which case they would be at risk of breast and ovarian cancer. This risk, however, does not become significant until the middle of the third decade. Therefore, genetic testing for hereditary breast and ovarian cancer is not recommended for children. Rather, they should be offered counselling and the possibility of testing when they have reached an age when they can make an informed choice.

See Chapter 41 for further information.

Case 6: Targeted treatment

1 The Philadelphia chromosome is created by translocation between Chromosomes 9 and 22 and is found in most cases of chronic myeloid leukaemia. Not all cases of CML are Philadephia chromosome-positive and it is also found in some other forms of leukaemia. The translocation juxtaposes the *abl* proto-oncogene on Chromosome 9 with the *bcr* gene on chromosome 22. This results in production of a fusion protein with abnormal kinase activity, which helps to drive the abnormal growth of the tumour cells (see Chapters 27 and 41).

2 *Imatinib* is a drug that was designed as a tyrosine kinase inhibitor (see Chapter 59). The drug binds to a site in the enzyme where ATP normally binds. It is a potent inhibitor of the abnormal enzyme that results from the *bcr-abl* fusion and has been found to be highly effective in the treatment of CML.

3 PCR testing for the *bcr-abl* fusion is done using PCR primers in the two genes that span the breakpoint. Normally, these primers would not cooperate in amplification, since the genes are on different chromosomes. In the typical translocation, however, the primers are sufficiently close for PCR amplification to occur and produce multiple copies of the sequence.

4 PCR is significantly more sensitive than cytogenetic analysis, and therefore able to detect abnormal cells in minute quantities. *Imatinib* can substantially reduce the number of leukaemic cells, but typically does not completely eliminate them.

5 Relapse occurs by proliferation of a small reservoir of leukaemic cells that undergo further mutation, resulting in a change in the conformation of the fusion protein, so that imatinib is no longer able to attach to the ATP-binding site. The period of remission can be prolonged if imatinib is used in combination with other chemotherapeutic agents.

See Chapters 27, 41, 59 for further information.

Case 7: Alzheimer disease

1 Alzheimer disease is a neurodegenerative disorder that presents with memory loss and behavioural changes. In about 2% of cases it is inherited as an autosomal dominant, but most cases are multifactorial. In families where autosomal dominant transmission does not occur, there is an empirical lifetime risk of Alzheimer disease of 20%. In first degree relatives of patients the risk is doubled.

2 The ApoE locus is known to be associated with risk of Alzheimer disease. This is a polymorphic locus, with three alleles known: ε2, ε3 and ε4. The ε4 allele is associated with increased risk of Alzheimer disease.

3 Testing for the ε4 allele is highly accurate, but has limited clinical utility and clinical validity. Relative risk of Alzheimer disease is greatest in homozygotes for the ε4 allele, but is increased also in those with just one ε4 allele. The test, which distinguishes just the presence or absence of the ε4 allele, is therefore of limited clinical utility, since the presence of an ε4 allele does not necessarily mean that a person will develop Alzheimer disease. There is, moreover, nothing that can be offered to carriers to modify their risk, making the test of limited clinical utility as well. This is why ApoE testing is not recommended on a routine basis.

4 Cheek brushing is a way to obtain epithelial cells from the lining of the mucous membrane of the cheek, and is a convenient source of cells for DNA analysis. A relatively small quantity of cells is obtained, sufficient to do targeted mutation testing. The major limitations are insufficient DNA for a large number of tests and lack of the RNA needed for some types of genetic tests. Cheek brushings, however, provide adequate material for apoE allele testing.

5 Larry has one ε4 allele, which does increase his risk of Alzheimer disease. ApoE is a pre-dispositional test, though, and not diagnostic, so there is still only a low risk that he will develop the disorder. There is no treatment so far available that will prevent Alzheimer disease, nor any special care plan based on the outcome of such tests.

See Chapter 32 for further information.

Case 8: A sleepy infant

1 Around 70–75% of individuals with Prader–Willi syndrome have a deletion involving 15q11-q13, invariably of the paternal chromosome (see Chapter 21). FISH should reveal such a deletion. Approximately 20–25% have uniparental disomy, with two copies of the maternal 15 and no representation of the paternal 15. The balance are thought to have mutations within the Chromosome 15 imprinting centre, an unknown cause, or are misdiagnosed. Methylation testing can distinguish the maternal and paternal copies of 15, which is abnormal in almost all cases of Prader–Willi syndrome.

2 Confirmation of suspected uniparental disomy is best done by obtaining blood from both parents and the child and using DNA polymorphisms to determine if the child has inherited Chromosome 15 markers from both parents. Finding genotypes inherited only from the mother would be indicative of maternal uniparental disomy.

3 Prader–Willi syndrome is thought to arise from lack of expression of a gene or genes on Chromosome 15 that normally are only expressed from the paternal chromosome. If both copies of 15 are of maternal origin, due to DNA methylation differences at this site in the two sexes, these genes will not be expressed even if they are present.
4 The recurrence risk of uniparental disomy is very low. It is thought to arise from two consecutive non-disjunction events. First, non-disjunction in maternal meiosis gives rise to a trisomy 15 zygote upon fertilization. A second postzygotic non-disjunction restores the normal number of chromosomes, but if the paternal 15 is lost, maternal uniparental disomy results. This probably relates to maternal age, since the frequency of maternal non-disjunction increases with age.
5 Kirsten's sister is not at increased risk of having an affected child, since uniparental disomy is only sporadic. Prader–Willi syndrome due to imprinting centre mutations can however be transmitted as a dominant trait.
6 Children with Prader–Willi syndrome are born with hypotonia, low birthweight and failure to thrive, but muscle tone and level of alertness tend to improve over time, as does feeding. In later childhood, however, a severe eating disorder usually ensues, along with behavioural problems and developmental delay. Without management, morbid obesity may result. There is now evidence that treatment with human growth hormone can result in control of the eating disorder, with significant improvement in somatic growth regulation and behaviour.

See Chapters 10, 21 for further information.

Case 9: Advance warning

1 The frequency of cystic fibrosis among newborns of northern European ancestry is about 1/2500. The carrier frequency can be calculated from the Hardy–Weinberg equation (see Chapter 35). If $q^2 = 1/2500$, $q = 1/50$, and the carrier frequency, $2pq$ is close to 1/25 (or 0.04).
2 There is no biochemical test for cystic fibrosis carrier status. The testing is done by mutation analysis on a panethnic group of patients, using a panel of multiple (25) mutations that includes the top 99.9% of pathogenic mutations known to be associated with the disorder (see Chapters 55, 57). Test sensitivity differs between populations, depending on the frequency of specific mutations in those populations.
3 Rita is found to be a carrier, but the testing is negative in Bill. There is still a chance that Bill carries a mutation not included in the panel (approximately 12% of cystic fibrosis mutations are not detected in individuals of northern European ancestry on the standard 25 mutation test panel). There is indeed a small residual risk to this pregnancy. The risk Bill is a carrier, calculated by Bayes' theorem, is

$$\frac{(0.04)(0.12)}{(0.04)(0.12) + (0.96)(1)} \cong 0.005.$$

4 The ΔF508 mutation leads to abnormal processing of the CFTR protein, causing it to fail to be transported to the cell membrane. The physiological result is lack of protein at the cell membrane and, in homozygotes, lack of chloride channel function.
5 If Bill carries a mutation, it was not one detectable on the standard mutation panel and the risk of transmitting it would be (0.005)/2. It would be possible to determine if the fetus has inherited Rita's ΔF508 mutation, of which there is a 50% chance, giving an overall risk for an affected child of $(0.005)/4 \cong 0.00125$, or 1/800. A carrier fetus would not be expected to show clinical signs of cystic fibrosis and it would not be possible in this instance to offer reliable prenatal testing for cystic fibrosis. There are laboratories that can perform more comprehensive sequencing analysis of the *CFTR* gene, but this is expensive and still would not absolutely rule out the presence of a pathogenic mutation. It is also possible to test for intestinal enzymes in amniotic fluid, which can be low in affected pregnancies due to intestinal blockage by thickened meconium, but the test is not done routinely due to questions about the reliability of results.

See Chapters 19, 55, 57 for further information.

Case 10: Enzyme replacement

1 The diagnosis of Fabry disease is confirmed by detection of deficient α-galactosidase enzyme activity in leucocytes or cultured fibroblasts. Although molecular genetic testing is possible, there is a wide variety of possible mutations, making molecular analysis more difficult than enzyme assay as a diagnostic test.
2 Fabry disease is inherited as an X-linked recessive trait, though some females manifest some signs of the disorder. Since Tom's brother is also affected, their mother must be a carrier. She has only one brother, who happens not to be affected. We do not have information about the generation prior to Tom's mother. Tom's father's death from myocardial infarction is ascribable to unrelated causes.
3 The pathophysiology of Fabry disease is based on deposition of the GL-3 glycolipid, globotriaosylceramide, in endothelial cells due to lack of adequate α-galactosidase enzyme activity. This leads to chronic ischaemia (deficient blood supply) in tissues and obstruction of small vessels, leading to peripheral neuropathy (causing weakness, decreased sensation, and pain), renal insufficiency (causing ankle oedema, proteinuria, and decreased creatinine clearance, indicative of decreased glomerular blood flow) and cardiac dysfunction. Deposition of storage material also occurs in corneal cells and the skin, leading to angiokeratomas.
4 Enzyme replacement therapy uses a purified, recombinant DNA-based enzyme synthesized *in vitro*. The infused enzyme is taken into cells by endocytosis before delivery to the lysosomes.
5 Other lysosomal storage disorders currently treated with enzyme replacement therapy include Gaucher disease (β-glucosidase deficiency), Hurler syndrome (α-L-iduronidase deficiency) and Pompe disease (α-1,4-glucosidase deficiency).

See Chapters 22, 45, 59 for further information.

Glossary

acrocentric: of a chromosome, with the centromere close to one telomere.
adenocarcinoma: malignant tumour of glandular tissue.
adenoma: non-malignant tumour of glandular tissue.
allele frequency: 'gene frequency'; the proportion of a given allele of all the alleles at a locus, in the individuals forming a specified population.
***Alu* repeat:** the most abundant repeat sequence in the human genome, found only in primates.
anticipation: onset of genetic disease at younger ages in later generations, or with increasing severity in each generation.
anticodon: sequence of three bases within tRNA that is the base pair rule complement to a specific triplet codon and is utilized as such in the translation of mRNA into polypeptide.
anti-sense strand: template strand of DNA.
apoptosis: programmed cell death.
ascertainment: recognition of individuals with a specified phenotype.
assortative mating: mate selection on the basis of specific characters.
atherosclerosis: arterial hardening with deposition of lipid.
balanced polymorphism: genetic polymorphism maintained in a population by opposing selective forces.
Bayes' Theorem: a mathematical approach that refines probabilities by taking into account all relevant knowledge.
benign tumour: abnormal, compact mass of cells that does not endanger life.
bivalent: homologous chromosomes while pairing during meiosis.
Blaschko's lines: clonal boundaries revealed in the skin in some disease conditions.
cancer: breakdown in homeostatic control of cell growth leading to metastasis.
candidate gene: genetic locus plausibly involved in causing disease.
carcinoma: malignant tumour of the skin or epithelial mucus membrane.
Caucasian: of Indo-European ethnicity.
cellular oncogene: proto-oncogene.
centimorgan: genetic map distance between two loci that are segregated on average in 1% of meioses.
Central Dogma: concept that genetic information is transferred in the cell in the direction: DNA → RNA → protein.
chiasma: connection between the chromatids of homologous chromosomes where crossing over is occurring at meiosis.
chromatid: one of the two strands which result from duplication of a chromosome, found during prophase and metaphase of mitosis and meiosis. Each chromatid contains a single, very long molecule of DNA. They separate at anaphase and are then known as daughter chromosomes.
chromatin: the material components of chromosomes.
chromosome abnormality: phenotypically significant change in chromosome number or structure.
***cis* conformation:** presence of alleles of different genes on the same strand of DNA, *c.f. trans*.
clone: two or more individuals (or cells) derived from one genome.
coarctation: narrowing of a vessel.
codominance: expression of both alleles in a heterozygote.
codon: a sequence of three bases within a gene, that corresponds to a specific amino acid in the corresponding polypeptide.
concordance: degree to which relatives, especially twins, share a particular trait.
consanguinity: genetic relationship.
consultand: individual who approached the clinician for genetic advice.
continuous variation: variation in a character which forms a continuous series from one extreme to the other.
coupling: *cis* conformation.
CRASH syndrome: corpus callosum hypoplasia, retardation, adducted thumbs, spastic paraparesis and hydrocephalus due to mutation in the L1 CAM cell adhesion molecule.
deletion: loss of some or all of a gene or chromosome.
diploid: having twice the haploid content of chromosomes, i.e. the normal full complement.
discontinuous variation: the existence of two or more non-overlapping classes with respect to a particular character.
DNA binding protein: protein which affects gene activity by becoming bound to the DNA.
DNA boost: computer-based method for distinguishing individual DNA profiles in a mixed sample.
DNA fingerprint: personally unique pattern of hypervariable minisatellite DNA repeats.
DNA hybridization: reassembly of complementary pairs of DNA single strands into a double-strand by base pairing.
DNA probe: small fragment of single-strand DNA with the same sequence of nucleotides as the section of native human DNA of interest, labelled with a radioactive or fluorescent tag.
DNA renaturation: reformation of double helical DNA from complementary, single strands; DNA hybridization.
dominant: an allele is said to be dominant over an alternative allele at the same locus when it, rather than the alternative allele, is expressed in a heterozygote.
dot blot: DNA, usually amplified by PCR, applied directly to a membrane without electrophoresis.
dynamic mutation: transient or progressive change in the DNA that affects its coding properties or degree of expression.
dysgenic: relating to a deleterious genetic change.
empiric risk: observed frequency of disease in a given situation.
endocarditis: inflammation of the inner lining of the heart.
ethics: the science of morals and human duty.
eugenic: relating to a beneficial genetic change.
eugenics: the use of genetic measures to improve the genetic characteristics of a population.
expressivity: degree to which an allele is expressed in an individual.
fibrillin: protein in connective tissue abnormal in Marfan syndrome.
fixation: elimination of alternative alleles in a population.
frameshift mutation: mutation involving loss or gain of nucleotides of a number not divisible by three, so that the translational reading frame is put out of register.
G-bands: pattern of AT-rich dark bands produced in chromosomes by special treatment followed by Giemsa staining.
gene: the basic unit of inheritance.

gene expression: creation of a phenotypic character corresponding to a gene. It is frequently (but erroneously) considered as synonymous with transcription.
gene flow: geographical movement of alleles by migration.
gene frequency: see 'allele frequency'.
gene map: physical representation of the relative positions of the genes in the genome.
gene therapy: correction of an inherited defect at the level of the gene.
genetic association: occurrence of a specific allele with a specific phenotype at frequency greater than expected by chance.
genetic code: set of correspondences between triplet codons of bases in mRNA and amino acids in polypeptides.
genetic drift: non-selective change in allele frequency.
genetic heterogeneity: similar genetic condition caused by different genes.
genome: genetic content of a haploid cell; the genetic makeup of a species.
genotype: genetic constitution of an individual.
germline mutation: mutation that can be transmitted to offspring.
Ghent criteria: accepted set of criteria used for diagnosis of Marfan syndrome.
haploid: possessing only one copy of the genetic material, as in a sperm or ovum.
haplotype: set of alleles of linked genes that tend to be inherited together.
heritability: the fraction of phenotypic variation that can be ascribed to genotypic variation.
heterozygote: individual with dissimilar alleles of a particular gene.
holoprosencephaly: failure of division of the forebrain into two hemispheres.
homeobox: characteristic DNA sequence found in genes for DNA binding proteins involved notably in pattern formation.
homozygote: individual with similar alleles of a particular gene.
human genome: theoretical concept that includes the genomes of all normal human beings, as well as the idea of an 'average' or typical genome for a human.
Human Genome Project: a major international collaborative effort to map and sequence the entire human genome.
hypervariable DNA: fraction of non-coding DNA consisting of repetitive sequences that shows a great deal of variation in repeat number between individuals.
hypotelorism: abnormally closely spaced orbits.
imprinting: acquisition by a gene of a semi-permanent modification that affects its expression. Imprinting can be changed in a subsequent generation.
inbreeding: breeding between individuals who share one or more common ancestors.
inbreeding depression: reduction in fitness caused by homozygosity of certain alleles due to inbreeding.
incest: sexual intercourse between close relatives, usually those sharing 25% or more of their genetic material.
inhibin: protein tested to screen prenatally for Down syndrome.
isochromosome: chromosome with two arms of equal length and identical sequence.
karyotype: a formula that describes the somatic chromosome complement of an individual or a photomicrograph of his/her metaphase chromosomes arranged in standard order.
liability: inherited predisposition.
linkage disequilibrium: co-occurrence of closely linked alleles in a population more frequently than expected by chance.
linkage phase: situation of alternative pairs of alleles with respect to one another on homologous chromosomes.
linked: of genes, close together on the same chromosome.
location score: the equivalent in multilocus mapping of the lod score in two-point mapping.
lod score: a mathematical score of the relative likelihood of two loci being linked calculated at the most probable degree of linkage.
lordosis: exaggerated forward convex curve of the lumbar spine.
macroorchidism: large testicles.
malignancy: ability of cells to sustain proliferation and invade other tissues.
malignant tumour: tumour with the capacity for unrestrained growth and shedding of invasive cells.
meiotic drive: any meiotic mechanism that results in unequal fertilization by the two types of gametes produced by a heterozygote.
Mendel's laws: set of rules governing inheritance of single-gene features discovered by Gregor Mendel, sometimes presented as the 'Law of Segregation of Genetic Factors' and the 'Law of Independent Assortment of Genetic Factors'.
metacentric: of a chromosome, with the centromere near the middle.
metaphase plate: arrangement of chromosomes that forms across the main axis of the spindle apparatus at metaphase.
metastasis: transfer of cancer cells about the body.
microsatellite DNA: category of repetitive DNA with tandem repeats of a very short sequence, e.g. 1–4 base pairs.
minisatellite DNA: category of repetitive DNA with tandem repeats of a sequence of intermediate length, e.g. 10–15 base pairs.
mitosis-suppressor gene: tumour suppressor gene; the normal allele of such a gene suppresses cell division, usually at the transition from G1 to S-, or G2 to M-phase of the mitotic cycle.
monosomy: presence of only one copy of a chromosome.
mosaic: existence in the body of more than one population of genetically distinct cells.
multifactorial trait: character that results from the joint action of several factors, including genes and environmental influences.
multipoint map: gene map based on several reference loci.
mutagen: environmental agent capable of causing damage to DNA.
mutation: process by which a gene undergoes a structural change to create a different allele; the new allele resulting from such a change.
mutator gene: faulty DNA repair gene.
myocardial infarction: death of heart muscle due to loss of blood supply.
neoplasia: ability of cancerous cells to proliferate in defiance of normal controls.
nodal: a gene concerned with body patterning.
nuchal transparency: visual appearance of accumulated fluid at the back of the neck in a 12-week fetus.
nucleoside: compound of a purine or pyrimidine base linked to the sugars ribose or deoxyribose, e.g. adenosine, guanosine, cytidine, thymidine, uridine.
nucleotide: compound of a purine or pyrimidine base linked to ribose or deoxyribose, plus phosphoric acid, e.g. d-adenosine triphosphate, d-ATP.
obligate carrier: individual who, logically, must be a carrier.
oligogenic: resulting from the joint action of a small number of genes.
oligohydramnios: defiency of amniotic fluid.

oligonucleotide: artificially synthesized DNA molecule.
oncogene: a modified proto-oncogene that contributes to a high rate of cell division, usually designated without a prefix, e.g. *myc*.
otitis media: middle ear infection.
outbreeding: breeding with an unrelated partner.
penetrance: proportion of individuals of a specific genotype that shows the expected phenotype.
pharmacogenetics: the aspect of genetics that deals with variation in response to drugs.
pharmacogenomics: use of genomics to design new drugs or select drugs to treat disease.
phase: of linkage, the state of association of alternative alleles at one locus with those at a genetically linked locus.
phenotype: visible, tangible, or otherwise measurable properties of an organism resulting from the interaction of his or her genes with the environment.
pleiotropy: phenomenon of a single gene being responsible for a number of distinct and often seemingly unrelated phenotypic traits.
point mutation: substitution, insertion or deletion in DNA that involves only a small number of nucleotides.
polygenic: resulting from the joint action of two or more genes.
polyhydramnios: excessive amniotic fluid.
polymorphism: presence in a population of two or more alleles at one locus at frequencies each greater than 1%; one allele of a polymorphic system, or its corresponding phenotype.
Potter sequence: a sequence of events that cause fetal abnormalities through oligohydramnios.
premutation: situation where there is expansion of triplet repeats beyond the normal range, but insufficient to cause disease.
preventive genetics: application of genetic insight for avoidance of disease.
proband: family member with specific phenotype who first came to the attention of the investigator or clinician.
progress zone: the region of the developing limb bud just behind the apical ectodermal ridge.
proposita: female proband.
propositus: male proband.
proto-oncogene: cellular oncogene; a normal allele that stimulates cell division, designated with the prefix '*c*', e.g. *c-myc*.
pseudo-autosomal region: homologous regions of the X and Y chromosomes where pairing and crossover occurs.
'rare': of genetic diseases, sometimes considered as occurring in less than 1/5000 births.
R-bands: reverse bands, GC-rich parts of chromosomes that do not stain darkly with Giemsa stain, *c.f.* G-bands.
recessive: an allele is said to be recessive to an alternative allele at the same locus when its expression is masked by that alternative in a heterozygote.
recurrence risk: risk a couple will have another child with the same disorder.
repulsion: '*trans*' conformation.
restriction endonuclease: enzyme that specifically cuts double-stranded DNA at a defined base sequence.
restriction fragment: portion of double-stranded DNA released when DNA is cut with a restriction endonuclease.
reverse transcriptase: viral enzyme that creates DNA copies from an RNA template.
sarcoma: malignant tumour of mesodermal tissue.
sense strand: DNA strand complementary to the template strand and of sequence similar to that in the RNA transcribed.
sex chromosomes: X and Y chromosomes.
sex limitation: sex-related expression of an autosomal gene due to sex-related differences in anatomy or physiology.
sex linkage: inheritance and expression of an allele in relation to sex, by virtue of the gene being carried on a sex chromosome.
silent mutation: mutation that causes no change in the corresponding polypeptide.
sister chromatids: two daughter strands of a duplicated chromosome joined by a common centromere.
somatic mutation: mutation that occurs in a body cell as distinct from the germ line.
SOX family: a family of gene transcription factors.
S-phase: DNA synthetic phase of the cell cycle.
START signal: triplet codon AUG that signifies where translation of mRNA should start.
statins: drugs that block cholesterol synthesis.
STOP signal: chain terminator, or 'nonsense codon'; triplet codon that indicates where on the mRNA translation should stop: UAA, UAG, UGA.
sub-metacentric: of a chromosome, with the centromere between the middle and one telomere.
susceptibility gene: gene with an allele that confers predisposition to a disease.
synapsis: side-by-side association of homologous chromosomes at meiosis.
syndrome: set of phenotypic features that occur together as a characteristic of a disease.
tandem repeats: two or more copies of the same sequence of nucleotides arranged in direct succession in DNA.
TCA cycle: tricarboxylic acid cycle.
telomere: specialized end of a chromosome.
template strand: anti-sense strand; the DNA strand along which RNA polymerase runs, producing an RNA molecule of complementary sequence.
test mating: mating with a recessive homozygote which reveals the genotype of that individual.
threshold trait: a character which shows discontinuous variation considered to be superimposed upon a continuously variable distribution of liabilities.
***trans* conformation:** alleles of two linked genes are said to be in *trans* conformation when they are on opposite chromosomes at meiosis, *c.f. cis*.
transcript: initially formed RNA product of the action of RNA polymerase.
translocation: mutation that involves transfer of a piece of DNA to an abnormal site.
triplet repeat: tandem repetition of a group of three bases in DNA.
Tumour suppressor gene: mitosis suppressor gene; a gene responsible for arresting mitosis at the G1 or G2 block.
viral oncogene: oncogene derived from a viral insert, designated with the prefix '*v*', e.g. *v-myc*.
xanthoma: yellow skin discoloration due to subcutaneous cholesterol deposition.
zinc finger protein: a protein of specialized structure stabilized by an atom of zinc, with the property of binding to specific DNA sequences.

Appendix: information sources and resources

Introductory general textbooks

Jorde, LB, Carey, JC, Bamshad, MJ and White, RL. *Medical Genetics*, 3rd edn. St Louis: Mosby, 2000.

Korf, BR. *Human Genetics and Genomics. A Problem-Based Approach*, 3rd edn. Oxford: Blackwell, 2007.

McLachlan, J. *Medical Embryology*. New York: Addison-Wesley, 1994.

Nussbaum, RL, McInnes, RR and Willard, HF. *Thompson and Thompson's Genetics in Medicine*, 7th edn. Philadelphia: Saunders, 2007.

Turnpenny, PD and Ellard, S. *Emery's Elements of Medical Genetics*, 12th edn. Edinburgh: Churchill Livingstone, 2005.

Westman, JA. *Medical Genetics for the Modern Clinician*. Baltimore, Philadelphia: Lippincott Williams and Wilkins, 2006.

Advanced texts

Childs, B, Beaudet, AL, Valle, D, Kinzler, KW and Vogelstein, B. *The Metabolic and Molecular Bases of Inherited Disease*, vols 1–4, eds: Scriver, CR and Sly, WS. New York: McGraw-Hill, 2000.

Pritchard, DJ. Cystic fibrosis allele frequency, sex ratio anomalies and fertility: a new theory for the dissemination of mutant alleles. *Human Genetics*, **87**: 671–6, 1991.

Pritchard, DJ. Genetic analysis of schizophrenia as an example of a putative multifactorial trait. *Annals of Human Genetics*, **60**: 105–23, 1996.

Rimoin, DL, Connor, JM, Pyeritz, RE and Korf, BR. *Emery and Rimoin's Principles and Practice of Medical Genetics*, vols 1–3, 5th edn. London: Churchill Livingstone, 2006.

Vogel, F and Motulsky, AG. *Human Genetics. Problems and Approaches*, 3rd edn. Berlin, Heidelberg, New York: Springer, 1997.

Specialized textbooks

Emery, AEH. *Methodology in Medical Genetics. An Introduction to Statistical Methods*, 2nd edn. Edinburgh: Churchill Livingstone, 1986.

Emery, AEH and Malcolm, S. *An Introduction to Recombinant DNA in Medicine*, 2nd edn. Wiley: Chichester, 1995.

Evett, IW and Weir, BS. *Interpreting DNA Evidence. Statistical Genetics for Forensic Scientists*. Sunderland, Massachusetts: Sinauer, 1998.

Gilbert, P. *A–Z of Syndromes and Inherited Disorders*, 3rd edn. Cheltenham: Nelson Thornes, 2000.

Harper, P. *Practical Genetic Counselling*, 5th edn. Oxford: Butterworth Heinemann, 1998.

Jones, E and Morris, A. *Mosby's Crash Course: Cell Biology and Genetics*. London, Philadelphia: Mosby, 1998.

Winter, RM and Baraitser, M. *Multiple Congenital Anomalies. A Diagnostic Compendium*. London: Chapman and Hall, 1991.

Internet databases

General sources and rare disorders

British Society for Human Genetics (BSHG): www//bshg.org.uk A useful startpoint with links to many other websites.

Clinical Genetics Computer Resources: http://www.kumc.edu/gec/prof/genecomp.html A valuable entry point to all the major genetics databases, for professional use.

GeneCards: http://bioinfo.weizmann.ac.il/cards/ Database of human genes and their products.

GeneReviews: http://genereviews.org An online genetics textbook with reviews and educational materials, including guidelines for diagnosis and management of genetic conditions and database of diagnostic laboratories.

Human Genome Epidemiology Network Reviews: http://www.cdc.gov/genomics/hugenet/reviews.htm Identifies human genetic variations and reports their frequency in different populations; describes associated disease risks and evaluates relevant genetic tests.

Human Mutation Database: http://www.hgmd.org A compendium of databases of mutations responsible for human genetic disorders.

Infobiogen Database Catalogue (DBCAT): http://www.pubmedcentral.nih.gov/articlerender.fcgi?artid=102454 A comprehensive public catalogue of biological databases.

National Center for Biotechnology Information: http://www.ncbi.nlm.nih.gov/ Provides links to many valuable genetic resources, including: http://www. ncbi.nlm.nih.gov/books/bv.fcgi?call=bv.View..ShowTOC&rid=gnd.TOC&depth=2 which gives access to the main genetic diseases by organ system and chromosome, with detailed disease maps of each chromosome.

National Organization for Rare Diseases (NORD): http://www.rarediseases.org/ Maintains a list of rare diseases and affiliated groups.

Online Mendelian Inheritance in Man (OMIM): http://www.ncbi.nlm.nih.gov/entrez/query.fcgi?CMD=search&DB=OMIM The standard and authoritative source of current knowledge of genes and single gene disorders. Presents links to relevant literature, map locations and clinical summaries.

POSSUM: http://www.possum.net.au/ Computer-aided diagnosis of genetic disorders and syndromes.

PubMed: http://www.ncbi.nlm.nih.gov/entrez/query.fcgi?db=PubMed A service of the National Library of Medicine giving access to 11 million MEDLINE citations of standard publications on medical topics.

Single gene disorders

Colour vision defects: http://www.mcw.edu/cellbio/colorvision/test1.htm

Cystic fibrosis: http://www.genet.sickkids.on.ca/cftr/

Diabetes: http://diabetes.niddk.nih.gov/index.htm

Haemophilia: http://www.hemophilia.org/home.htm

Muscular dystrophy: http://www.mdausa.org/

Sickle cell disease: http://www.scinfo.org/

Thalassemia: http://sickle.bwh.harvard.edu/menu_thal.html

DNA-based techniques, gene mapping and gene therapy

DNA microarrays: http://www.ncbi.nlm.nih.gov/About/primer/microarrays.html; http://science-education.nih.gov/newsnapshots/TOC_Chips/toc_chips.html

European Bioinformatics Institute (EBI): http://www.ebi.ac.uk/ Access to nucleotide and protein databases.

Gene Almanac: http://www.dnalc.org/ddnalc/websites/ Provides access to websites on many relevant issues.

Gene therapy:
http://www.nature.com/gt/progress_and_prospects.html
Human Genome Project Information: http://www.ornl.gov/TechResources/Human_Genome/home.html General information on the quest to sequence the human genome.

Chromosomal errors
Down syndrome: http://www.nlm.nih.gov/medlineplus/downsyndrome.html; http://www.nads.org/
Klinefelter syndrome: http://www.nlm.nih.gov/medlineplus/ency/article/000382.htm
Turner syndrome: http://turners.nichd.nih.gov/
Other trisomies: see **SOFT**, below.

Mitochondrial defects
Mitomap: http://www.mitomap.org

Embryology, development and birth defects
Common disorders of infants: http://www.marchofdimes.org
Images of normal and abnormal embryos: http://www.med.unc.edu/embryo_images/
International Clearinghouse of Birth Defects:
http://www.icbdsr.org/page.asp?p=9895&l=1

Cancer
General: http://cancer.gov/cancerinformation; http://www.massgeneral.org/cancer/

Populations and screening
Allele Frequency Database (ALFRED): http://alfred.med.yale.edu/alfred/index.asp
Frequency of Inherited Disorders Database (FIDD): http://archive.uwcm.ac.uk/uwcm/mg/fidd/background.html
Human Genome Epidemiology Network Reviews: see above.

Ethics
American College of Medical Genetics: http://www.acmg.net
American College of Obstetrics and Gynecology:
http://www.acog.org
American Society of Human Genetics: http://www.ashg.org
American Society of Reproductive Medicine:
http://www.asrm.org
International Federation of Gynecology and Obstetrics:
http://www.figo.org
Research program on Ethical, Legal and Social Implications of the Human Genome Project (ELSI):
http://www.nhgri.nih.gov/ELSI

Laboratory services
Clinical Molecular Genetics Society (UK): www.cmgs.org
European Directory of DNA Laboratories: www.eddnal.com
GeneClinics (USA): www.geneclinics.org
GeneTests: http://www.genetests.org
GeneReviews: see above.

Family support
Family Village: http://www.familyvillage.wisc.edu/ Information on medical disorders, targeted at the general public.
Genetic Alliance (USA): http://www.geneticalliance.org A good source of information on family support groups for genetic disorders.
Genetic Interest Group (UK): www.gig.org.uk A national alliance of patient organizations.
NORD: see above.
Support Organization for Trisomy 18, 13 and Related Disorders (SOFT): http://www.trisomy.org

Index

Note: page numbers in *italics* refer to figures and tables